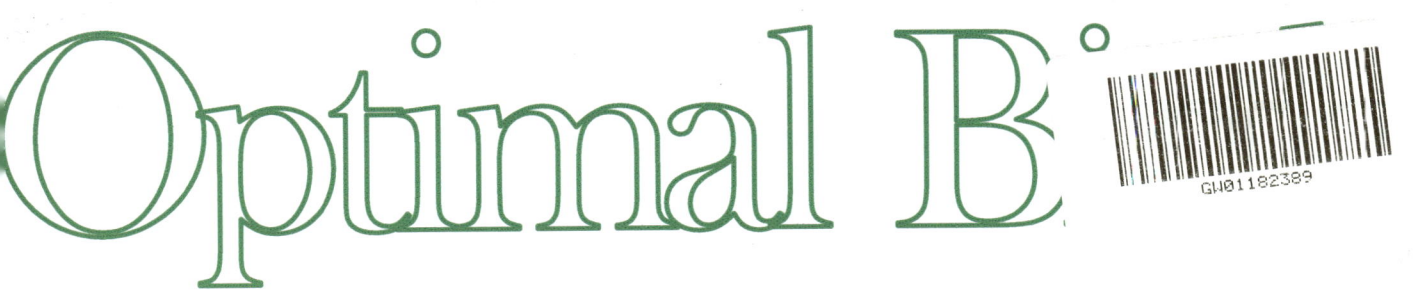

Comments from a few professionals who've provided feedback:

"I have read the book from cover to cover. I must say that I was very impressed with the contents."

A midwife

"I bought this book as both a midwife and a very sceptical first-time mum-to-be. After reading it, I feel quite empowered and am keen to give all the suggestions for optimal birth a try. I have already informed my care givers (to be!) of what to expect. Thank you."

A midwife and mum-to-be

"This book reaffirms my professional and personal experiences. Thank you so much for sending me a copy."

Senior Lecturer in Midwifery at a British university

"I thought I would peruse the book prior to a session to 3rd yr students on control. I must admit I was easily captivated. I found the narrative style of the book easy to read and the stories compelling, in fact I found it difficult to put down. This is a useful book for all midwives and students to enable them to get a feel of a totally different culture of childbirth which they need to support."

Principal Lecturer in Midwifery (British university)

"I think the content is very moving and insightful. I think your strategy of publishing in this area is very useful in moving the normal/optimal birth agenda forward. All the very best with your work for now and the future."

Professor at another UK University and Director of a Midwifery Research Group

Please note:
The second edition of this book is now in development. If you would like to give feedback on the current edition or contribute material or ideas to the second one (due out in 2010) please contact Fresh Heart Publishing via www.freshheartpublishing.co.uk (click on 'Contact us') or write to Fresh Heart, PO Box 225, Chester le Street, DH3 9BQ.

The What, The Why & The How

Optimal Birth
The What, The Why & The How

Optimal Birth
The What, The Why & The How

Sylvie Donna

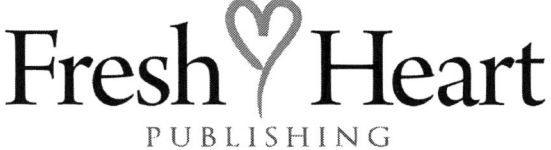

First published in Great Britain in 2009 by
FRESH HEART PUBLISHING
a division of Fresh Heart
PO Box 225, Chester le Street, DH3 9BQ
www.freshheartpublishing.co.uk

© Sylvie Donna 2009

The moral right of Sylvie Donna to be identified as the author of this work has been asserted in accordance with the Copyright, Designs and Patents Act 1988.

All rights reserved. No part of this publication may be reproduced, stored in a retrieval system, or transmitted, in any form or by any means, electronic, mechanical, photocopying, recording or otherwise, without the prior permission of the publisher. Nor may this publication be circulated in any form of binding or cover other than that in which it is published and without a similar condition being imposed on the subsequent purchaser.

A CIP catalogue record for this publication is available from the British Library

ISBN: 978 1 906619 04 6

Set in different fonts to reflect different 'voices' as follows:
- Franklin Gothic Book—for all the author's commentary
- Bookman Old Style—for all commentary from experts
- Comic Sans MS—for all other contributors' commentary

Designed and typeset by Fresh Heart Publishing
Cover design by Fresh Heart Publishing
Front and back cover trees are by Nina Klose; the baby is Jumeira, one of the author's 'optimal' babies

Printed and bound in Great Britain by Jasprint, Tyne & Wear

Disclaimer
While the advice and information contained in this book is believed to be accurate and true at the time of going to press, neither the author nor the publisher can accept any legal responsibility for loss, damage or injury occasioned to any person acting or refraining from action as a result of information contained herein. The advice is intended as a guideline only.

DEDICATION

For all the professionals working in health care who are fighting to give families the right to safer, more effective and more compassionate care

CONTENTS

Acknowledgements ix

Introduction 1

Optimal Birth: The What 3

- **The physiological processes 5**
  Pregnancy ◆ Labour ◆ Birth ◆ Postpartum ◆ The natural norm ◆ Life-saving intervention ◆ Grey areas

- **Caesareans 44**
  Optimal or not? The facts... ◆ The operation itself ◆ The fashion ◆ The feeling ◆ Are caesareans really necessary?

Optimal Birth: The Why 52

- **Reason No. 1: Research suggests it's safest to minimise interventions 52**
  Pregnancy ◆ Labour ◆ Birth and beyond

- **Reason No. 2: All drugs for pain relief have side effects 53**
  Gas and air ◆ Pethidine ◆ Diamorphine ◆ Epidurals

- **Reason No. 3: Babies are being disadvantaged, perhaps far into the future 54**
  The baby's perspective ◆ Hard data ◆ What about a baby's capacity to love?

- **Reason No. 4: Women end up feeling disempowered, upset and depressed 57**
  Negative emotions postnatally... ◆ But do you really want an empowered woman?

- **Reason No. 5: The natural processes are simply too easily disturbed 61**
  The hormonal cocktail of pregnancy ◆ The hormonally-triggered switchover to 'instinctual' ◆ The hormones of labour and birth ◆ Hormones produced shortly after the birth

- **Reason No. 6: Intervention is an uncontrolled experiment 64**
  From the birth of time... ◆ 1800-1900 ◆ The 1900s and 1910s ◆ The 1920s and 1930s ◆ The 1940s ◆ The 1950s ◆ The 1960s ◆ The 1970s ◆ The 1980s and 1990s ◆ How much takes place now? ◆ How much intervention is needed?

- **Reason No. 7: Optimal is more beautiful... 69**
  The dignity and experience of optimal birth

Optimal Birth: The How 73

- **A few questions to contemplate 74**
  Training ◆ Experience ◆ Research ◆ The Law ◆ Power ◆ Protocols ◆ Optimality

- **The antenatal period 75**
  What's the purpose of antenatal care? ◆ What are the potential problems? ◆ What are the potential opportunities? ◆ What are the potential risks? ◆ The chance to develop an even better relationship ◆ The importance of an accurate due date ◆ The importance of a balanced view ◆ Requests for home birth ◆ The risks of risk assessment ◆ Testing protocols ◆ Monitoring procedures ◆ Ultrasound ◆ Antenatal checks ◆ Psychological preparation for birth ◆ The importance and role of birth plans

- **Intrapartum care 91**
  The importance of non-disturbance ◆ Disturbance vs. negligence ◆ The prevalence of accidental disturbance ◆ The reality of working within protocols ◆ The reality of non-disturbance ◆ Using water ◆ What if labour goes on and on? ◆ What if your client has brought along a doula? ◆ Typical birthing positions ◆ Unexpected events

- **The puerperium   109**
  Postnatal scenarios ◆ Cord-cutting ◆ PPH ◆ Prematurity ◆ Breastfeeding ◆ Mothering ◆ Postnatal lifestyle adjustment

Your input!   120
Birthframes index   121
Useful contacts   122
Bibliography   124
Recommended reading   125
Index   126
Order form   129
Testimonials from three well-known figures   130
Who is Sylvie Donna? Who is Michel Odent?   131
Why this book?   132

ACKNOWLEDGEMENTS

I would like to thank all the people who made this book possible by helping me and contributing to this project on behalf of all the women, men and babies who might be helped by it. I am particularly grateful to five professionals who provided support or reviewed and commented on this new edition: a Head of Midwifery, a former Head of Midwifery (both in the NHS), a midwife working in a private London hospital, an independent midwife and a midwife who is a consultant for a legal firm, which deals with litigation and dispute management, amongst other things. Of course, I am responsible for any omissions or errors... I hope that for the second edition of this book I will be able to add your own name to thank you for helping me improve this first version!

Many other people also contributed material to this book. I consulted with all of them on how material would be used. Even the rather critical or analytical introductory blurbs and commentaries you will see did get approved. My reason for writing blurbs was to place birth stories in the context of the book and make the overall message of the book consistent and clear. My consultation with contributors was useful in many cases because it allowed me to identify misunderstandings, which might otherwise have been left unresolved. Of course, I also took the opportunity to request many explanations and additions, which is why some accounts, which had initially appeared elsewhere, appear in this book in much longer form. Most of the accounts and comments are original, though. I did, incidentally, eventually decide to anglicise the spelling (and occasionally the wording) of accounts for easier reading.

As you will see, many of the contributors were very happy to be named. Initially, I thought almost everybody would want to be anonymous. Then, one day, very early on in the process, I received an email from a woman who stated in very bald terms, "I don't want or need to be anonymous!" Other contributors said, "I'd love to be named", or similar, and explained why they wanted to contribute towards this project. In the words of one contributor: "I would be really pleased for you to use my story. I do think that it's important for other mothers, who may be in the same situation, to feel that they can be in control and make their own decisions about what they want for their birth." It soon became clear that this was a subject on which people wanted to 'stand up and be counted'. Perhaps, also, they wanted it to be clear to readers that their contributions were totally authentic.

In cases where contributors did request anonymity this was sometimes at the request of husbands or children and sometimes because the content of what had been written was sensitive or potentially embarrassing in some way. I must admit, there were cases where I suggested to people that they should be anonymous where they simply refused. In other cases where I expected a request to come for anonymity (in particular because of the surrounding text, which I'd also shown the contributor), I was told it was fine to use the name. Of course, I respected people's decisions on this, but I have taken two names out for legal reasons.

I requested many explanations when consulting with people who contributed

Birth stories were contributed by Debbie Brindley, 'Tina C from the UK', Ruth Clark, Krisanne Collard, Pauline Farrance, Sarah-Jane Forder, Sarah Hobart, Nina Klose, Liliana Lammers, 'Christina from the UK', Ashley Marshall, Nathalie Meddings, Nuala OSullivan, Clare O'Ryan, Jenny Sanderson, Maria Shanahan, Jo Siebert (and Dr Lawrence Impey), Fiona Lucy Stoppard, Rachel Urbach. A special thank you to Michel Odent for allowing me to print his comments on the birth of his daughter and the other birth stories he told me (and later also checked in writing).

Other birth stories, which appear in the companion volume for pregnant women *BIRTH: Countdown to Optimal*, which are mentioned in this book here and there, were contributed by Bhavna Amlani, Ph Anderton, Helen Arundell, Janet Balaskas, Elaine Batchelor, Sarah Buckley, Emma Cameron, Sarah Cave, Marion Chatfield, Jeannette Clark, Kathryn Clarke, Esther Culpin, Mave Denyer, Beth Dubois, Amanda Fergusson, Helene Gee, Elise Hansen, Janet Hanton (along with Caroline Flint and Pam Wild from www.birthcentre.com), Jenny Hodge, Tracy Hoekema, Angela Horn, 'Iona and Laura from California', Deborah Jackson, Jennifer Jacoby, Tanya Kudryashova, Nicolette Lawson, Alan Low, Cara Low, Steve and Olga Mellor, David Newbound, Sue Pakes, Gaia Polliri, Monica Reid, Justine Renwick, Justine Rowan, Joanne Searle, Laura Shanley, Debbie Shaw, Gemma Shepherd, Sarah Stanley, Fiona Taylor, Georgina Taylor, Jan Tritten, Caroline Turner, Ulrike von Moltke, Janet Walshaw, Caro Walton, Michael White, Liz Woolley, Rebecca Wright, Heba Zaphiriou-Zarifi and several anonymous contributors.

Extracts from birth stories, diaries, birth plans, letters or emails, interviews, self-standing comments or information texts (some of which were used in these pages, all in *BIRTH: Countdown to Optimal*) were contributed by Helen Arundell, Celina Barton, Elaine Batchelor, Paula Bays, Wendy Blumfield, Debbie Brindley, Bill Bryson (with CARE International), Sarah Buckley, Emma Cameron, Amanda Chalfen, Ruth Clark, Kathryn Clarke, Kathy Cleere, Rachel Cockburn, Janine DeBaise, Beth Dubois, Sarah-Jane Forder, Mary Frankland, Jill Harradine, Jenny Hodge, Kris Holloway, Angela Horn, Eleanor Jackson, Jennifer Jacoby, Libby Kelly, Eliza Klose, Nina Klose, Liliana Lammers, Dr Nicolette Lawson, Julia Lockwood, (and Melanie Milan), Karen Low, Liz Perry, Anne Phillips, Ashley Marshall, Shari Henry Rife, Justine Rowan, Hazel Rymell, Katya S from Moscow, Jenny Sanderson, Kay Sawford, Claire Saxby, Amanda Sealy, Joanne Searle, Gemma Shepherd, Teri Small, Sarah Stanley, Fiona Lucy Stoppard, Clare Swain, Fiona Taylor, Georgina Taylor, Jan Tritten, Jill Unwin, Rachel Urbach, Juliana van Olphen-Fehr, Ulrike von Moltke, Carol Walton, Julie White, Clare Winter, Sonia Winter, Rebecca Wright and by numerous anonymous contributors. A very special thank you to everyone who asked to remain anonymous!

Thank you, too, to everybody who contributed photographs. Particular thanks to Nina Klose, Jenny Sanderson, Jill Furmanovsky (www.jillfurmanovsky.com), Nuala OSullivan, Elaine Batchelor and John Huson, as well as to my pregnant models Sarah Morris, 'Sue' and 'Linda' (who both asked me not to reveal their surnames), and to one anonymous, naked, pregnant woman.

Other photos (of babies, midwives, children, etc.) were contributed very generously by numerous people, including Richard Bailey, Sarah Cave, Melissa Deas, Anita Khemka of UNICEF India and Ashley Marshall. Quite a few people contributed photos asking for them to be used anonymously or separately from a birth story, even though they had usually put their name to the other material they had contributed. In some cases, intentionally, the positioning of photographs or the caption underneath makes the identity of people clear and in others photographs are used to break up the text or illustrate points in a general way.

I would also like to thank Nina Klose, Sarah Buckley, Esther Culpin, Liliana Lammers, Angela Horn, Sheila Kitzinger and Dr Claire Robson for practical support. I am particularly grateful to Dr Sarah Buckley for allowing me to use adapted extracts from her excellent research articles. Thank you too, to Dani Zur of *Mother and Baby Magazine* for letting me use some of the results from the survey conducted in association with Persil in 2002.

A very, very special thank you to my original reviewers and editors—i.e. the people who gave me feedback on the original book *BIRTH: Countdown to Optimal*. In alphabetical order they were: Nina Klose, Liliana Lammers, Michel Odent, Theresa Prentice, Nancy Radford, Clare O'Ryan, Jenny Sanderson, Liz Woolley and Rebecca Wright. (There was also one other, who was a key person in the development of this book, who asked to remain anonymous... Thank you, mystery mother of four!) Thank you also to Nancy Radford for her invaluable advice and technical support, to Clare O'Ryan for acting as a perfect sounding board to my ideas, either face-to-face or over the phone. An enormous thank you to Michel Odent for all the material he contributed and for all the queries and requests he answered.

I would also like to mention the obstetrician who attended the birth of my first child in Sri Lanka and all the staff who supported me. Thank you! I am also grateful to Elaine Batchelor for helping me to work out a backup programme for my second labour (in Reading) for the period when Michel wasn't available, and to the NHS for providing my routine antenatal and postnatal care. Thank you in particular to Jo Farrington for one long, wonderful, reassuring antenatal chat and to my GP for not striking me off his list! Thank you to the NHS midwife, who helped smooth the path to my third and final labour by not hassling me and at the same time offering me invaluable support... it's a great shame you weren't able to attend the actual birth. My thanks to the NHS midwives who did arrive for the last few minutes and went along with my requests. A big thank you to Dr Lawrence Impey in Oxford and Dr Donald Gibb in London, who appeared out of the blue in birth stories. Along with all the other supportive professionals I came into contact with while researching this book, you really do seem to be working to optimise conditions for mother, father, baby, family and society at large each and every time a new child is born.

Perhaps my first obstetrician was right when he said he was convinced that violent births result in a violent society, while gentle births result in gentle, loving societies. Let's hope we find out the outcome of a mass move towards gentle birth over the next few decades. Our world needs a bit more peace and harmony.

Sylvie Donna

The publisher would also like to thank the following for the use of previously published material:
- Clairview Books for allowing the reproduction of extracts from *Birth and Breastfeeding* by Michel Odent (Forest Row, 2007)
- Souvenir Press for material extracted from *Birth Reborn* by Michel Odent (Souvenir Press 1994)
- Shufu no Tomosya for the photographs of Liliana Lammers which were originally published in the Japanese-language magazine *Balloon* (pp 21, 56 and 69)
- *Reader's Digest* for information and ideas which appeared in an article in the July 2003 edition of *Reader's Digest* magazine (p81)
- *LLL GB News* for allowing the publication of an adapted and extended version of an account which appeared in the magazine (Birthframe 30)
- *New Beginnings* for allowing the publication of a longer version of an account which originally appeared in the May/June 2003 issue (Birthframe 14)

If any material has accidentally been used without appropriate acknowledgement, or if any details are incorrect, please contact the publisher so that amendments can be made in future editions. Every possible effort has been made to ensure that all details of contributions are correct.

INTRODUCTION

I decided to write this book after writing another book called *BIRTH: Countdown to Optimal* (which is for pregnant women) and after various conversations with midwives. Although numerous books about midwifery are available, there doesn't seem to be one which has a clear focus on ways of supporting women who opt for safest approaches, according to research. (Of course, based on WHO guidelines, which in turn are based on research, this means going through pregnancy and birth with as few drugs and interventions as possible.) Somehow, the advice which would be relevant when caring for at least 95% of pregnant women (if they chose a physiological birth) has got lost amongst the advice which relates to the other 5% or less, who are likely to need drugs or interventions from the point of view of safety. The focus on pathology has meant that fewer and fewer midwives feel confident about supporting normal labour—although thankfully this is now a major focus of midwifery training. Needless to say, perhaps, it really is vital that all midwives know how to support normal labour and birth (following the physiological processes) because women who choose this safest route need a high standard of care. This book has been written for midwives who want to consider (or reconsider) best ways of providing support for women who want to have a natural birth, if at all possible.

In the recent past the emphasis on pathology over normality has meant that 'normal' almost came to mean 'abnormal', because women who were hoping for a straightforward, but safe physiological labour and birth were being treated as unusual. Unnecessary interventions had become so commonplace in the labour ward and delivery suite that a woman who insisted on having none (unless they were needed for safety) was branded an extremist, even though research was very definitely on her side. Hopefully, this situation has changed radically!

In some places there may still be midwives who are shocked or cynical about requests for a 'natural birth', despite the Royal College of Midwives' campaign to reinstate normal birth in British labour wards and delivery suites. Perhaps there are two very understandable reasons for this. Firstly, they may never actually have witnessed a truly 'normal' birth, i.e. a physiological one with no complications. (Of course, this is because many women are requesting pain relief, or are consenting to it when it's offered. And while some midwives may have witnessed a normal birth—without any anaesthesia or analgesia—they may not have witnessed one which has proceeded in optimal conditions, according to the true physiological processes.) Another reason why certain professionals may react negatively to any request for a 'natural birth' is perhaps their worry about things going wrong. Although even the most superficial study of statistics will make it clear that there is *always* a maternal and fetal mortality rate to take into account, the reality of an individual death is horrifying, particularly given the high risk of litigation. In fact, the risk of a criminal investigation might be what puts many midwives off supporting other women. They may be concerned that their superiors may fail to support them if there are not sufficient records, which will in turn lead to excessive (and probably intrusive or invasive) monitoring. Perhaps it's time a 'normal birth' consent form was introduced, requesting non-disturbance!

Whatever your own views, feelings or experience, the aim of this book is to support you if you want to help improve the safety of the births you facilitate and if you want to help women *actually have* the natural births they request. While I have tried to avoid giving patronising advice, I have made some tentative suggestions which are all based on research, feedback and suggestions I've received and/or my own experience as a mother who has given birth three times, entirely physiologically. Of course, I have at all times tried to take NICE guidelines into account and typical protocols. In any cases where I suggest changes or extensions to these I hope you will view these in the spirit they were intended—as a springboard for thought, discussion and possibly even action!

If, as you embark on reading this book, you doubt the value of supporting physiological birth (perhaps because you have seen so many women request pain relief after all), please suspend your disbelief for as long as it takes you to read the whole book. After all, we have to recognise that while Queen Victoria set in motion a hope for painfree birth in 1853 (when she agreed to try out chloroform for the birth of her eighth child), this hope has not yet become a reality. Even women who have the best of anaesthesia complain of pain beforehand or afterwards, and side effects are unfortunately all too common. As we all know, but maybe sometimes prefer to forget, the use of any unnecessary drugs or interventions during labour and birth compromises safety. For this reason alone it's well worth knowing how to make labour and birth as good as possible for women who opt out of this artificial approach, perhaps after reading research evidence or simply because they trust that the natural, physiological processes will be pretty effective, thank you very much! From personal experience and from the extensive research I've carried out (over a period of almost twelve years now), I'm convinced that the physiological processes are much more effective than we often assume. I'm also sure that they're worth 'enduring' because outcomes really do seem to be better for both mother and baby, not to mention families and the midwives who provide care.

Before I sign off—in case you're wondering who on earth I am—I'll give you a little background to this project. Formerly a teacher in adult education, I chose to write about birth after experiencing three entirely physiological births myself and after hearing about other women's experiences. I include my own birth stories in this book for information and also because I think it's important to convey how difficult it was to arrange my natural births. After deciding that 'physiological' was safest during my first pregnancy, I had to fight long and hard to exercise my right to have an 'optimal' birth. Plenty of professionals doubted the research evidence and many were worried about the idea of supporting a woman who was labouring without drugs... When writing, not being a midwife myself, I wanted to add 'weight' and authority to my own words, so I also conducted a great deal of research—both academic and personal. As you will see, I had no trouble finding midwives and consultants who would contribute material. Michel Odent is mentioned here and there because he attended the birth of my second baby. Comments from mothers or midwives are included so as to provide a window into the world of increased safety and satisfaction.

2 *Optimal Birth: The What, The Why & The How*

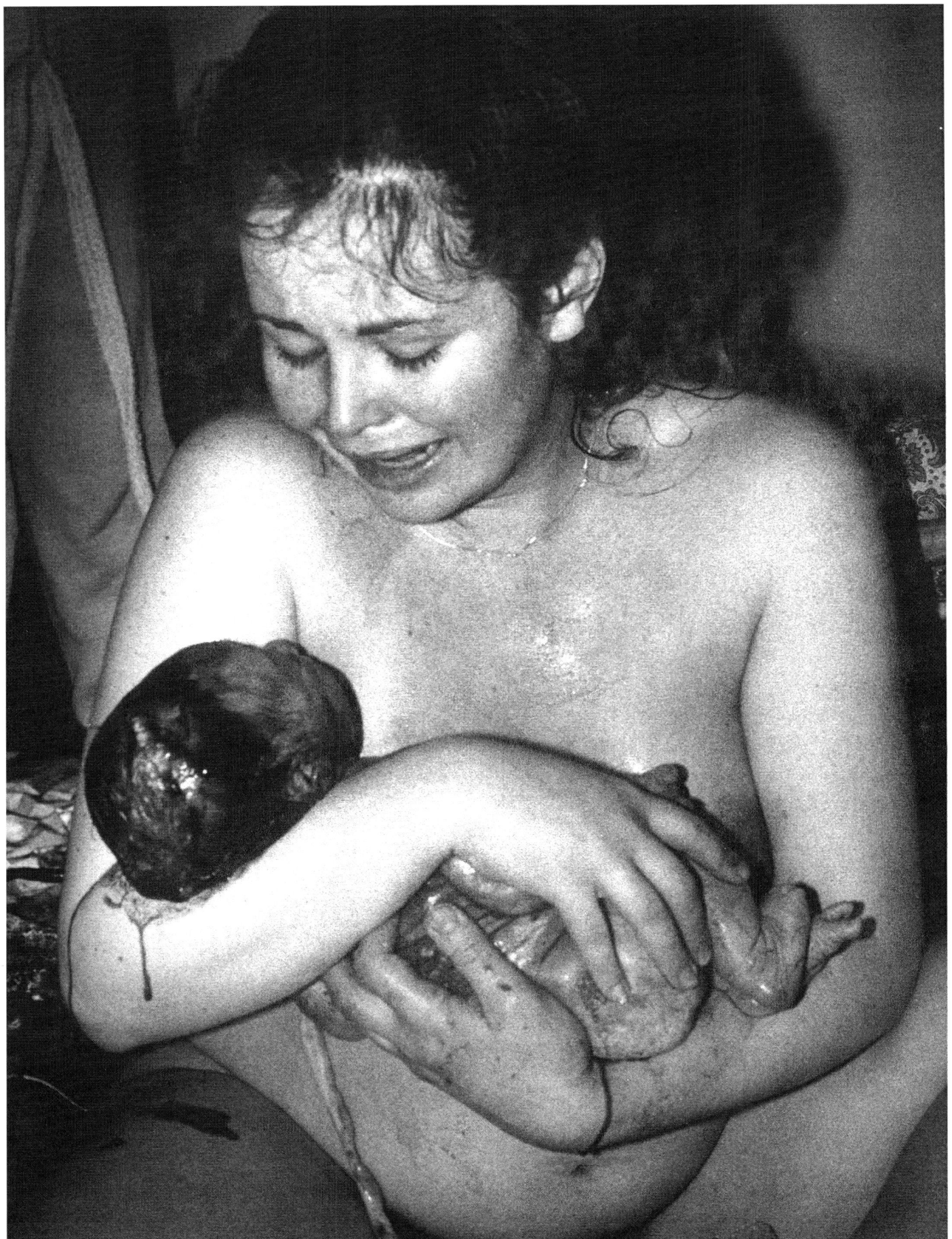

Nuala OSullivan, a mother from London, fully conscious and actively participating during her entirely physiological birth
Photo © Jill Furmanovsky (www.jillfurmanovsky.com)

OPTIMAL BIRTH: THE WHAT

The simplest way of defining an optimal birth is to say it's a birth which is as good as it possibly can be, for both mother and baby—and hopefully for midwives too!

Optimal birth is actually a little different from *natural* birth as it's been understood over the last few decades. I like to use the phrase 'old natural' to describe that... It's often meant a great departure from the real physiological processes because interventions have merely changed from being pharmacological to being New Age. Instead of drips and jabs, women in the 1970s, 80s and 90s typically had whale music playing in the background while they allowed themselves to be prodded by their acupuncturist's needles (or shiatsu therapist's fingers) and shouted at (or 'coached') by a committed birthing partner. Occasionally, a beautiful birth occurred after all this 'natural' intervention, but most of the time it resulted in huge amounts of disappointment and feelings of failure. More often than not, women would give up on the idea of 'natural' after a few hours of excruciating contractions and would willingly accept pethidine, an epidural or gas and air. Others would be diagnosed with dystocia (or 'failure to progress') and after being put on a drip to augment contractions would end up having either forceps or an emergency caesarean. Afterwards, these mothers were forced to admit they'd been wrong to assume it was all so possible and many of them felt disillusioned, disappointed, angry and even guilty. As you know, this is not just an historical scenario, it's still happening every day in maternity wards all over the country. What a shame these mothers haven't heard of 'new natural'...

As you may have guessed, 'new natural' (another term for 'optimal'), means allowing the physiological processes to proceed without *any* kind of interventions, whether pharmacological or New Age. It means natural, as in giving birth like a cavewoman, with full midwifery back-up and ready access to life-saving intervention in case it's needed. In a nutshell, optimal means an ultra-natural approach, backed-up by all the best our society has to offer.[1] [Numbers refer to notes on the next page.] Your expertise as a midwife is crucial to the optimality of this kind of birth because obviously, without it, maternal and fetal risks are much higher.

In an optimal birth no pain relief or intervention is used, unless absolutely necessary, because any interventions (of any kind) are likely to disturb the physiological processes and consequently the level of risk to both the labouring woman and her baby.[2] In case you question this, consider for a moment how an epidural immediately puts a woman at risk because it inevitably results in a lowering of blood pressure; and consider how the use of artificial oxytocin for augmentation immediately necessitates higher levels of monitoring because no-one can be sure precisely which dose is ideal (or dangerous) for any one particular woman. And—to make sure we're clear about this—let me say that no interventions means no induction, electronic fetal monitoring, TENS, gas and air, pethidine or epidurals. It even means no complementary therapies such as shiatsu, acupuncture and homeopathy, precisely because they can all be so incredibly powerful.

Unlike 'old natural', which didn't facilitate the natural processes, 'optimal' really is possible for most women, as long as a few basic principles are respected. It's not only possible, it's desirable...

- My own research has made me conclude that an optimal birth usually means far less pain is experienced overall by the mother, if postnatal pain is taken into account too.[3] When a woman is fully alert and undistracted she is likely to have a shorter labour, a fast second stage[4] and she's far less likely to sustain a bad tear, or indeed any tear at all.[5] Any pain experienced is also likely to be more manageable because of the endorphins which are naturally produced and the subsequent unusual state of mind which results when the physiological processes remain truly undisturbed.[6] Postnatal psychological pain is likely to be less too, which brings us to the next point...
- After optimal births, bonding can proceed more smoothly not least because both mother and baby are extremely alert.[7] Higher rates of breastfeeding are also likely to result—sometimes even when the mother has planned to formula-feed—because many drugs used for pain relief (in particular opiates such as pethidine or diamorphine) weaken a baby's suck. With a normal suck, a newborn can easily get the colostrum and milk he or she needs, without hurting the mother through ineffectual sucking.
- Babies face far fewer risks, both perinatally and postnatally—into adulthood and old age. (We'll come back to this in more detail later.)[8]
- Babies experience high levels of alertness at birth, which may have enormous repercussions in terms of bonding and formative experiences. If these two types of early experience are at all important, experiencing an optimal birth may have an enormous impact on a baby's later psychological development.
- Higher levels of satisfaction are experienced by mothers because they experience the endorphins which are spontaneously produced postnatally.[9]
- Midwives have greater job satisfaction because fully natural births have a strangely compelling atmosphere...

In short, 'optimal' means a less painful experience for the mother, both physically and psychologically, fewer health risks and a better deal for the baby[10], not to mention satisfaction for you, the midwife. If you question this last point, let me ask you to consider for a moment why it is that midwives who have witnessed many completely physiological births are often prepared to go to great lengths to safeguard their right to attend women as they feel is right (e.g. by becoming an independent midwife)... Fortunately, the situation in Britain is fairly supportive of a woman's right to choose, and a midwife's right to support her, in particular since the Royal College of Midwives is promoting 'normal' birth once more. (I'm sure you know about the Campaign for Normal Birth. On the RCM website (www.rcm.org) it says: "Intervention and caesarean shouldn't be the first choice—they should be the last.") It's time we reminded ourselves what 'normal' really means.

We need to remind ourselves what 'normal' really means in birth

Notes

1. For a review and comparison of obstetric approaches (either 'managed' or natural) see the book co-authored by seven researchers (Enkin et al) *Guide to Effective Care in Pregnancy and Childbirth* (Oxford University Press 2000), Jadad and Enkin's book *Randomized Controlled Trials: Questions, Answers and Musings* (Blackwell 2007), *Normal Childbirth: Evidence and Debate* (Churchill Livingstone 2004), *Home Birth* (Pinter & Martin 2006), *Born in the USA: How a broken maternity system must be fixed to put women and children first* (University of California Press 2006) and *Pushed: The painful truth about childbirth and modern maternity care* (DaCapo Lifelong 2008).
2. For an exploration of this see: Odent M. The second stage as a disruption of the fetus ejection reflex. *Midwifery Today*. Int Midwife. 2000 Autumn;(55):12.
3. Quite a few contributors to my original book *BIRTH: Countdown to Optimal* mentioned their surprise at the lack of pain in their labours or the surprising nature of the sensations. Others experienced intense pain but found they could travel through it, thanks to the strange hormonal processes taking place, which inevitably have an effect on the mind as well as the body.
4. See: Odent M. The fetus ejection reflex. *Birth* 1987; 14:104-5.
5. For more on this subject read *Is there sex after childbirth?* by Juliet Rix (Thorsons 1995) and Michel Odent. The perineal preoccupation. In: *The Caesarean* (p96-101). Free Association Books. London 2004.
6. See: Odent M. New reasons and new ways to study birth physiology. *International Journal of Gynecology and Obstetrics* 2001; 75:S39-S45 and Goland, R. S. et al. Biologically Active Corticotrophin-releasing Hormone in Maternal and Fetal Plasma during Pregnancy. *American Journal of Obstetrics and Gynecology* 159 (1984): 884-890.
7. If you're interested in considering how a baby's ability to love might develop also see: Niles Newton. The Influence of the Let-Down Reflex in Breast Feeding on the Mother-Child Relationship. *Marriage and Family Living* 1958; 20: 18-20.
8. If you would like to explore this issue yourself, see the Primal Health database at www.birthworks.org/primalhealth. To consider the possible link between the use of analgesics in labour and later drug use in the grown baby see: Jacobson B, Nyberg K. Opiate addiction in adult offspring through possible imprinting after obstetric treatment. *BMJ* 1990; 301: 1067-70 and Nyberg K, Buka SL, Lipsitt LP. Perinatal medication as a potential risk factor for adult drug abuse in a North American cohort. *Epidemiology* 2000; 11(6): 715-16.
9. For an exploration of related issues see: *Evolution's End: Reclaiming the Potential of Our Intelligence* (San Francisco: Harper 1995): 178-179; Odent, M. Orgasmic states, Ecstatic states and Mystical emotions. In: *The Scientification of Love* (pp 75-79). Free Association Books. London 1999.
10. If you're interested in filling in gaps, note that in general randomised controlled trials are impossible in many cases in the perinatal period. Women would refuse to participate in the process of randomisation because they usually have strong preferences at this time. This is why there is a lack of valuable hard data on several issues.

Also note that in *BIRTH: Countdown to Optimal* I do recommend a few well-tried and 'sensible' interventions:
- The use of folic acid preconceptually and in the first trimester so as to prevent spinal malformations.
- The use of vitamin supplements (e.g. Sanatogen's *Pronatal*) from the second trimester onwards and Omega-3 supplements in the third trimester. This is because many modern women have inadequate diets.
- Drinking 1-3 cups of raspberry leaf tea per day during the third trimester—a tried and tested uterotonic.
- The prophylactic use of homeopathic Arnica 30 in the last month of pregnancy, which is at worst harmless, but may help prevent or heal bruising during the birth.

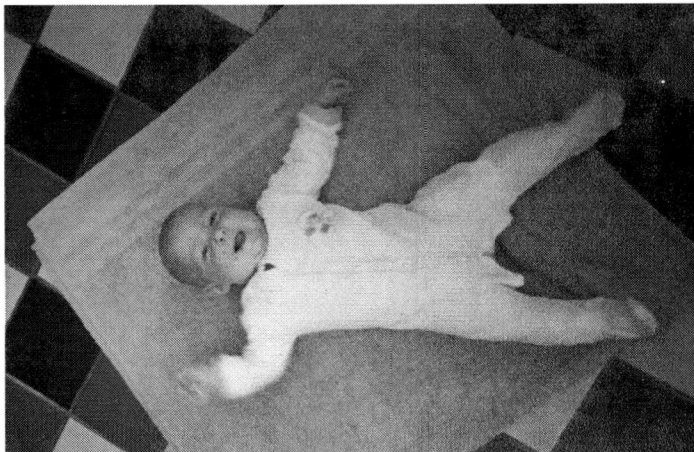
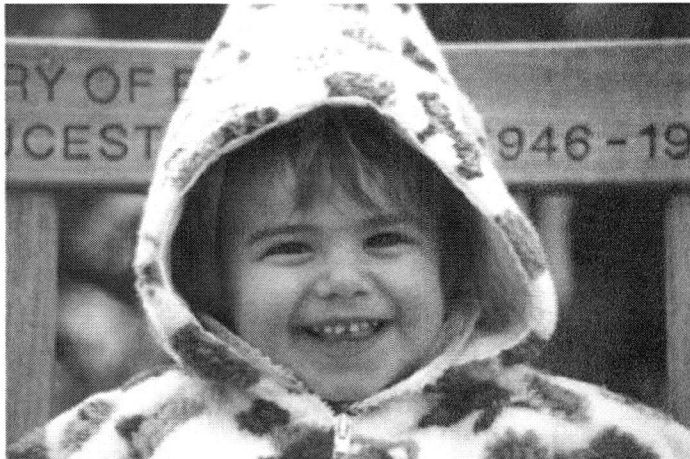
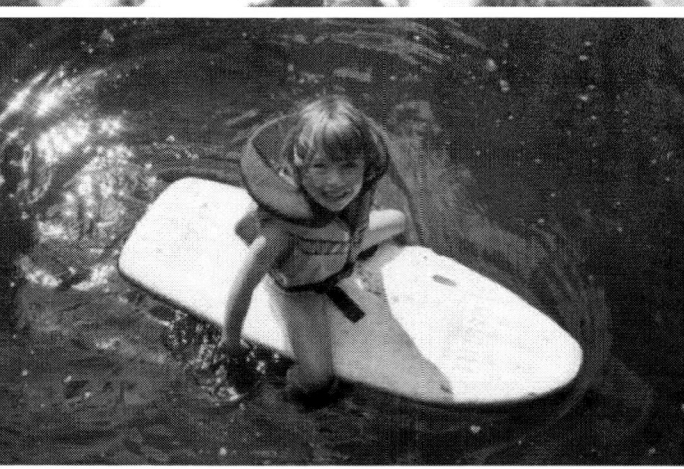

A few optimally-birthed children

THE PHYSIOLOGICAL PROCESSES

Of course, you know what happens in pregnancy and birth—you're a midwife after all... But can you make a clear differentiation between processes which are natural and those which are typical when analgesia, anaesthesia or complementary therapies are used, or when non-essential interventions or even disturbance take place? If you're used to supporting women who are using anaesthesia, analgesia or complementary therapies you may have become so used to dealing with risks caused by unnecessary interventions and may have forgotten the characteristics of a truly undisturbed physiological birth. Research over the last few decades has needed to relate to the use of drugs and interventions for legal reasons. As a result, relatively little attention has been paid to documenting the undisturbed processes and some midwives have never even witnessed them.

The effect of emotions on the natural processes of conception, pregnancy, labour and birth may also have been neglected in recent decades. As we know from the simple effect fear has on the production of a hormone such as adrenaline, a person's emotional state can have an enormous impact on physiological states. The effect of emotions is also obvious if we remember that adrenaline usually inhibits the production of oxytocin—the hormone which stimulates contractions—which in turn is produced by the simple act of sharing a meal with a friend or loved one.

Since adrenaline and oxytocin are usually antagonistic the role of emotions is clear

Neglecting the physiological processes or even underestimating the importance of something like emotions is dangerous if an appropriate decision tree for watchful waiting is to be developed and understood. In order to provide appropriate and helpful support for women labouring naturally—so as to produce optimal outcomes—it is therefore vital that the processes of an entirely physiological pregnancy, labour and birth are well understood.

Understanding the natural processes is the key to developing a good decision tree

Pregnancy

Of course, a woman's experience of pregnancy is likely to vary according to her health, personality, emotional responses, social environment, geographical location, antenatal care and culture. This means not only that each woman starts from a different point than any other woman on the planet, but also that she can influence the course of her own pregnancy according to what she does, and what she allows other people to do to her mind or body. And we need to remember in all this that whatever happens or is done to her is also likely to affect her baby too. Of course, this has enormous implications for care.

Whether the woman perceives pregnancy as something positive or negative—or as a neutrally interesting change in her circumstances, or even as a life-threatening situation—may well depend on her experience of birth so far and even on how the professionals she encounters speak to her...

THE FIRST TRIMESTER (WEEKS 1-12)

The first three months are often a time of heightened emotions and physical unease due to occasional bouts of nausea and tiredness, and unfamiliar bodily changes. Of course, the upheaval is caused by the different hormones circulating and the effect of the growing placenta. Emotions are often triggered by thoughts about pregnancy and birth and they might even stimulate shockingly vivid dreams. Women might experience an overwhelming need to sleep at any time of the day and they usually also need to go to the toilet more often because of pressure on the bladder. It's in this period that the baby is going through its most crucial development—all the major body organs are being formed.

THE SECOND TRIMESTER (WEEKS 13-28)

Most women experience fewer discomforts during this second three-month period. Any nausea usually disappears completely by Week 13 or 14 because the placenta should now be fully functioning. Hormones settle down and fewer trips are needed to the toilet. Most women perceive the slowly emerging bump positively because it's tangible proof of the pregnancy, which is usually considered a good thing. Many, though, will still be grappling with odd thoughts and feelings and some will not have come to terms with the fact of being pregnant.

More blood is now circulating around the woman's body (meaning more work for her lungs, kidneys and heart), thanks to the work of the placenta. This will sometimes mean that women are mistakenly diagnosed as suffering from anaemia, when really the lower percentage of haemoglobin in their blood is simply an indication that the placenta is functioning normally. (More on this later.)

Typically, women feel much more alert and energetic in this trimester but they sometimes worry about the idea of giving birth or about impending motherhood. They may also have all sorts of fears about the welfare of the baby at this stage. All this is perfectly normal because it's a sign the woman is tuning in to her baby and his or her needs. From the 18th or 20th week onwards, most women can feel the baby kicking and moving about now and then.

THE THIRD TRIMESTER (WEEKS 29-40+)

Often women experience no particular changes as they enter the third trimester, except for a dramatically increasing girth. The fact of getting bigger may bother some women, especially if poor posture is causing backache or if they are afraid of giving birth. Tiredness may also be a big problem because of the woman's increased weight and uncomfortable or disrupted nights, caused by difficulty finding a good position and a bladder which is being pushed out of the way! The woman may well feel a need to drink more water than usual, which is logical considering that the amniotic fluid is constantly being replaced. Stretch marks may appear and nipples are likely to look different.

Most women find themselves thinking a lot about the upcoming birth. Changing hormones in the woman's body are gradually preparing both her and her baby for the birth. Labour will begin spontaneously, the timing being affected by genetics, health, diet, lifestyle, psychology, circumstances... as well as an incorrectly calculated due date.

Week by week...

It's useful to consider pregnancy week by week because this information may easily be forgotten or changed by an overly interventionist view of birth. The following guide is intended to help you talk to pregnant women in such a way that they bond with their growing babies as well as possible, which might hopefully motivate them to do as much as possible for their babies' good. For this reason, instead of distancing terms such as 'fetus', more personal words such as 'baby' have been used. Obviously, if you use this guide with your clients you will need to change 'the' to 'your' when referring to 'the baby', for example.

THE FIRST TRIMESTER

The first trimester is very important because this is when all the baby's organs and bones are being formed.

Weeks 1 & 2

During these first two weeks one or more ova (eggs) mature inside the woman's ovaries. Meanwhile, the endometrium (the lining of the womb) builds up so as to provide a suitable place for the ovum to nestle in, after it's been fertilised. This will happen after the ovum is released from one of the ovaries and one of the woman's partner's sperm comes up to meet it. (In previous months when no ovum was fertilised, the endometrium was eventually released in the form of a menstrual period.)

Of course, some women may not realise that half of the developing baby's chromosomes (its genetic make-up) will be from herself and the other half from her partner.

Week 3

Conception takes place either at the beginning of this week or later if the woman usually has a long cycle. (When women ovulate later, their due date is also later because it takes a baby around 266 days—or 38 weeks—to develop.) If only one baby is growing (instead of twins or triplets!), only one of a possible 200 million sperm fertilises the ovum in this third week so all the sperm released into the vagina when the man had an orgasm were in competition with each other. It takes about 45 minutes for the sperm to reach the newly released ovum and some people say that lying down for half an hour or so after sex helps this process. It's helpful if the woman is already taking folic acid supplements by this stage because this is a nutrient many people are deficient in.

During conception the pronucleus of the sperm which unites with the ovum is drawn into the ovum itself. Very quickly, the cell membrane around the ovum closes to seal out all the other sperm. This process is only successful 40% of the time when sperm and ovum meet so it's an especially fortuitous month when a woman becomes pregnant. An incredible series of processes are taking place successfully.

Within 24 hours the newly fertilised cell, which is called a zygote, divides into two (a process called 'cleavage'!) and becomes a 'morula'. As the morula develops and fluid enters the mass of cells it becomes a 'blastocyst', which continues dividing so that after nine months it will consist of several hundred billion cells. The one fertilised cell transforms and differentiates itself to make a new person, thanks to the DNA inside the genes in the ovum and sperm.

> Note: At times in the text I make suggestions as to what you might do. Please don't take offence—I realise you're the expert. It's just that imperatives ("Do this! Do that!) are shorter than carefully-worded suggestions and I've tried to be brief throughout this book. Also, it wasn't always easy to separate 'The How' from 'The What'...

Week 4

On the tenth or eleventh day after fertilisation, having successfully travelled along one of the woman's fallopian tubes, the blastocyst implants itself into the lining of her womb. From this point onwards the tiny baby is called an 'embryo'. It is nourished by tiny blood vessels called chorionic villi in the lining of the womb. These villi were produced by the embryo itself, even though it is still only the size of a pinhead.

If the woman has conceived identical twins or triplets (or more!), by the end of this week the single blastocyst will have already divided up to form two, three or more separate embryos. If she is expecting non-identical twins or triplets, etc., more than one egg will have been released, fertilised and implanted two weeks ago.

Week 5

By the end of this week many women spontaneously realise they are pregnant and confirm this using one of the widely available home pregnancy tests. It's good if a pregnancy is confirmed early on because knowing for sure motivates many women to do everything possible for the good of the developing baby. If a first test is negative but the woman's period still hasn't started, you may need to tell a woman that she may still be pregnant. Explain that the negative result may be due to low levels of hCG—human chorionic gonadotrophin, the hormone manufactured by the blastocyst which the test tries to detect. Also, tell her that levels may be low if she ovulated late in her cycle and encourage her to do another test in a few days' time and again after a week or so, if she still thinks she's pregnant.

Of course, taking at least 400mg of folic acid per day is particularly important this week and over the next few weeks because folic acid is crucial in ensuring healthy development of the neural tube, which eventually becomes the spinal column and brain. It's also vital that the woman drinks enough water. Requirements vary according to height, weight, activity levels, climate, etc, so I won't give any precise recommendations, but do encourage your client to drink plenty of water. Remind her to check bottled water for sodium levels and to only drink water when the label says the level is lower than 10mg per litre. (It's useful to tell her that levels in sparkling water tend to be dramatically higher, so it's probably best if she drinks mainly still water.)

The embryo's brain already has two separate lobes. In appearance, the embryo is a bit like a grey, jelly-like, translucent tadpole, with a head and a tail. It's only a few millimetres long—perhaps as long as a grain of rice. It swims around in a miniature yolk sac and amniotic sac which protect it from harm.

The woman's future baby is already connected to the woman by a miniature umbilical cord and cells are beginning to differentiate so as to form the baby's skin, intestines, a primitive nervous system and bones.

Week 6

Several crucial developments take place this week. By the end of the week, the umbilical cord, digestive tract, kidneys, liver, heart and bloodstream are already forming and beginning to function—the heart will start beating during this week—and all these organs and systems are helping the embryo to get and use food from the rich lining of the woman's womb. The mouth and jaw are also developing now and ten discrete dental buds are growing in each jaw. The four shallow pits which have already appeared on the little embryo's head will later develop into eyes and ears.

The most important development this week sounds unimpressive but is actually crucial. A groove appears down the embryo's body; this will soon form the spinal cord and the brain. Of course, the folic acid which is routinely recommended up until approximately 12 weeks after conception ensures this process takes place smoothly. It is essential to ensure that this neural tube develops successfully because it consists of 125,000 cells. This is amazing when you consider that the embryo is still only the size of a pea.

Week 7

The woman's baby is still developing at a phenomenal rate. To get an idea just how fast this is, consider that while the embryo's limb buds will have developed by the 30th day after conception, by the 31st day (which is in the middle of this week) these same buds will have become subdivided into hands, arms and shoulders. The brain will be 25% bigger than it was just two days earlier.

By the end of this week, the embryo is the size of a small grape, growing at a rate of 1mm a day. If we could see it, we might think its head looked big in relation to its body, but this is normal. Already a face is forming, with tightly closed eyelids over dark-looking eyes. The embryo also has rudimentary arms and legs and is making its first movements. At the end of each limb small indentations which will later become fingers and toes are already discernible. Bone cells are also appearing.

The development of the woman's future baby's lungs, intestines, liver and kidneys continues and sex organs begin to form. (At every stage when you talk to women, make sure you say 'he or she' when referring to the baby inside them, so that they can get used to the idea of having either!) The pancreas and thyroid are already in place. The embryo's heart, which recently started beating, is currently beginning to form its four separate chambers.

The nervous system, including the embryo's spinal cord and brain, is almost completely formed. In about a week's time (41 days after conception) the complex structure of the mature brain will already be in evidence, albeit in miniature. The embryo is becoming so complex, that it will soon be known by a different term!

> Note: In most of the text, references to research are not provided. These will be included in a future edition. (Time constraints have limited what was possible for this first discussion document.) You will find some references in the books recommended for further reading.

Week 8

By the end of this week (six weeks after conception), the embryo technically starts being called a fetus—a word, which means 'little one'. It is no longer dependent on a yolk sac for nourishment, so this has already disappeared.

The little one's face is continuing to form: its nose is now pointed and already has nostrils; its eyes and ears are growing; and the two sides of its jaw will have joined together to make a mouth. Inside its mouth, there is a tiny tongue and taste buds will begin to appear on it in two weeks' time. (The palate will also begin to form at that time.) Since the inner parts of the ears are developing the growing baby will soon have a sense of balance. This is useful because it is already moving around a lot in its sac, even though the woman won't be able to feel this yet.

The little one's tiny skeleton is now fully formed out of soft cartilage; this will later develop into bone. All the internal organs are in evidence, even though they are not yet fully developed or in their final positions. The arms and legs have grown longer in the last week and if only it were possible to take a peek, we would be able to discern shoulders, elbows, hips and knees. Even fingers and toes are beginning to form, although they are joined by webs of skin for the time being.

There is evidence that the baby's brain is working by this stage, as electrical activity can now be measured. By the end of this week the baby will be around 2½cm long.

Week 9

The baby's limbs are continuing to develop rapidly and its fingers and toes are becoming more clearly defined.

Movements which were initially merely floating are gradually becoming a form of exercise for newly forming muscles. Movements will increasingly synchronise with the woman's own movements as her baby's vestibular system (which is concerned with gravity and balance in space) starts to develop. Periods of activity will alternate with periods of rest from now on until the birth, when a pattern of nighttime rest and daytime activity will eventually become established. The baby's brain, which coordinates all this movement, is continuing to develop: by now the brainstem (the lower portion of the brain) will be fully developed and the midbrain and forebrain (a little higher up) will start to expand. The wrinkles on the outer surface of the forebrain (the cerebral cortex), which are so characteristic of human beings and which allow us to accommodate vastly more brain cells than other species, are now also beginning to appear. Oxygen is being pumped round the baby's tiny body in red blood cells, which are already being produced by the liver. Beta-endorphins are already detectable in this blood, which suggests the woman's tiny baby can already experience pleasure.

The baby's face, eyes, nose, lips, tongue and the first signs of teeth and bone would be clearly visible to us with ultrasound, although this is not advised, as will be explained later. By the end of this week urogenital development begins for both sexes. If the baby is to be a boy, a penis would now also probably be visible.

All this is happening in miniature because the baby still only weighs little more than a grape.

Week 10

Just eight weeks after the woman's baby was conceived, tactile sensitivity has developed in the face. If the cheeks were to be stroked gently with a hair, the growing baby would move its head away, bend its trunk and pelvis and extend its arms and shoulders enough to push the hair away. (Don't ask me how researchers know this, but they claim that they do.) Sensitivity on other areas of skin will develop gradually over the next few weeks.

Chest movements, which are now detectable to researchers, might well be practice exercises for breathing after birth. Inside the baby's chest, the heart has finished dividing into four chambers and each is connected to the others by tiny valves.

The placenta, to which the baby is already attached, begins to produce progesterone around this time. The woman's tiny baby is still being nourished entirely by the so-called corpus luteum, although this will soon change.

Fingers, hands, wrists, toes and ankles are well-defined and the face is even more recognisably human. The baby is now roughly the size of a large strawberry.

Week 11

Either by now or in a few days' time (depending on when the woman conceived), all the little one's major body organs will have finished forming. Even miniature ovaries and testicles will have finished forming and the baby's circulation will be functioning properly. This all means the most critical period of development is over. For some reason, this means the risk of miscarriage also decreases sharply around this time.

> When the baby is getting all his or her nourishment via the placenta any nausea should disappear

---

The first time I found out I was pregnant, we were on an Easter holiday above the Arctic Circle in Finland. My first noticeable sign of pregnancy was terrible insomnia. I crept outdoors at 4am, as a pink spring dawn broke over a wide, flat snowscape. I felt overwhelmed with the knowledge that I was not alone. Although still only a microscopic ball of cells, my future offspring was already with me. What would this dawn of a new life be like, for me and for this child?

Three months later, my husband and I took the ferry to Bruges for the weekend. As our wake churned behind us towards Dover's chalk cliffs, I thought about how this point in my life was a metaphysical departure, too, towards a time in my life when I would come to know the new human beings who would enter my life through my own womb.

I never stop wondering at the journey that begins with a particular event of copulation—perhaps specifically remembered, perhaps not—into a single cell, into ten billion cells born months later as a fully-formed human baby.

Nina Klose

Week 12

The tiny baby living inside your client is beginning to look more human. Its head is becoming more rounded, even though it would still look rather large in proportion to her body. The eyelids are now formed, but are closed over the eyes, and the external ears even have earlobes.

By the end of this week the growing baby is getting all its nourishment via the placenta, which should now be fully functioning. The blood vessels in the umbilical cord carry food and oxygen to the tiny baby and then take carbon dioxide back out again. The little one can now open and shut its mouth and swallow; it uses this new skill to continuously take in amniotic fluid. Doing this will help its lungs develop, so that they are ready for breathing, as soon as he or she is born.

The kidneys are now beginning to function, which means the growing baby will urinate into the amniotic fluid. Reassure the woman that this is nothing to worry about—her womb constantly replaces this fluid so that her baby's environment stays fresh. Amazing as it might seem, a complete change of amniotic fluid is effected once every twenty-four hours. (This rate will even gradually increase over the next few weeks.) Any waste products in the urine from the growing baby are automatically dealt with by its own kidneys; other waste products which do not come out in the baby's urine are stored in its own intestines, ready to be excreted soon after birth as meconium, which will be the newborn baby's first 'poo'. This early poo is different from normal poos, as you probably know, in that its tar-like consistency actually acts to block the baby's bowel before birth; only if a baby becomes distressed while in the womb is this secreted into the amniotic fluid.

The baby's muscles, having further developed over the last couple of weeks, now allow for much more vigorous movement. In experiments, babies have been observed rolling from side to side, extending and then flexing their backs and necks, waving their arms and kicking their legs—straight into the side wall of the amniotic sac! The usually graceful and apparently voluntary and spontaneous movements the baby now makes are thought by some to be an early example of initiative and self-expression. Such creative gymnastics seem to demonstrate quite sophisticated brain activity, which only a few decades ago would have been considered impossible. Movements of the face—frowns, pursing the lips, opening and closing the mouth—all seem to indicate an emotional response to whatever's going on, given that the pituitary started producing pleasurable beta-endorphins a few weeks ago.

Babies in the womb at this age who have had their genitals stroked under experimental conditions (accidentally, I hope) have shown a clear response, which suggests a high level of sensitivity. Small, well-coordinated movements of tiny fingers and toes (which are both growing miniature finger- and toenails) suggest further sensitivity and emotional response.

The woman's baby now weighs about 14g and is perhaps 7 or 8cm long. Clearly, a lot more growth and development is needed before this little being can survive independently, outside the safety of the womb. At least it is now a little less susceptible to harm from infection or chemicals circulating around the woman's own body.

THE SECOND TRIMESTER

When the woman enters this second period of development her 'baby' will be much more of a being in its own right and its support system, the placenta, should be functioning effectively, thanks to the production of progesterone. This means that if the woman suffered from nausea or vomiting in the first trimester, it's likely to disappear now or at least fade very soon.

Week 13

The baby now begins to do more and more things which seem more recognisably 'human'. It might suck its thumb, for example, extend its fingers, or even yawn when it's tired. Tiredness is perhaps understandable given that its periods of movement are extremely frequent, with rest periods extending no longer than 15 minutes until around Week 20. The baby's neck is also longer, which makes it look much more human.

Being completely formed, the baby is now focusing on growing (at an even faster rate than before), so good nutrition with plenty of protein is extremely important.

Its skin sensitivity is increasing to the point where even the palms of its hands would respond to strokes; its arms and legs would certainly be sensitive to hair strokes. Some primitive reflexes are also either already present or will develop over the next four weeks.

Some people believe that personality is also beginning to develop at this stage because at least two research projects have concluded that exposure to influenza during the second trimester (between the third and seventh months of pregnancy) results in increased susceptibility to schizophrenia, so it might be especially important for your client to avoid people who are snuffly over the next few months.

Week 14

Almost three months since conception, the growing baby is now approximately 9cm long and will definitely be receiving all nourishment from 'its' placenta, which some young children have referred to as a kind of friend in the womb. It looks like a large, liver-like organ and it will be born separately, just after the baby.

The baby's eyes have now moved away from the side of the head to the front, and the baby's ears have moved up from the neck to their proper position on the head, but they're still fused shut for the time being. The baby has eyebrows now, as well as a small amount of hair on its head. The basic parts of the spinal cord and brain are in place, and the baby's respiratory tract, which starts at the nose and branches again and again on the way to the lungs, is now ready for the growing baby's first breathing movements. As for other movements, the baby may now start moving its arms and legs rhythmically. Increased skin sensitivity means that if it were possible to stroke the baby very gently on the cheek, we would see it turn its head and start searching for something, probably a nipple to suckle from!

The next four weeks are a period of rapid skeletal development. We know this because some researchers have tracked it on X-rays.

Week 15

It is in this week that the baby's sex organs will mature. Its nose will also be better formed and its head and eyebrow hair will gradually start to become coarser. If your client's baby has a gene for black hair, the pigment cells of the hair follicles are now beginning to produce black pigment.

It seems likely that taste buds are also functioning by now. We know for certain that no essential changes take place in taste receptors after this point, except for the fact that they multiply and spread themselves more widely. This means that the growing baby will be having taste experiences based on what the woman eats and drinks herself from now until the birth. It's possible that these experiences may affect the little one's preferences in childhood and possibly also beyond—I've certainly observed this in my own children! Based on the contents of amniotic fluid which has been tested, we know that the baby will be tasting glucose, fructose, lactic, pyruvic and citric acid, fatty acids, phospholipids, creatinine, urea, uric acid, amino acids, polypeptides, proteins and salts, amongst other things. It doesn't sound very appetising but it certainly indicates that the baby is having a wide range of gustatory experience.

As well as sucking its thumb, the baby may also suck its fingers, hands and toes and hold its own umbilical cord by this stage.

Week 16

By now, the baby will weigh about 75g and will be about 11½cm long. If we could look at it, we would see transparent skin, with fine networks of blood vessels underneath.

Hard bones are beginning to develop and the baby's legs will have become longer. Both arms and legs will now have joints. The baby already has well-formed fingernails and toenails and its fingers would already produce a unique fingerprint. It can now coordinate all its movements and it will be moving around energetically, although the pregnant woman probably won't be able to feel this just yet.

Even though the baby's ears are not yet fully formed, the baby is already responding to sound, probably by feeling vibrations through its skin. Its eyes are now open and quite expressive. During invasive procedures, expressions such as squinting and sneering have been filmed at this stage of pregnancy. Researchers who observed these expressions felt certain they represented meaningful reactions to what was happening.

The baby's eyebrows and eyelashes are growing and the baby will already have fine downy hair ('lanugo') on both its face and body. This lanugo usually disappears by the time of the birth, but it can still be seen on premature babies.

Although the major organs are now fully developed, the baby will continue to grow rapidly this month and in the rest of the pregnancy so that it will be capable of independent life. Already, it will be making breathing movements as practice movements for after the birth.

Notice I've said nothing about scans here. (See pp 85-86 for a detailed discussion on ultrasound.)

Week 17

By now, the baby will measure about 15cm, which is approximately the length of a pen. It will weigh about 175g. These are landmark measurements because for the first time, the baby weighs more than its support system, the placenta. The baby is still becoming increasingly sensitive... fetal abdomens and buttocks have responded to hair strokes in experiments at this stage and different responses have been recorded when babies were exposed to different kinds of music: Beethoven, Brahms and hard-rock music made them restless, while Vivaldi and Mozart calmed them down. Perhaps the woman should bear this in mind when deciding which music to listen to, although of course her own tastes are also important.

Week 18

The baby may now be as long as 20cm and your client may soon notice her moving around inside her. By the end of this week, you should be able to hear the baby's heartbeat with an ordinary fetal stethoscope (a Pinard), i.e. with a device which doesn't use ultrasound (unlike the Sonicaid).

The baby will be drinking amniotic fluid through a perfectly formed mouth and lips. This is a practice exercise so that breathing takes place without undue effort or fatigue after the birth. Sometimes this exercise will make the growing baby develop hiccups, which the might notice as a jerking of her abdomen. The baby will also be practising sucking, maybe using its thumb, which is obviously preparation for feeding after birth. The growing baby may also be making other sounds quite voluntarily by now, which is perhaps the first step in language learning.

Bones are still continuing to form rapidly and the baby's nasal septum will now have fused with the palate.

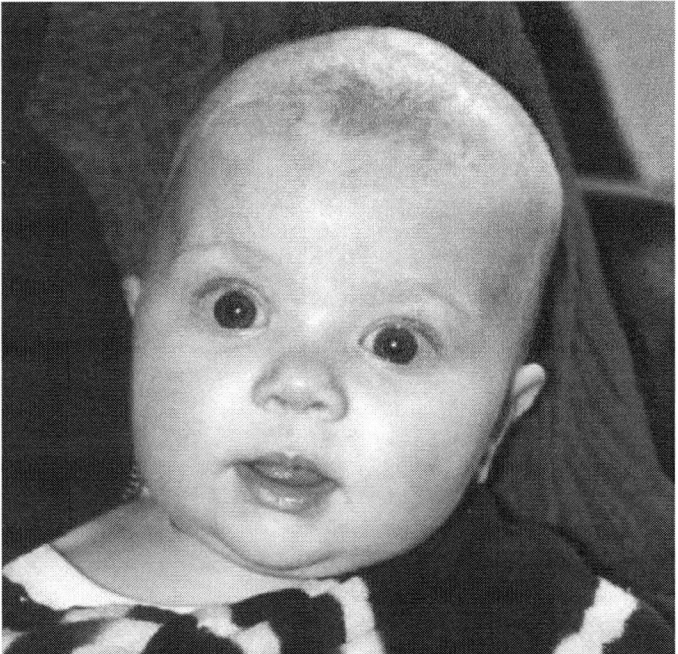

If the woman seems receptive, explain during antenatal appointments about the advantages of avoiding drugs during birth... Of course, babies are more alert if they're born naturally. Also ask her to consider whether she really wants a 'routine' scan, whose effects we can only guess at. (More on this later...)

Week 19

This week, buds for permanent teeth are forming behind those which have already formed for the milk teeth. The baby's sense of touch is also still developing: the baby would respond if touched almost anywhere on its body.

The growing baby will now be making stronger and better coordinated movements, which might even include back flips, rolls and little punches. These gymnastics are only possible because its nervous system is now much more sophisticated.

By the way, in order to ensure optimal outcomes, don't recommend that women simulate pain in any way in order to practise for labour. Nowadays it's been well-established that hormones (which are affected by emotions) pass across the placenta—so the woman's own nervousness, tension, pain or fear would probably be shared with her developing baby if she were to do this.

Week 20

The baby has been growing fast, so by now its body will have reached its correct relative proportions. The baby is now about half as tall as it will be at birth; it will only weigh about 340g, though—about the weight of a grapefruit. Ear development is continuing, with myelin insulation taking place in the ear nerve (the cochlear nerve). This no doubt means the baby is hearing even more sounds—those of the woman's body as well as a muffled version of any she hears herself. Her voice and that of her partner are likely to be a particular focus...

The parts of the system which allow a person to register head and body motion and the pull of gravity are all fully grown by now. This means the baby will probably already be aware of its own movements. For some reason it is common for babies to have a quiet period at this stage, in terms of bodily movements.

Hair could probably be seen on the baby's head, and sebum from sebaceous glands mixes with skin cells so as to begin to form 'vernix caseosa'. (This is the greasy covering over the lanugo which protects the little one's skin while it is in the womb.)

The baby can now also grip firmly with its hands and would reach out for a source of light (such as a torch beam panned slowly across the woman's abdomen), even though its eyes are still fused shut.

It's possible that from now on protective substances may pass through the woman's blood, through the placenta to her baby, so as to help the baby resist disease in the first few weeks of its life.

Week 21

The baby now weighs about 450g. Hair growth is a prominent feature of the next four weeks. It is also over this period that the baby's permanent teeth buds finish forming and that it will develop so-called 'brown fat', which is an important source of heat and energy for the newborn. It will also begin to make crying motions over the next few weeks and will continue to practise sucking.

The woman should by now feel very definite strong kicks sometimes high up in her tummy and sometimes low down near her pubic hair.

Week 22

At 22 weeks, the baby is about 30cm long but will still be very red and wrinkled in appearance. The gradually increasing levels of fat in its body should be noticeable to your client through her increasingly rounded form!

She may by now be able to feel the differences between different parts of her baby's body as it kicks, jumps and turns around. Sometimes she may feel a hand, sometimes a foot, the head or the buttocks. These movements may actually usually take place when she herself is trying to rest because her baby is likely to be at its most active then. (Perhaps it finds the movement of its mother's body soothing and sleep-inducing.) Your client's partner will also be able to become more aware of his baby this week because if he puts his ear to his partner's abdomen, he should hear a distinct heartbeat.

Over the next four weeks, most organs will become capable of functioning. By this early stage of gestation, the baby will also have started renewing its own skin cells. The growing baby's eyelids and eyebrows will be well-formed, even though the eyes will still be fused shut, and the baby's face will be even more expressive. In experiments, puckering of the lips, scowling and muscle tension around the eyes have all been associated with audible crying at this stage of pregnancy. (The sounds can actually be heard by the mother and researchers under certain experimental conditions.) These appropriate facial expressions are interesting in that they suggest that the baby has by now developed clear links between body and brain.

Also, only 20 weeks after conception, research has revealed that hearing and memory are becoming increasingly acute. Researchers have shown that newborn babies remember voices and music which they heard in the womb at this stage of pregnancy. This means that any lullaby the woman sings and any music she plays from now on may have a noticeably calming effect on her newborn later on. The same applies to her partner's voice so it's a good idea to tell the woman to encourage him to speak to their growing baby—and for her to do the same, of course.

When the growing baby is 20 weeks old, it will be able to hear its mother's voice

Week 23

The baby's arms and legs are now well developed. It can now grip with its hands... ultrasound scans have clearly shown this by this stage of pregnancy. The fine hair (the lanugo) which covers its body is beginning to darken. The woman may find that Braxton Hicks contractions (painless tightenings of the womb which began around Week 6), now become more pronounced. You might point out to her that this means her baby is regularly getting practice hugs and massage sessions! If she makes love with her partner, her body's own response may also have an effect on her baby. Research experiments focusing on this period of pregnancy have demonstrated that an unborn baby's heart rate either shoots up or slows down when the mother has an orgasm.

By 24 weeks the baby will look and behave much the same as a newborn

Week 24

In the UK, the baby is considered legally viable at the end of this week, which means its birth would need to be registered if it should happen to take place prematurely. The baby will now probably weigh over half a kilo and will be about 33cm long. Encourage the woman to imagine her curled up in her womb, cushioned by the bag of waters that surrounds the baby and totally dependent on the placenta for food and oxygen, as well as the disposal of its waste products. Everything she might ingest (food, drink, drugs, other chemicals, air, smoke, etc.) would still cross the placenta and would still be shared with her baby, so you need to continue to make her aware of this.

Since the amniotic fluid is now changed every four hours, it's a good idea for the woman to drink lots and lots of water. Amniotic fluid is very important because not only does it provide important liquid for the baby's digestion (enabling it to wee), it also regulates its temperature and protects it from infection and any sudden bumps the pregnant woman may experience.

By now the baby will actually look and behave much the same as a baby at birth. It is continuing to make breathing movements (practising for life outside the womb) and it coughs spontaneously whenever it needs to. It continues to kick and punch and even turn somersaults, so as to build up its muscles for life outside the womb. It might also sometimes make a fist, which indicates that it is developing its grasping reflex, which would be useful if we human beings still carried our babies round on our backs—without back-carriers!—like chimpanzees. However, the baby is unlike a newborn in that its eyes are still a bit bulgy (because of its thin face) and they are still sealed shut.

The baby is making great progress in other respects too: its skin is getting thicker; its sweat glands (so important for temperature control) are forming in the skin; and its responses to its environment are becoming even more obvious. Awareness of sounds may have increased to such an extent that any sudden noise makes it jump and it is likely to react to sounds it finds unpleasant by moving in different ways. Loud music is likely to wake it up, if it's asleep. The baby may continue to suck its thumb in an apparent attempt to comfort itself. Over the next four weeks, the part of the baby's brain concerned with personality and intelligence is becoming much more complex so we can guess that its personality may be developing over this period too.

In some countries the baby is already considered legally 'viable' by the end of this week, even though its lungs are not yet sufficiently developed for independent survival outside the womb. Premature baby care is developing and some remarkable babies already survive.

The part of the baby's brain concerned with personality and intelligence is becoming much more complex

Resting while pregnant...

Advise women to be careful about how they rest from now on. Although no research has as yet confirmed that there is anything behind 'optimal fetal positioning', common sense and anecdotal accounts confirm that it's worth taking seriously—not to mention the increase in posterior labours.

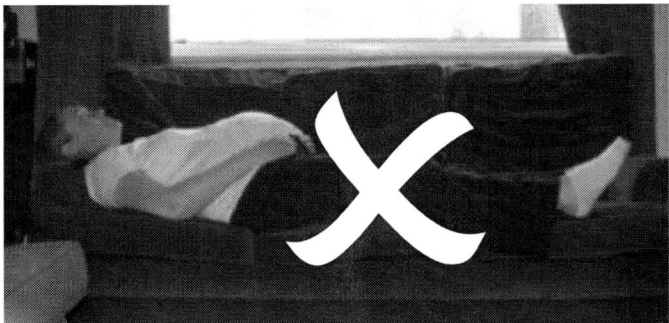

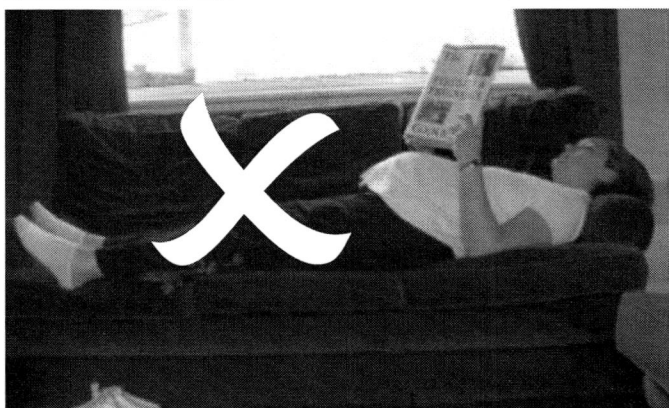

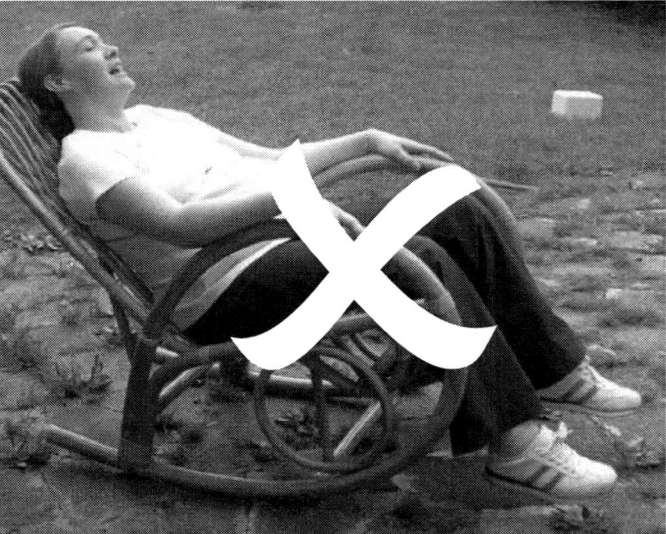

Some positions pregnant women should avoid

If the woman lies in these positions, the baby is likely to be deprived of oxygen because lying on the back depresses the vena cava, which takes blood from the placenta, and therefore the baby. Lying back also does nothing to help the baby get into a good position for the birth. How about doing most antenatal checks with the woman lying on her back, but propped up, so there's no pressure on the vena cava? Auscultation can even be done with the woman sitting up straight.

In any case, tell the woman not to lie down on her back or lean back in any sitting position, including in the bath, at any time outside her antenatal appointments. She can still have a bath, but she needs to sit up and lean forward—or she can stick to showers while she's pregnant. In any case, a woman's bump should not be exposed to very hot water because it can result in stillbirth. In other words, *never* encourage a woman to 'lie back and relax'!

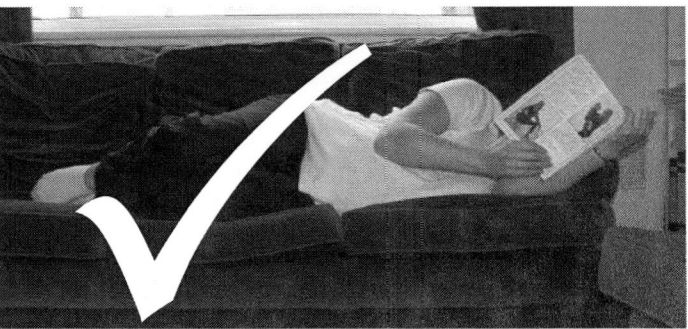

Here's a position to recommend for relaxation. Of course lying on the *left* side is much, much better for the baby (from the point of view of getting enough oxygen) than lying on the right side. As well as optimising oxygen flow, it also lowers the woman's risk of getting high blood pressure. Lying on her left side, she can read, sleep, read to children (they're usually very happy to climb on top), chat to friends...

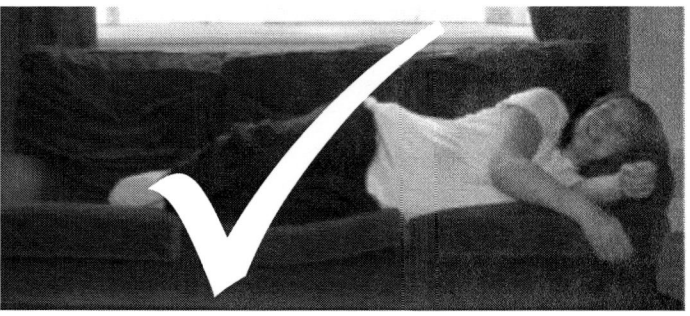

Here are above: *A good all-purpose position for a pregnant woman*

... or even watch TV! Suggest she stick to gentle comedy or romantic films, though, because frightening or hilarious films might cause her to produce excessive amounts of hormones, which might have an impact on the baby or start labour off. I've heard of a few labours that started after over-strenuous laughter or something noisy or frightening happening nearby. Beyond an awareness of these risks, encourage pregnant women to relax, of course. Whenever you do so, please do repeat the reminder about not lying back, though! Perhaps encourage the woman to prop herself up with a small cushion placed under her bottom, at the base of her spine, or to use a triangular cushion or piece of foam. (Of course, these are also fantastic for helping women to sleep comfortably while lying on their left side.) Also encourage women to use a 'pregnancy rocker' or 'kneeling chair'—(see www.backinaction.co.uk)— to optimise outcomes all round for both mother and baby.

This is something to take seriously... Getting into good habits can help the woman avoid a difficult posterior labour and optimise oxygen flow for the baby

Week 25

Over the next month, the growing baby's eyes begin to open and shut, it gets significantly longer and puts on a substantial amount of weight. Its ears are now structurally complete so it can hear its mother's voice clearly. This means she should perhaps be aware of the way she talks about the baby while it's living inside her, and afterwards too. (Some surprising perinatal memories have come out under hypnosis.) Encourage her to remember it's a person to be treated with respect and sensitivity. If she questions this, suggest she consider how easily babies cry when a person is around who seems unsympathetic to them.

Her baby's reactions to loud noises may still be quite dramatic: she will simply feel a sudden jolt as the baby moves. Some sounds will be less alarming to the baby because it will be used to hearing many of them, e.g. the continuous sloshing and squelching of the mother's stomach and bowels. Apparently, noises from these places peak at 85 decibels, which is really quite loud. (One researcher found it was the volume which his vacuum cleaner made at his ears when he was vacuuming a carpeted floor.) Sounds which are heard at around 55 decibels include the constant rumble of the mother's blood in the arteries which supply the uterus and placenta, which move in synchrony with her heart. (To give her an idea how loud this is, tell her that normal speech is usually about 60 decibels.) As a result of her baby's development in hearing ability, some experts believe it's a good idea for her to sing to her baby from now on, as well as talk to him or her.

On a more physical level, the baby's bone centres begin to harden this week.

> I felt absolutely great, energised with the life force running through me—sounds weird, I know but it really was like that. I'd never felt better. My skin, nails and hair were all glossy and smooth. A lot of my hair fell out and I had to grow it longer in an attempt to cover up the bald patches (it grew back a year later). For the first time in my life I loved my body, it was doing things automatically and I felt impelled to feed it lots of things I don't like eating—meat, milk, porridge, custard (all foods my child loves). It did feel a bit like hosting an alien who was driving me around from the inside like I was a car.

As you've probably realised—or found out by reading the Introduction—comments like the one above appear here and there in boxes like this. The idea in including them was to give you a glimpse into women's experience of physiological birth or its alternatives.

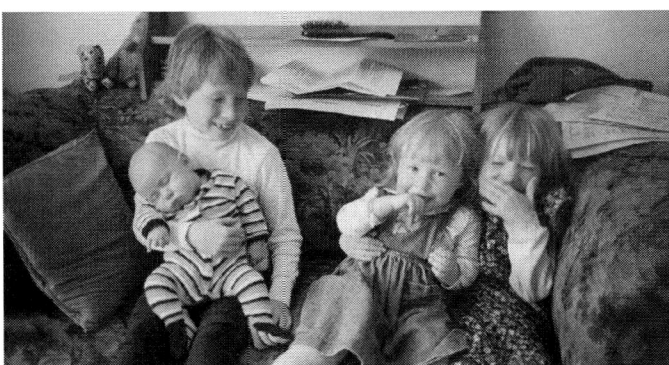

A family of optimally-birthed children

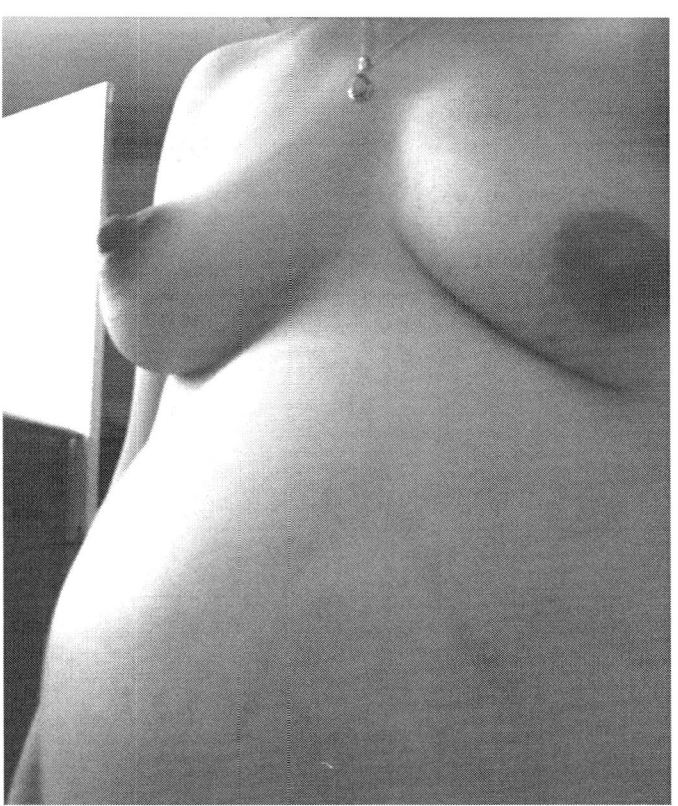

Encourage women to love their growing bump

Week 26

The baby is now growing at a rate of 1cm a week and every extra centimeter is making it stronger. By now, it will weigh almost a kilo. The ongoing increase in length means that the baby's positioning in the womb needs to change. It will find itself either the right way up or upside down in the womb, depending on how it flexes or extends its knees. These movements must require an enormous amount of brain-to-body coordination and it's interesting that they won't be possible outside the womb until 2-3 weeks after birth.

Other changes are taking place this week. Firstly, the baby's skin, which was previously paper-thin, is now becoming thicker and opaque. Secondly the baby's eyelashes are lengthening. Thirdly, the number of its tastebuds is increasing. Research from as far back as 1937 shows that if something sweet is introduced into the amniotic fluid, a baby will swallow more rapidly. This of course means that the mother needs to consider carefully whether or not both she and her baby really need that chocolate bar or ice cream, before she eats it... Remind your client of the importance of a good diet.

By the end of this week, the baby's chance of survival outside the womb would be much higher, although every extra week spent inside its mother helps to prepare it for the outside world. Nature did not intend babies to be born at this early stage of gestation, but if the woman's baby is born prematurely, she can perhaps use kangaroo care. (See the Birthframe 35 for more on this.)

The baby is growing stronger every week and now weighs almost a whole kilo!

Week 27

The baby is still growing very fast and will probably weigh just over a kilo by now. Its eyes are now open and will have blue irises (slate grey, in fact—the colour of muscle), but this colour may change after the birth. The nostrils are open and the baby is practising breathing.

If your client wants to try and visualise her baby, remind her to include a very wrinkled skin, coated in creamy vernix. The wrinkling is no doubt due to the watery nature of her baby's present home. Its creamy white covering is there for its own protection. It's a bit like staying in the bath, covered in protective, nourishing, moisturising cream so as to avoid having waterlogged skin!

The baby's heart will now be beating at a rate of 120-140 beats per minute, which is double the speed of an adult's heart rate.

The baby's heart will now be beating twice as fast as the woman's own heart

Week 28

Most countries consider a baby legally viable by the end of this week. Paediatricians are optimistic about a premature baby's survival at this stage—some even put it at 95%.

Assuming that your client is going to carry her baby to term, she is now well on her way to having a full-term birth as long as she avoids liquorice, shocks and inadequate diets. (That's what research suggests!) The third trimester (which officially starts next week) is her 'home run', so to speak. Encourage her to enjoy the last few months of her pregnancy so that her baby has a happy emotional environment to swim around in. Research suggests this is important, so it's good if she avoids all stress at this stage.

The baby's length and weight will have increased even more. However, the variety of birth weights and lengths make measurements increasingly difficult to generalise so I shall not mention them from now on. The ever-increasing size of the baby means that it is nearing the end of the time when it can lie stretched out. Perhaps because of an increasing lack of space, the volume of amniotic fluid in the womb will reach a peak between now and Week 32. As a result of this increase in size and a decrease in the amount of liquid to move about in, the baby will find it more and more of a challenge to find a position that feels comfortable over the next few weeks... so it will not be the only one who is shifting and twisting about in an effort to find the ideal position for a peaceful sleep!

The baby is definitely listening to its mother's speech patterns very carefully now. A study in 1975 which analysed the cries of premature babies born at 28 weeks clearly showed that babies were copying their mothers' basic speech patterns. Obviously, this requires a sophisticated level of filtering on the part of the baby. As well as screening out its mother's body's squelching and gurgling, the baby will also be filtering out louder ambient sounds in order to focus on its mother's voice. Obviously, this is another important stage of language development.

The baby will also be appreciating tastes more, as it gets used to differentiating between whatever the mother eats. Research has shown that babies can now respond to sweet, sour and bitter tastes. The growing baby will actually have more taste buds at this stage in its development than it will have at birth, so its palate really might be quite discerning.

Difficult as it might be to believe, the baby will probably also start having another range of new experiences around this time: sexual feelings. Quite by accident, some American researchers observed male babies having an erection while analysing a series of sonograms; in fact, six babies at about this stage of gestation were observed in this state! These erections doubtless prove that the appropriate nerve pathways are working by this time and they probably also indicate that unborn babies experience some of the feelings that adult men experience along with an erection. We can guess this because all six babies who were having erections were also thumb-sucking—which is almost certainly a pleasure-seeking pastime.

On a more general level, the thinking part of the baby's brain has now become much bigger and more complex. By now, it is possible for preborns to feel pain and they respond in much the same way as full-term babies. Muscles in the baby's body are also becoming even stronger, which the mother will notice in the form of assertive kicks from within! Her partner will almost certainly be able to feel the baby move too, if he puts his hand on his partner's bump. The couple may be able to watch the shape of a foot or a bottom travel across the woman's middle, as the baby changes position.

Finally, from this time onwards, the growing baby will be laying down fat underneath its skin in preparation for after his or her birth.

The thinking part of the brain is bigger

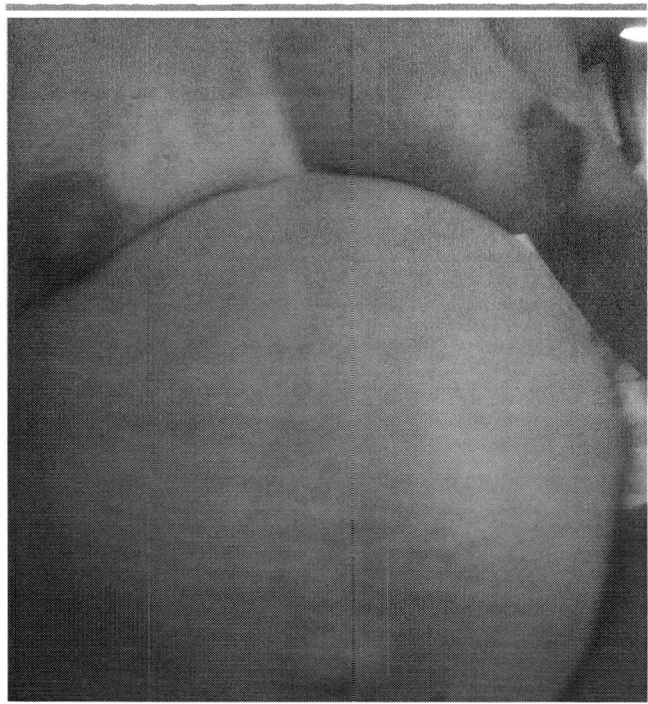

Be sympathetic when women complain! Often they need a friendly ear, rather than drugs or treatments.

THE THIRD TRIMESTER

Different books mark this trimester as beginning at different points. Assuming it begins at the beginning of Week 29, the woman is now entering the last phase of her baby's development. The main focus now is on growth and lung maturation, so the baby can breathe well when it's born. Growth is very important over the next few months because heavier babies tend to be stronger and healthier. That explains why it really is vital for the woman to eat well over the next twelve weeks or so—even if she feels huge!

It's vital that the woman eats well

The woman also needs to be careful about her stress levels. Many mothers I've heard from seem to make a connection between a stressful third trimester and a difficult birth. But while some women find it stressful having to continue working, others have reported stress caused from boredom and having too much time to think. While a house move is too stressful for some women, for others it signals a joyous new beginning. The key is probably self-awareness: whatever your client does, she should not cause herself too much *negative* stress. Part of this—whatever her approach to rest, work and leisure activities—is to try to maintain harmony around herself so that she's in a good state of mind when her due date approaches. Instead of getting embroiled in a disagreement, she should consider either stepping down with dignity, or asserting herself amicably and respectfully. If she's still working, she'll need to be particularly careful she doesn't allow the stresses of the job to affect her. She should do what she can in a methodical way, remembering that nobody is indispensable. She's got a much more important project on the go! However, if something really is upsetting her, she should get it sorted so her mind is at rest. Self-awareness should be followed by action.

Week 29

By now the baby may already have quite an impressive head of hair and its brain will have become more sophisticated. The two halves of its brain have developed a degree of asymmetry, the left side being stronger. Of course, this is the hemisphere that controls the right side of the body, which is why most people are right-handed.

A lot of other things are happening around now... The fat deposits which are being laid down between now and the end of Week 32 are smoothing the growing baby's body contours, although its skin will still be covered with thick white vernix. Rhythmic breathing motions continue as practice for breathing after the birth.

Reassure each woman that her partner may well find her beautiful and awesome! Remind her of all the miracles happening on a moment-by-moment basis inside her body and of the baby living inside.

The growing baby's experience is becoming more intense. Some young children remember these last few weeks in their mother's womb...

The baby is also still growing fast, thanks to the nutrients which pass across the placenta and the amount of amniotic fluid it is drinking. We know from studies which have used radioactive tracers that growing babies drink from 15 to 40 milliliters of amniotic fluid every hour from now on until they're born. This nourishment adds up to 40 calories a day when a baby is swallowing normally and is supplemented by the nourishment which is provided via the placenta. Large, well-nourished babies swallow at a higher rate than small, grossly malnourished babies. This is why your client needs to avoid smoking, alcohol, junk food and bitter tastes, such as coffee. After all, studies have shown that when a bitter-tasting substance is injected into the amniotic fluid, babies suddenly stop drinking it. In the same studies, when saccharine was injected, some babies even doubled their rate of swallowing. No, this does not mean your client can eat loads of cakes and sweets! Her baby needs her to provide a balanced diet. She should persuade her baby to swallow fast by providing it with lots of good quality, tasty food. That way, it will get into a good pattern of growth in the last few weeks before its birth.

Week 30

The baby's facial features will now be well-developed. Other aspects of its appearance are also continuing to change this week: the lanugo (the fine layer of hair on its skin) is disappearing from its face and its skin is becoming paler and less wrinkled. This is mainly because of the fat which is continuing to build up underneath its skin and which will help keep it warm after it's born. As well as storing fat, the growing baby is now also storing up iron reserves for after the birth. Finally, male babies' testes will descend into the scrotum during this week.

The baby's experience of the physical world is probably becoming much more intense. A startle reaction would already be recordable to researchers. It's also very likely that the baby will be aware of any Braxton Hicks contractions your client is spontaneously having. Perhaps the experience of these intermittent tightenings in the womb is what gives us a liking for cuddles in later life—who knows? The baby may also be becoming increasingly aware of its restricted environment. I remember one of my own children recalling her time in my womb, saying, "It got very crowded in there at the end." (Comments from young children about their 'wombhood'—their time *in utero*—have been reported by quite a few mothers. It's obviously not possible to ascertain whether these are 'real' memories or only imagined ones, but some children do give the impression of being able to remember their pre-birth experience up to the age of 2.) Perhaps the strong kicks your client now feels are kicks of frustration as well as attempts at exercise! The constant wriggling she will be aware of is almost certainly a sign that her baby is trying to get comfortable.

Getting the baby well-positioned...

As we've already noted, although there's no official proof, it does seem to be a good idea to encourage women to help their baby get into a good position for the birth. Midwives Jean Sutton and Pauline Scott have written about this at length in their book *Optimal Foetal Positioning*, published by Birth Concepts in New Zealand in 1996). As they explain, not only is an anterior labour likely to be easier (because the woman will get breaks between contractions), it's also far less likely to result in a caesarean. It is surely possible that the dramatic increase in posterior labours is due to our lifestyle these days, as compared to our ancestors, who were more likely to be on their hands and knees, scrubbing the kitchen floor, than lazing back on the sofa, watching TV and reading a pregnancy book.

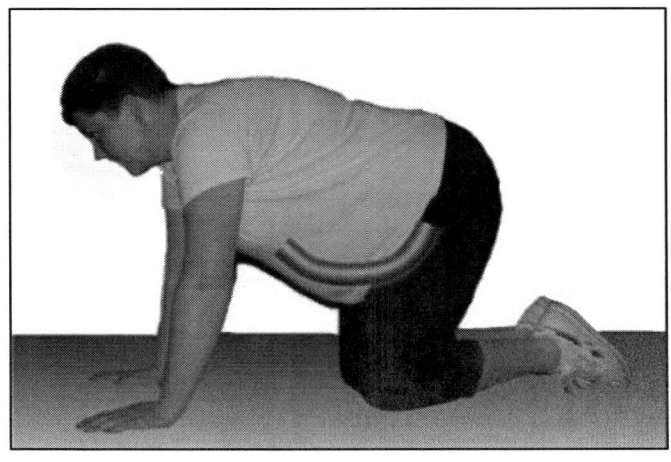

An anterior labour will probably be easier and far less painful

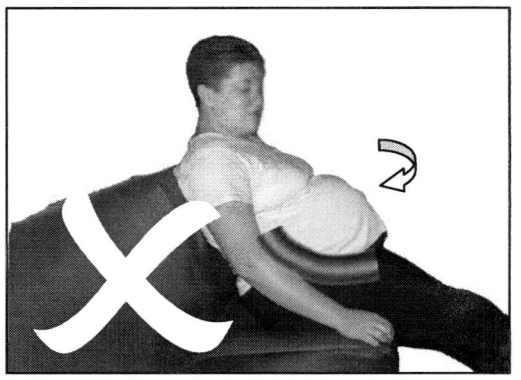

If you imagine the dark line being the baby's back, it's easy to see how lying back is not helpful in the last few weeks of pregnancy. The baby's back will tend to flip down because of the pull of gravity. This would result in a posterior labour, which would probably be much more painful.

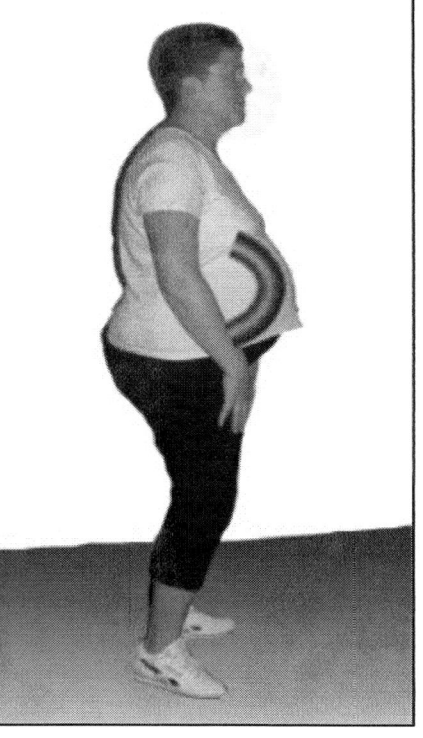

Tell the woman to kneel down as much as possible, for 10-15 minutes at a time, at least three times a day, especially in the last six weeks of her pregnancy. Make sure that when she does this she keeps her back straight. (She can even arch her back slightly, but mustn't let it sag.) Encourage her to think of things she can do in this position. She can pick things up off the floor, vacuum clean using the hand attachment, wash the floor, help a child with a jigsaw...

All this will also help her avoid backache!

When the woman is standing up, ask her to imagine herself bouncing from the knees. This will help her to carry her weight well and avoid strain to her back. Her baby is also likely to get into and stay in a good position for the birth if she does this.

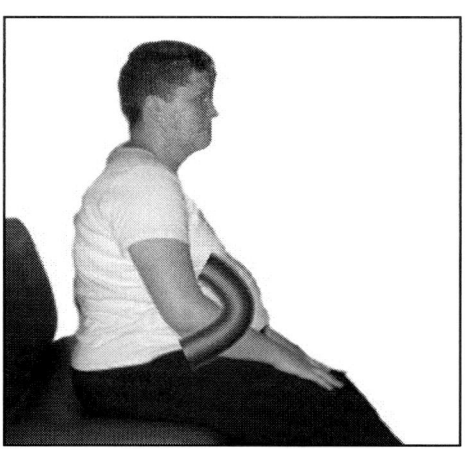

The woman needs to make the effort so as to have a better birth

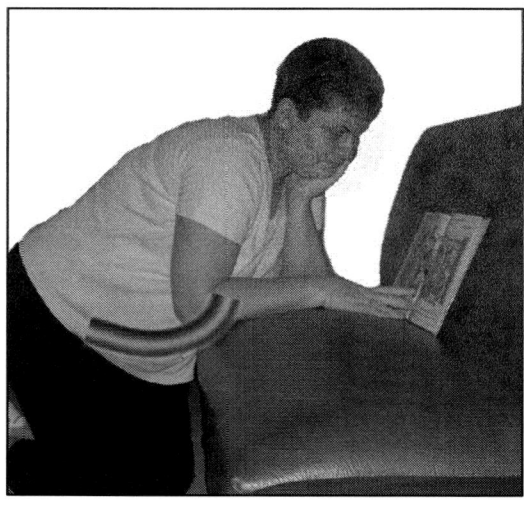

In this more upright sitting position, the baby's back is more likely to stay round the woman's front. With any type of chair, it's best to sit on the edge. Reassure the woman that it really is worth the effort!

A helpful reading position is kneeling down by the sofa and reading the book or magazine propped up. As well as requiring relatively little effort, this also involves leaning forward. This is a great position for reading to a toddler.

Week 31

Little by little, the growing baby will be getting plumper. It should now have gained around 50g of fat, which represents 3.5% of its total body weight. By the time it's born, body fat will account for 15% of its total body weight. (The percentage of body fat to body weight for an average-sized woman is around 27%.) The additional accumulated fat means it would no longer be possible to see the blood vessels beneath the baby's skin—if only we could take a peek. The shadowy images which represent the baby's growing bones would also no longer be visible now.

By this stage in the pregnancy the woman may occasionally feel very breathless, but the baby will certainly be getting plenty of oxygen from its mother, thanks to the flow of blood through the placenta, along the umbilical cord. Of course, this oxygen is essential for the baby's survival and brain development so the woman needs to make sure she does nothing to compromise it. This means she should continue to avoid smokers (and smoking) and not lie on her back unless you ask her to at an antenatal check-up! (Remember to prop her back up, so there's no pressure on the vena cava, and check the fetal heartbeat while she's sitting up...)

Remind women to stand and sit well so as to get their baby in a good position

Week 32

By the end of this week the baby will be completely formed and its body will be in perfect proportion, taking into account the fact that the proportions will be that of a baby, i.e. large head and skinny limbs! It will be building up its immune system, taking antibodies from its mother so as to be able to fight off disease and infection after it's born. It will also have beautifully formed miniature eyelashes and eyebrows, so must look very cute!

The baby is continuing to gain weight... In fact, from now on until the time when it is born, it will gain at a rate of about 250g a week. This means it's more important than ever that your client continues to eat well.

By now, the baby will have curled up into the well-known fetal position. Its head will probably already be pointing downwards, simply because the head is the heaviest part and gravity is likely to draw it downwards. If this isn't the case, reassure your client. Before 32 weeks, as you know, 50% of babies will be in a breech position but as these babies' heads become heavier than their bottoms, they usually spontaneously turn cephalic around now, or at least by the 36th week of pregnancy. Even if a baby stays breech, a normal optimal birth is still possible, so you might consider attending a vaginal breech birth.

Encourage women to experiment with interesting clothes combinations... She needs to see her increasing size as a positive development because it means her baby is growing, as he or she should

The unborn baby may like classical music! Suggest that women experiment...

Week 33

As the baby continues to become chubbier, its skin smoothes out even more. If it has turned to a head down position by now, it will probably stay like that now until its birth. After all, it no longer has the luxury of being able to perform somersaults.

It will be going through some important development during the next few weeks. Its lungs will begin to produce surfactant (a substance similar to detergent), which will help them to expand and withstand pressure. It will also prevent the baby's lungs from collapsing at birth. Its brain will also develop some new abilities. According to French research, a baby in the womb at this stage of gestation can be taught to recognise a nursery rhyme or simple piece of music and respond to it after the birth, as long as it's played daily for a month. Mozart and Vivaldi were the composers babies responded to best. I don't recommend you recommend your clients attempt any artificial exercises like these themselves, though, as I've already said. Doing what they spontaneously want to do is probably the best thing for their babies, who will benefit most from having contented and healthy mothers and an uncontrived environment. Babies can have interesting tastes in music, in my experience.

Week 34

This week the growing baby is becoming more rounded. The lanugo, the fine covering of hair all over its body, begins to disappear and the growing baby's skin will be getting pinker. Its ear cartilage is still soft, though, and the so-called plantar creases—creases on the soles of the feet—are still visible. Over the next four weeks, the hair on the baby's head will get longer and the baby's nails will grow long enough to reach the tips of its fingers.

The movements the pregnant woman will now be feeling will probably be much gentler than a few weeks ago. The increasing lack of space which we've already mentioned makes those vigorous kicks and punches she felt before a near impossibility. She shouldn't worry about this apparent decrease in movement but should nevertheless continue to be aware of how and when her baby is moving about. If there is a change of pattern or a long absence of any movement, she should contact you so you can check the baby's OK, preferably with your Pinard! (I've already mentioned the idea of avoiding ultrasound.)

The woman should avoid any potentially stressful over-stimulating events, e.g. carnivals, theatre performances, violent movies or sports events. Loud music, overly prolonged and hearty laughter and energetic dancing are also things she should be careful of. Of course, this is because of the close link between emotional and hormonal states and the possibility that upsetting the balance could trigger labour. If she is at a concert or play (or other event) and suddenly feels her baby moving around vigorously in response to some of the sound effects or music, she should leave immediately or at least move to a seat at the back of the hall or theatre. Her baby might be truly upset!

Optimal fetal positioning...

Back to that subject again! I would like to share with you something of my own experience here, as a pregnant woman. Although in my second pregnancy I was convinced that the way I stood, sat and lay could have an effect on my baby's positioning, I still hadn't taken any action by the time I was 38 weeks' pregnant. I only acted when my midwife told me my baby was ROA, which I knew from my reading could easily mean my baby would 'flip' into a posterior ROP as I went into labour—as had happened at the end of my first pregnancy, in fact.

Two days later, having still made no significant changes, I realised the only way I would persuade myself to turn my baby to a firm LOA position was to get down on my hands and knees for 10-15 minutes, at least three times a day, using a chart to record that I had done so.

It was definitely worth doing this because my baby soon turned to LOA and I had a very straightforward two-hour labour afterwards. Much better than the first time!

10-15 mins on hands and knees	Mon 3/10	Tue 4/10	Wed 5/10	Thu 6/10	Fri 7/10	Sat 8/10	Sun 9/10
1st time	✓	✓	✓	✓	✓		
2nd time	✓	✓	✓	✓	✓		
3rd time	✓	✓	✓	✓			

A tracking chart for ensuring that women really do get down on their hands and knees!

Week 35

If, for whatever reason, the baby were to be born now—anything from 34 weeks and 2 days' gestation onwards—she would have an excellent chance of survival.

During her last few weeks in the womb the baby is now doing an impressive amount of weeing... a remarkable 600ml every day. The wee initially goes into the amniotic fluid, of course, and then the waste products are filtered through the placenta into the mother's own bloodstream. Eventually, the baby's waste products are dealt with by the mother's own kidneys, along with her own waste. Since the mother's kidneys need to function very efficiently in order to deal with all this waste, it's very important for her to continue to drink plenty of good quality drinking water.

As well as weeing, the baby will be doing a lot of sucking practice now. If she is sucking her thumb or her hands (which is likely), she may even already have some sucking blisters! Developing a strong suck now and in the weeks to come is, of course, extremely important because it's necessary for successful breastfeeding.

As the baby sucks and manoeuvres carefully inside the mother, she will carry on trying to decipher sounds coming from outside her little world and will continue responding to tastes and changes in light.

Week 36

If your client is one of the 1 in 80 mums carrying twins you will probably have noticed this by now when you have palpated her abdomen. You can perhaps help her to consider her options carefully because many mothers have managed to carry their twins to term and even have them vaginally. (Again, we'll come back to this later.) Even if your client is carrying 'just' one baby, she may be interested to know that twins at this stage of gestation have been filmed hugging, stroking and patting things in the womb. This leads me to guess that growing babies may have emotional needs at this stage of development, so it might be a good idea to suggest your client tenderly strokes her expanding bump, if she isn't already doing so! You never know, it may well be reassuring for the baby inside. Remind her too that she can talk to her baby with the expectation that it will be listening, and possibly even understanding... who knows?

In normal circumstances, your client can imagine her baby gaining about 14g of fat a day at this stage. Tell her that this even rises to about 28g a day during the last four weeks of gestation. Her baby is piling on the pounds (or grams, actually) so as to be able to cope with the lower temperatures outside the womb, after its birth. The woman should keep eating substantial quantities of good, wholesome food to help this process along.

The baby is almost fully mature now, even in terms of lung maturation. (Obviously, this is important because the baby must be able to breathe when it's born). It may have quite long hair—it may be up to 5cm long. If the woman is carrying a boy, his testicles will probably already have descended at this stage.

Ideally the baby's position should be LOA, which you can explain to her means head-down and with its back round at her own front, on the left side of her bump. If the baby is in a different position, explain what it is to the woman so that she is aware of what's happening. If her baby is in another position (ROA, LOP, ROP or one of the breech positions) ask her to consider how she is using her body during the day and at night.

For ideal positioning, as I've already mentioned, my research has led me to conclude that it's best for the mother to sleep on her left side and to avoid leaning back while she's awake. This will facilitate an anterior, rather than a posterior position, and will result in LOA, rather than ROA. Explain to your client that the reason to take note of the baby's position is so as to optimise the chances of the birth being easy... and safe, of course. Explain how with anterior positioning (LOA or ROA) she will get 100% painfree breaks between contractions (which may in any case not be painful). With posterior positioning she is likely to have no breaks at all—just varying degrees of intensity—which I know from my own first labour is *extremely* hard work! Also explain that if a baby who is initially posterior doesn't 'turn' to an anterior position by the time the mother reaches the second stage of labour, the birth is much, much more painful. (Unfortunately, I know this first-hand too from my own first experience of giving birth!) If the baby is anterior, this stage can be completely painfree (as I also know), apart from that famous 'ring of fire'.

If the woman is anxious about all this, reassure her, explaining that many women still go on to have optimal births, even when their babies are not ideally positioned.

Week 37

Of course, for some midwives this is a landmark week because a woman is normally required to have completed 37 weeks if she wants to have a home birth because of the risks associated with prematurity. (Is her due date accurate though? Perhaps it's worth checking.)

The growing baby's vernix (the thick creamy coating covering its body) is disappearing now and it may have almost reached its birth weight, whatever that's going to be. Your client can imagine her baby with a thicker neck and with eyelids that open and close easily. The baby will continue to rehearse breathing movements—even though no air will be going into its lungs as yet—and the repeated hiccups the woman may be aware of coming from her bump are still ongoing proof of this. (It's a sign that amniotic fluid has passed into her baby's trachea.)

If your client's baby is lying in a breech position, it's still possible her baby may turn round spontaneously before the birth so she may still be able to have a cephalic birth. She may also want a vaginal breech birth.

If this is your client's first baby, and it's cephalic, as you know, its head will probably drop into her pelvis very soon, ready for the birth. (I assume you'll explain the term 'engaged'.) If it's her second or subsequent baby it will probably descend just as your client is going into labour.

At the end of this week, the baby is generally considered to be 'term'. As you no doubt know, a baby is considered term when she is between 37 and 42 weeks' gestation (between 259 and 294 days since the LMP).

Week 38

The growing baby's contours are now very well-rounded and its skull is firm. Its size will be even closer to its birthweight.

The baby is now spending as much as 60% of its time asleep and its sleep is now falling into clearly detectable patterns. Now it even dreams like an adult. We know this because of the rapid eye movement (REM) associated with the dreaming state, which has been observed in babies in the womb at this stage of gestation. (REM sleep has been recorded from as early as 23 weeks' gestation.) Since it is thought that dreaming encourages brain development, we can guess that the baby is continuing to develop in terms of emotions and general intelligence. Measurement of brain waves increasingly shows more organisation, steadier activity, and greater synchrony between the left and right halves of the brain. Research has also shown that the baby is by now uttering a much more definite cry (only audible in research conditions). Since crying is an essential means of communication for babies, this isn't bad news. If a baby couldn't cry when it was born, how else would it be able to get its mother's attention? Of course, it needs to fit in a little crying practice before its birth day.

Don't tell your clients to put their feet up! That might be bad for the baby and might also result in a more difficult birth

Week 39

The baby's rate of growth is slowing down, which is just as well really because there is very little room left in its mother's womb. Phenomenal development has taken place over the last 37 weeks (from conception onwards, remembering that the woman's baby only really started growing from Week 3). The original fertilised cell has become a well-organised bundle of two hundred million cells and these cells now weigh approximately six billion times more than the original fertilised egg!

The amniotic fluid around the baby is being renewed every three hours, so your client needs to keep drinking water. If the baby remains undistressed, the amniotic fluid will remain clear because the waste products which aren't released in its wee will remain in its bowel. The sticky greeny-black substance which results from the storage of these waste products, which as we've already mentioned is called meconium, is a mixture of excretions from the baby's alimentary glands, bile pigment, lanugo and cells from its bowel wall. When this original gestational waste has been cleared in the first few nappies, the newborn's poos will become an interesting and pleasant-smelling orange colour if he or she is being breastfed. (Bottle-fed babies' poos are browner and have a stronger odour.)

Whether or not your client's baby is ready to be born this week or next will depend not only on individual variation but also on the precise date this baby was conceived. (Does the woman know precisely when ovulated in the month she conceived?) I would encourage you to resist attempting to hurry the baby along at this stage... Nature can cope very well without our interference; in fact, disturbance usually results in worse outcomes, not better ones. The woman will go into labour and give birth spontaneously when her baby is sufficiently mature and when her body has prepared precisely the correct balance of hormones to make the birth possible. (Postmaturity is a rare phenomenon and is perhaps worried about too much.)

Encourage your client to enjoy these last few days of life without a tiny baby to care for. Babies are much easier to look after when they're inside us! She should relax, walk, dance, paint, write, sing, bake cakes, contemplate the beauty of nature... If she's happy and contented, her baby is likely to be relaxed and happy too—because it's sharing its mother's hormonal environment. Virtually everything crosses the placenta, of course. True intimacy.

However, while focusing on her well-being your client should also spend some time preparing for her baby's arrival. Does she have everything she needs... soft towels, receiving blankets, baby clothes?

Week 40

If your client hasn't already done so, she may now be nearing the time of her labour. However, since only 3% of babies arrive on their due date she may still have a fair wait. 80% of babies are born within 14 days of their due date, either before or after. The rest are born either earlier or later than 42 weeks—perhaps because they were conceived at the end of a very long menstrual cycle.

If your client's baby has now been growing inside her for a full 38 weeks, it will certainly be as heavy as it is to be at the time of its birth, and as long. Its fingernails may be so sharp that it scratches itself with them.

Although most of its lanugo (fine hair) and vernix will have disappeared by now, at birth a little lanugo may still be seen over its shoulders, back, arms and legs and some traces of vernix (cream) may remain in skin folds.

The temporal lobe of the baby's brain—the part to which the ear sends its data—will now be fully myelinated. Other parts of its brain and nervous system will only be partially insulated at birth, so it's clear that the baby's hearing is given full priority. In this respect, it's worth remembering that under hypnosis in later life, people can often recall comments which are made around the time of their birth which have affected them in some way.

The baby's nose is also fairly well-developed now, meaning that it will display a decided preference for certain smells as soon as it's born. It's interesting that a newborn will express these preferences even with no practice or experience. The smell of its mother's own breasts—and armpits, actually!—will be particularly attractive to the newborn baby. So whatever your client does, she shouldn't worry about body odour just now!

The part of the baby which is to be born first—its 'presenting part'—will probably be in the lower segment of the woman's womb, pressing through the already softened, partially opened cervix. If this baby is a second or subsequent baby, it is likely to engage at the onset of labour. Obviously, the timing of engagement varies.

If indeed the baby is ready to be born, it will send a hormonal signal to your client's body calling for an end to the pregnancy. (This is a signal scientists would like to know more about!) Your client's body will respond by releasing oxytocin (the 'hormone of love') to make her uterus contract. The irregular and then regular contractions which follow are an inevitable part of labour—so she should try and view them very positively. They are there to help her baby exit her womb, descend through her pelvis and enter this world...

Of course, it's a dramatic business coming into this world from the baby's point of view. The journey itself involves travelling down a long, narrow and unfamiliar passage. Your client shouldn't worry about her baby getting damaged, though. Its body will now be very flexible, thanks to fluid intervertebral disks and joints which can fold neatly in tight places. Even the head plates which guard the baby's brain will yield to pressure by overlapping, which may result in a pointed head or 'pixie' look at birth. (Reassure the woman that these plates will gradually reposition themselves again.) The baby may well be shocked at birth... the reassuring hug of the womb will be gone, temperatures will no longer be constant, and supplies of food and drink won't be on tap any more. It will need plenty of tender love and care. How will all this affect your own approach to care at the birth?

I knew that the way in which due dates are calculated in England is about two weeks shorter than elsewhere in Europe, and medics get twitchy and start wanting to induce births here, when in Sweden they wouldn't consider it at the same point. Plus first babies are routinely late—probably because the calculations are wrong. My dates could not be accurate as I'd not known I was pregnant in the first place, but anxieties always seem to grow in the last two months. My way of avoiding them was to keep working and keep to a minimum contact with the world of pregnancy.

Week 41

It's worth noting, if your client is still pregnant, that only a baby born after 41 weeks and 6 days is technically overdue—that's 293 days—because human gestation can be anything from 37-42 weeks. However, following NICE guidelines, you will probably be monitoring her more closely from now on. Despite this, given the wide variation please do make an effort to reassure your client.

Encourage her to reconsider the precise date of conception if you haven't already done so, taking into account the length of your client's normal monthly cycle and of course also her sexual activity around the time she thinks she conceived. If her cycle is irregular, this could explain things, of course... How many days late has her period been in the past? The birth could be the same number of days late. For example, a 33-day cycle would mean she could only expect her baby 5 days after the EDD given in the official charts. Also, ask her if her partner was away on business at any time in the month she got pregnant. She could only have become pregnant when she made love! Help her to think through dates and reassure her in any case...

At this potentially worrying time, remind your client just how amazing her body is, managing to conceive a baby and get it grown this far. Of course it should know precisely how to get it born too! It's a process which takes usually takes place with no help... Watchful waiting should involve an absolute minimum of disturbance, so that the physiological processes can take place smoothly. Encourage your client to tune into her baby and talk to it too. She will soon know if the 'it' is a girl or a boy.

While your client is waiting, it's a good idea if she keeps thinking about her baby, imagining what he or she might be like. It's not possible to calculate how heavy or tall he or she will be, no matter how large or compact the mother, but here are a few interesting facts about babies' weights and heights around the time of their birth...

- A typical birth weight is 3.5 kilos. (That's 7½ pounds, if metric means nothing to you).
- Only 5% of babies weigh less than 2.5 kilos or more than 4.25 kilos.
- If the baby's a boy, it's likely he will weigh about 200 grams (½lb) more than a girl would.
- Whatever the newborn's weight, it will decrease in the first three days after the birth. As you know, this is nothing to worry about—it really is perfectly normal as the new baby adjusts to life outside its mother's body.
- By about 10 days after the birth, the baby should have regained his or her birth weight and the long-term process of growth will have re-established itself.
- The newborn's height will be just under a third of that of a typical adult, i.e. 51cm (or 20in).
- 95% of babies fall within the range of 46-56cm.

Only a baby born after 41 weeks and 6 days is technically overdue since human gestation can be anything from 37-42 weeks

Here are a few more interesting facts for you to pass on, to keep your client's mind off her wait...

- A newborn's body is made up of approximately 70% water, 16% fat, 11% protein and 1% carbohydrate.
- Despite the fact that her new baby's heart will weigh less than 30g at birth, the baby's pulse rate will be about 180 beats per minute during the actual birth and it will then average 140 beats per minute in the first few weeks. During the first year of the baby's life, the rate will gradually decrease to 115 beats per minute, by which time the baby won't even have doubled in weight.
- Your client's new baby's eyesight will already be fairly well-developed at birth: her baby will be able to focus over the distance from her breast to her face and it's likely he or she will be attracted its mother's face, rather than to less complex, less curvaceous, less mobile, inanimate objects.
- At birth, the baby will be ideally predisposed to bond with your client, provided of course there are no drugs in his or her system. If your client were to have any drugs in her system that would also be a disappointment for her baby, because her face would be less responsive. After all, research into the behaviour of babies just after birth has revealed that babies typically spend up to an hour staring intently at their mother's face, if given the chance, before they fall asleep for the first time outside the womb. This is a first exchange which your client should look forward to and cherish and it's one of the reasons why it's best for her to opt for an optimal birth, i.e. a birth which involves an absolute minimum of intervention and no drugs whatsoever. The aim is to make her baby's birth as gentle and as trauma-free as possible so that she and her baby can both start off their relationship well.

Week 42

Your client really shouldn't worry. She probably ovulated later than she thinks. Perhaps that particular month when she conceived was a strange one in terms of her normal cycle. The baby is probably developing as he or she should. He or she is probably soon going to start the birth process. Beyond carrying out non-invasive checks to confirm the baby is still OK and after making sure the woman is aware of any potentially dangerous symptoms (e.g. bleeding), make every effort to reassure your client. Don't pressurise her to accept an induction. Too many inductions prove to be unnecessary and unsafe, not to mention traumatic for the women giving birth. Remember that only 1% of babies who are thought antenatally to be 'postmature' actually turn out to be so when they are born (and even then symptoms are not usually life-threatening). The other 99% show no signs of postmaturity and clearly weren't yet ready to be born.

Also encourage the mother to monitor her baby's movements herself. She can even keep a kick chart if she wants to, which may provide you with useful information. Remind your client that the process of labour and birth often begins very suddenly after a seemingly interminable wait! Strange and wonderful things are happening within her body. Encourage her to continue to trust her baby's ability to get itself born, while continuing to talk to him or her, perhaps asking him or her to hurry up! They're going to meet up properly soon.

Week 43

If you're still reading this on behalf of your client, note that female babies spend on average one day longer inside their mother's bodies than males. And white babies on average spend five days longer inside the womb than black babies. Apparently, these differences are purely racial and have nothing to do with individual size variations, wealth or even poverty. Until now, nobody has been able to explain why these variations occur.

In any case, if your client is still pregnant now, she probably just miscalculated her LMP (last menstrual period), or maybe she ovulated very late in the month she got pregnant. If you find she is worried, encourage her to focus on this feeling and try and work out why... Are there any psychological issues she needs to resolve before she gives birth? Does she need to make any other preparations? Is she happy with the arrangements she's made with her birth attendants, friends and family?

She should also consider whether she really, intuitively, feels there's something wrong. If she feels pretty confident that everything's basically OK with both herself and her baby, she should consider what's been happening lately... Has there been any diarrhoea? Any loss of appetite? Any increased sexual desire? Any impatience or a deep need to tidy up and organise things? Of course, these are all signs of imminent labour, so she should relax if the answer is 'Yes!' When she does go into labour, as she will, she should continue to imagine what her baby might be experiencing. This is the beginning of its life!

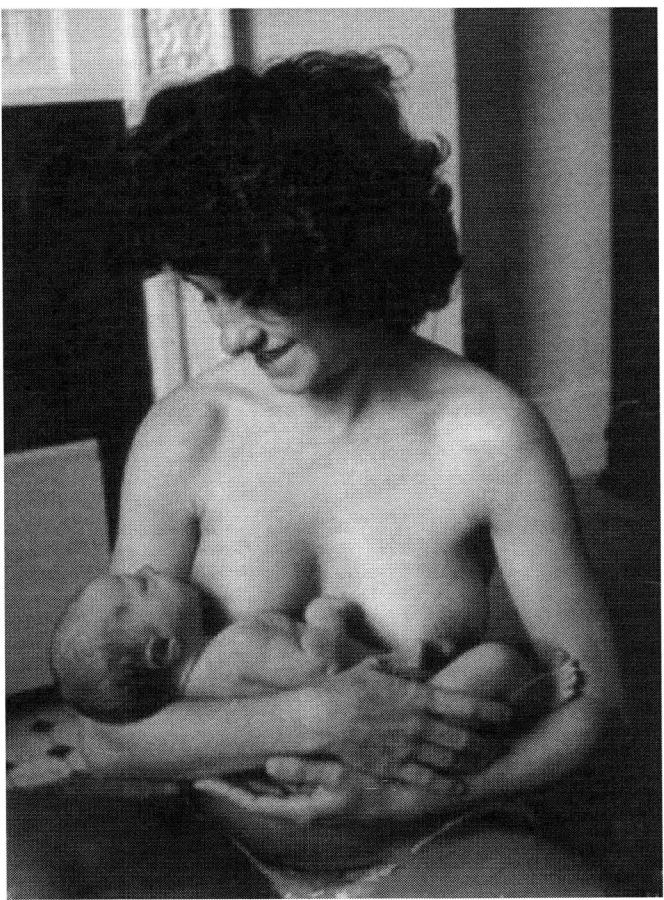

Liliana Lammers moments after giving birth physiologically [see Birthframe 20]

Labour

As you know, it's not always easy to know when a woman is really in active labour because the latent phase may seem very similar. To make matters worse, many women experience 'false' labour, or stop-start labour. And there also seems to be little agreement in the literature as to when precisely labour begins or even how fast it should progress, so as to be considered 'normal'. The Friedman curve, once so closely followed, is now widely disregarded—and even the originator, Emanuel Friedman, expressed horror at the way in which it came to be used.

Michel Odent, who has observed 15,000 labours, many of which must have been entirely physiological (because of his preference for this), joked to me that he only ever diagnosed labour in retrospect—when a baby had been born! Other practitioners who have been over-keen to diagnose have often ended up feeling the need to augment labour in one of the usual ways, because it has often not progressed as expected. Midwives who have not done this have later described a labour as lasting for 'five days', or similar. In Michel's view, these were not actually cases of five-day labours, but cases where a woman simply had a long latent phase, or where she had a stop-start labour. In any case, he prefers never to confirm to a woman that she is actually *in labour* because he says that doing so can put her under pressure to 'deliver'.

Despite this uncertainty about how or when labour begins, in very broad terms we can make some observations about the onset of labour and of course it's important for pregnant women to understand these too. When there are no attempts at induction, there might be various signs that labour is beginning.

- A woman will become aware that something is changing within her body. Perhaps she suddenly has either a bigger or a smaller appetite; she may become restless and have a sudden spurt of energy; she might experience a bout of diarrhoea, which will indicate that her body is 'clearing the way' for the new baby.
- Sometimes, the pregnant woman might notice a 'show', a discharge of a jelly-like substance, which may be smeared with blood. Seeing this jelly would be a sign that the cervix is beginning to open so as to eventually release the baby into the outside world.
- Sometimes, but less frequently, a woman might experience a gush of 'water' from between her legs.
- Of course, in all these cases, eventually the woman will notice that her uterus is gradually—or suddenly—becoming active as it flexes so as to fully open up the cervix and push the baby down through her pelvis, out into the world.

Of course, the rhythmical 'flexes' of the uterine muscles are usually—rather unhelpfully, it must be said—called 'contractions' in most books on childbirth, or 'rushes' in some others, which is again sometimes an undescriptive, unhelpful term because at some points during her labour a woman may not feel that things are 'rushing' anywhere. Having said this, if a woman has not interfered with the physiological processes taking place within her at any point during her pregnancy or labour, she is certainly likely to feel that an enormously powerful, absorbing, irreversible process is taking place, and 'sweeping' her along towards a predetermined biological end. That end is, of course, the birth of the baby... or babies, in the case of a multiple birth.

Are the sensations of labour and birth painful? As you no doubt know they are to most women, but not all. Some only experience pain for a short part of their labour and some don't experience any pain at all during the birth itself. A few women experience some or all of the process as being interesting or absorbing, rather than painful. Some even report labour and birth as 'orgasmic' (which makes sense when you consider that the hormone which opens up the cervix in labour—oxytocin—is the same one as is responsible for orgasm). Even when women experience contractions as outrageously painful they usually go into an interesting state of mind if they're completely undisturbed. This means they become totally absorbed by the labour and birth and find they are able to cope as long as they take the contractions one by one.

It's vital not to disturb the woman

Most midwives, it must be said, have never witnessed this because their behaviour or speech (either with the best intentions, or as a result of hospital-imposed protocols) cause a disturbance. Instead of providing a safety net, the midwife then becomes a disruption to the smooth proceeding of the labour (and birth), which is rather tragic, really. When, on the other hand, midwives give the labouring woman the feeling of being secure and when they monitor so unobtrusively that the labouring woman isn't even aware of it happening, they provide the perfect conditions... because of course they can intervene at any point if it is necessary, for safety. In most cases, though, women experiencing a fully physiological labour in a safe, but undisturbed environment find the resources within themselves to withstand all difficult sensations. And relatively quickly they have dilated to the magical 10cm, ready to proceed to the second stage.

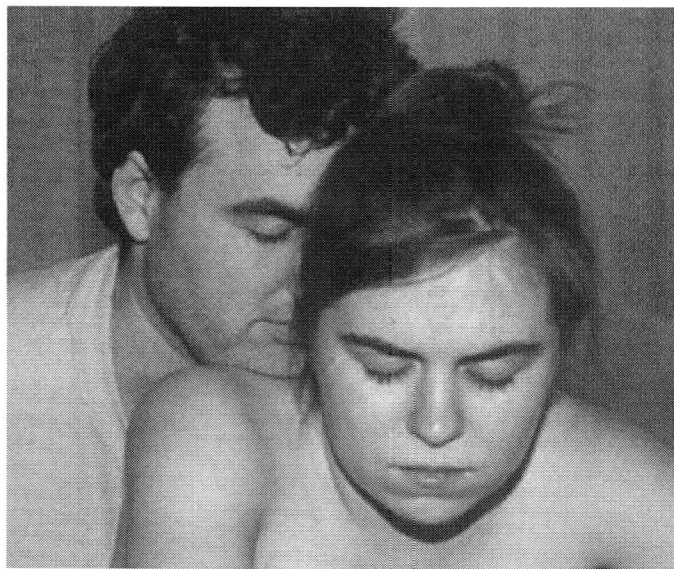

Because of the importance of not disturbing women in labour (which is easily done with a camera) I refused all photos of women in labour and actually giving birth except this one and one other from Ashley Marshall, a doula in America. It's vital that no-one uses a camera until after the placenta has been born—because it may well cause a life-threatening disturbance.

Since, as we've already noted, many midwives have never witnessed a completely physiological labour and birth or experienced them first-hand (while giving birth to their own babies) I am including some comments from contributors. I hope these will give you some insight into how the physiological processes are typically experienced in an optimal labour and birth.

> I had a whole night of very strong, regular contractions 24 hours before Asya was born. I was sure this was the real thing, but at 6am they petered out. Apparently this kind of 'false labour' is very common, because the body produces the most oxytocin at night. It didn't feel false! The good news is that false labour does help to open the cervix, so your labour will probably be that much shorter when it does get going for real.

> The night before Arion was born I had an innate sense that it would be the following day. I woke a few minutes to 6pm and had to go up to go to the loo. Shortly afterwards, I had a show and things started to happen. I felt a tightening in my stomach that felt like a contraction. I had been unaware of anything up till this point. Very soon, I was having contractions every five minutes, lasting approximately 30 seconds.
> [Arion was in fact born a few hours later.]

> I woke up needing to pee, and made it to the loo with clear liquid coming down my legs. The odd thing was that I had no control over this liquid, it just sort of fell out when I stood up.
> [The baby was born the same day.]

> Well, time went on. Due to finish work soon. On Sunday 25 June 2000 I was a little off, and I slept like a baby. Must have needed it, as Darren could not believe I had slept so well due to the noise going off outside—neighbours. Thought nothing of it. On the Monday, I took my son to school, as normal, and waddled off to work for my last week. I was up and down like a yoyo, going back and forth to the loo. Well, something was happening and I was just not ready. Rang the midwife, but by the time I had finished talking I was huffing and puffing...
> [Twins were born just after 3pm the same day.]

> At 32 weeks I had an antenatal check-up and was told the babies were roughly 6lb each in weight, so you can imagine my surprise and shock. The next few weeks I got bigger and bigger and everyone was hoping for an early delivery... even the doctors at the hospital couldn't understand after 36 weeks how I was still carrying them. Then 40 weeks approached and my due date. I attended another antenatal clinic, where I saw the consultant. He told me there was still plenty of room for them to grow so he would not induce me! 40 weeks + 3 days, my contractions started and I went to hospital, where they told me it was the first time they had ever seen a twin pregnancy overdue. By 6am the first baby was ready to arrive; I pushed for about 15 minutes and Megan Victoria was born at 6.19am, weighing 7lb 1oz, then six minutes later after pushing came Thomas William, weighing 7lb 12oz, both perfectly healthy.
>
> *Clare Swain*

> Perhaps what I experienced was false labour, or perhaps it was interrupted labour. All I know is that my strong, regular contractions suddenly stopped after I'd been talking to my mother on the phone for five minutes. She sounded horrified that I was in labour when I answered the phone. She then immediately switched to a totally boring, irrelevant topic for the rest of the conversation... er, monologue. No amount of relaxation exercises could restart the contractions when I came off the phone. However, the next day, when my contractions started again, they were even more purposeful and my 'real' labour lasted less than two hours.

> I did not want to leave the top floor of our house, I did not want the curtains open, and I did not want the lights on. Almost as soon as labour had begun I had started to withdraw into what I see as a sort of animal protective state.

> At the beginning my temperature perception was going up and down, so during a contraction all my clothes came off, then I was freezing in between, and they all had to go on.

> In the middle of the night my waters broke. I was asleep. It was about one o'clock in the morning and I woke up and I was just lying in bed and it was all wet. I called the nurse and she said, "No, you've probably just wet yourself," which made me feel really bad—it was really horrible. But I was certain it was my waters that had broken and so I insisted and she came and checked then called the doctor who was on call that night. He examined me and I was already 7cm dilated. But I hadn't felt any pain or anything—just pressure. I'd been feeling that for some time when I was standing up.

> Before my labour I ate voraciously. Part of my first stage I then spent throwing up into the toilet! This felt fine, actually. Afterwards, I rationalised that I must have digested most of the food I'd had beforehand anyway.

> You asked how I felt about shouting but to be honest it was more like a cow 'mooing'. It felt good to me and I reached a point where I stopped even caring what anyone else may have thought of it.

> Found standing up and leaning over the bed on a beanbag, rocking and having someone massage my lower back excellent for pain relief.

> Baby turned from posterior position to anterior a short time after I adopted an all-fours, bottom-up position.

> When they checked me over, I was 9cm dilated. The twins wanted out. There was nothing I could do but go with the flow.

> I had now been on my feet for about 9 hours with nothing to eat since the night before (my breakfast having hit the stairs some time before), and I really wanted to lie down. I did not care if labour stopped for half an hour; I just wanted a rest.

> Instead of putting on the Julian Cope compilation tape I had made specially for the labour, I knew I had to listen to music from my ancestors, from my soul, and put on some Welsh male voice choir albums... which then played for the next five hours. An email sent by a friend after the birth said, "After 5 hours of Welsh singing, the birth must have seemed a breeze."

> I went from Stage 1 to Stage 2 in about five minutes. From being able to hold a normal phone conversation one minute, I was suddenly only capable of screaming blue murder the next. My husband has never shown a cooler nerve as he drove me to the hospital. By this time I was screaming so loudly I was sure the whole of London could hear me. Incapable of sitting in the car I was raging around the back seat like a werewolf. I was in the grip of elemental forces that were telling me to go find a lair, a den, a quiet place to do this really important job. An overwhelmingly strong instinct was telling me to get my trousers off so that this being could come out. I would have done it in the lift. I would have done it in front of a million people. As it was, they found me a room and a couch and I was told the very encouraging news that I was already fully dilated.

> My midwife used a Sonicaid (a waterproof one bought especially for my water birth), but I can hardly recall it. I think she only listened once to the heartbeat at the same time as she examined me internally.

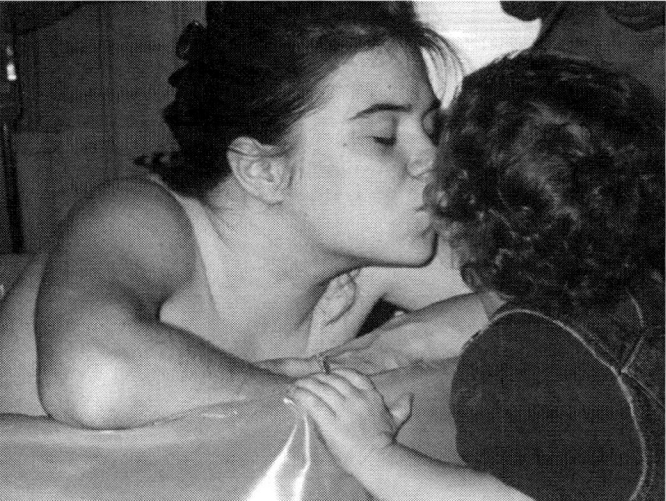

This is Ashley Marshall again. Incidentally, when I explained my policy of not using photos of women in labour to Ashley, she said: "I'm sorry to say that I was in very active labour when this photo was taken. It was at my request, though, as I wanted the event to be documented. I just love birth! I think a simple statement about children at birth would justify using the photo. Sometimes it is in fact reassuring for older children if they can be there when the baby's born—and this may be OK for the mother as long as she's not disturbed by having them around.

Birth

Towards the end of a physiological labour, without any intervention at all, the cervix will have opened up fully to about 10cm dilation, so as to allow the passage of the baby's head. Then, thanks to the powerful rhythmic muscular contractions which have been taking place and which still continue, the baby descends through the woman's pelvis and down through the soft, fleshy folds of her vagina. (There is sometimes a break of 20 minutes or longer between the cervix becoming fully dilated and the baby descending. During this period—or a shorter period—the woman experiences no contractions whatsoever. Other women continue on without a moment's break.) One of the bones which would normally block the baby's downwards passage—the tailbone (or coccyx)—moves out of the way when the woman is in an upright position. (It is much more likely that this will happen during an optimal birth because the woman will be entirely conscious and responding to her body's cues.) When the baby's head stretches the perineum the woman usually experiences a sudden burning sensation, often called the 'ring of fire'. Then suddenly, first the baby's head, then its body emerges through the woman's vagina. Of course, if it is a breech birth, the baby's bottom or feet will come first, followed by the rest of the body.

She will suddenly flick her hips forward

If the woman has not been disturbed in any way during her labour, she is likely to be in a pleasant 'submerged' state of mind and just before the moment of birth it is possible she may experience what Michel Odent calls a 'fetus ejection reflex', i.e. a sudden and compelling rush of energy which automatically makes birth simple, safe, active and intuitive. (This is when—mysteriously—adrenaline and oxytocin are successfully and only momentarily produced simultaneously. Instead of being antagonistic, as they normally are, they are both facilitative at this particular and very specific moment of birth.) The woman will typically pull herself to an upright position and spontaneously flick her hips forwards so as to facilitate the birth of the baby's head.

Again, since so few professionals have seen or experienced this kind of entirely physiological birth, here and overleaf are some comments from women who have...

> I have done some exciting stuff like parachute jumps, wing-walking, trips to war zones, but giving birth was definitely the most intense thing ever. My body felt totally out of control.

> For me, the most important thing was to take things moment by moment. If I hadn't done I would almost certainly have been overwhelmed... Actually, I was overwhelmed but I always kept going for another minute. When I experienced the fetus ejection reflex my body seemed to act on its own, although thoughts were still going through my head. It was very sudden and spontaneous and came after great feelings of 'not being able to do this thing of birth' successfully. But I could actually.

I felt overwhelmed but just kept going...

My body seemed to know when I should push, to pant or hold back

In second stage my body seemed to know when I should push, to pant or hold back, and I didn't need the midwife's help to control the delivery.

At the next contraction I said that I could feel the head crowning; I don't think anyone believed me. My next comment was "Ah that's better, the head's out." I then remember someone saying that they needed to get me off the toilet; once again I had my own ideas. I also had another contraction and the body was born. With this contraction I lifted myself off the toilet seat and caught our baby. I brought her up between my legs and sat back down to cuddle her for the first time. It was 10.30am, and she straightaway went to my breast.

I had gone from no baby to baby in about 3 minutes. This was a truly shocking experience, and I remember screaming as this thing fell out of my body.

As I lifted the baby up, just after he'd been born he didn't cry, just opened his eyes and looked around curiously. I felt like superwoman—amazed, empowered and overjoyed that birth could be such a wonderful experience!

My daughter Isabel was born on 9th December 1999, at 8.43pm. She was born in my bedroom just by the door. I had told the midwives I would make it to the end of the bed but when push came to shove I didn't want to get any further into the room.

I asked for an enema during my first labour because I felt blocked up. I was given a pessary and just a little poo came out a short time later. At the time, I didn't feel I'd been disturbed by this procedure but looking back I wonder whether I was in fact because I had a very long and difficult second stage. In my second labour, I again felt constipated, but my request for an enema was ignored. A few minutes later, I suddenly decided I'd stand up and do my 'poo' straight onto the floor! As I pulled myself up I also knew I was going to have a baby—not do a poo at all—so I think I wasn't really the least bit confused. The baby came out easily—she was obviously ready. It didn't even hurt!

From what I'd read about births, I had expected pushing to feel good. It didn't feel good to me. But it was really weird and interesting. The best part was definitely the moment after the pushing ended, when here she was at last, a whole new person!

Rebecca was delivered in a supported squatting position, Ros in a leaning forward crouching position, Juliet and Natasha in a kneeling position. Third stages were all in the kneeling-up position except for Rebecca, when I was lying down (and it was the least comfortable).

Keeping upright keeps the tailbone out of the way making the pelvic area wider so that the baby has a little more room to get out.

This time I wasn't lying down when I gave birth. I was squatting. Michel asked David to hold me under the armpits while I squatted—which was, in fact, difficult for him to do. I think Michel wanted me to get into that position because he knew she was going to be a big baby. But I didn't have to do any pushing at all. There was never any need to push... it was all just coming slowly but surely—and then fast.

A midwife's account:

As the last few barriers to Jenny's relaxing disappear (the last of the children are taken out), contractions become more painful, impinging on her concentration. Contracting strongly, every four minutes for 30-40 seconds. Jenny feels she needs to move away from things happening around her. Darkened bathroom, candles. I remove all offensive smells (cooking in the kitchen). She's out of the bath kneeling now, leaning over. Tim's applying pressure to Jenny's back. Things have hotted up. 15 minutes later: Pressure increases, intensity increases. Jenny thinks it's a boy—only a man would muck her about like this! Tim looks on, not making any comment. 30 minutes later: Shoulders and baby and all. Together Tim and Jenny investigate what their new baby looks like. "A girl," says Tim. "I'm glad you're a girl". Tears! Placenta born into the washing up bowl. All present and correct. Jenny has a bath with herb infusion. Baby checked and all there—not a *little* girl at 9lb 5oz (4.22 kg)!

I felt no pain at all during the second stage, just an incredible surging strength.

With two clear pushes the baby came down the birth canal. I did this in about 2 seconds, between two contractions. I'd say it was like doing a very easy, but big poo—not diarrhoea exactly, but very easy and even more satisfying than producing two long, plump turds. What I produced, after I'd then felt the 'ring of fire' and had flicked my hips forward twice, with the next two contractions, was a beautiful, baby, who now lay at my feet on a crumpled up sheet, looking up at me with rapt attention. When she suddenly burst into tears, I picked her up and put her to my breast. She seemed relieved and suckled with gusto.

As I pushed the baby out, my whole body was rising up in the water. That took me by surprise, but it did not make the birth difficult. The midwife said, "Julia, get ready to catch the baby," and I said, "but what should I do with it?"

I found the whole experience of a natural birth very exciting and satisfying. It hurt like hell, but it was bearable (just). I would be happy to go through the whole thing again next week if I could. It was a real peak experience for me.

I felt no pain at all during the second stage, just an incredible surging strength

26 *Optimal Birth: The What, The Why & The How*

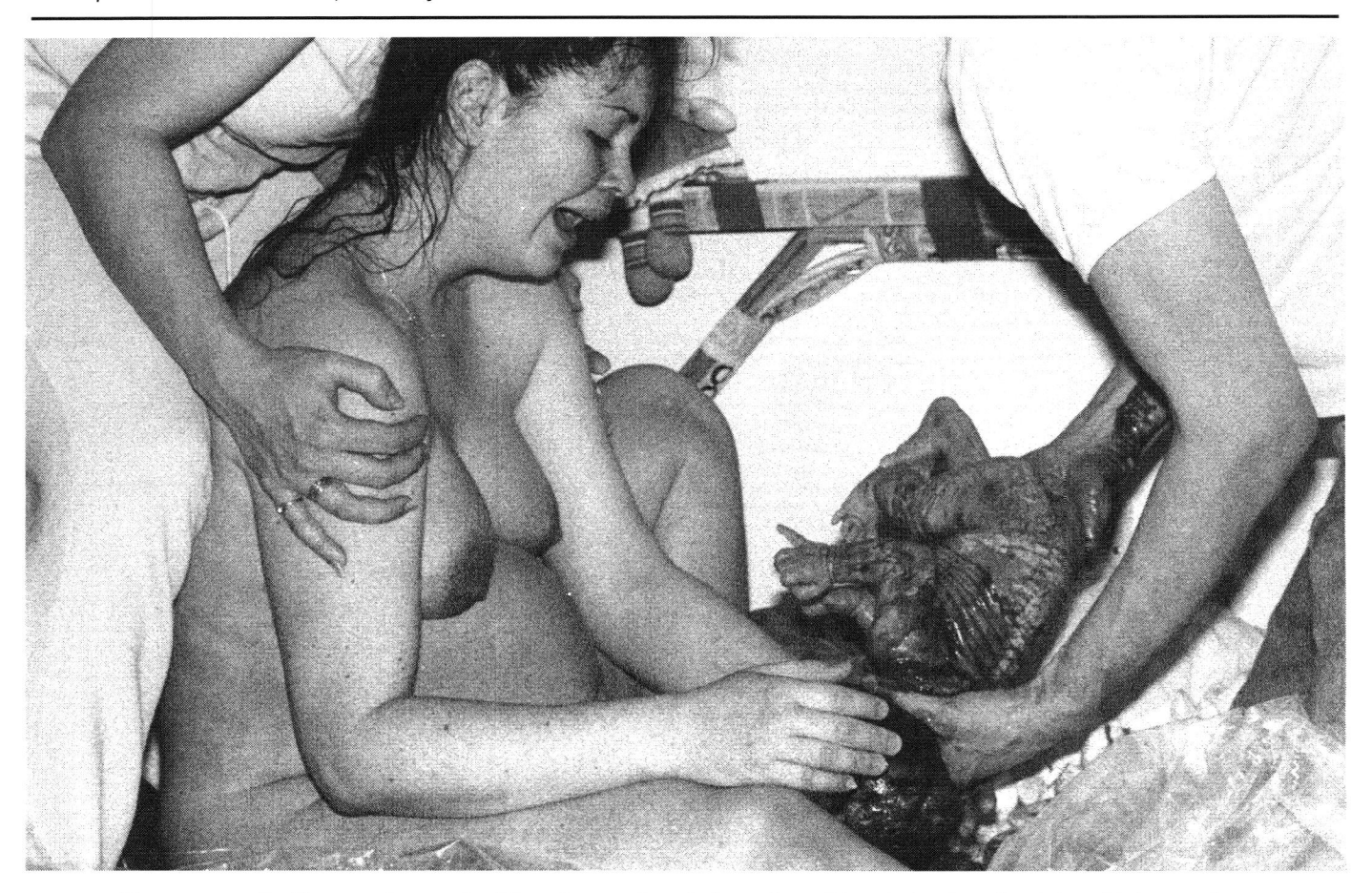

The woman will either spontaneously pick up her newborn baby, or have it handed to her silently by a birth attendant
Photo © Jill Furmanovsky (www.jillfurmanovsky.com)

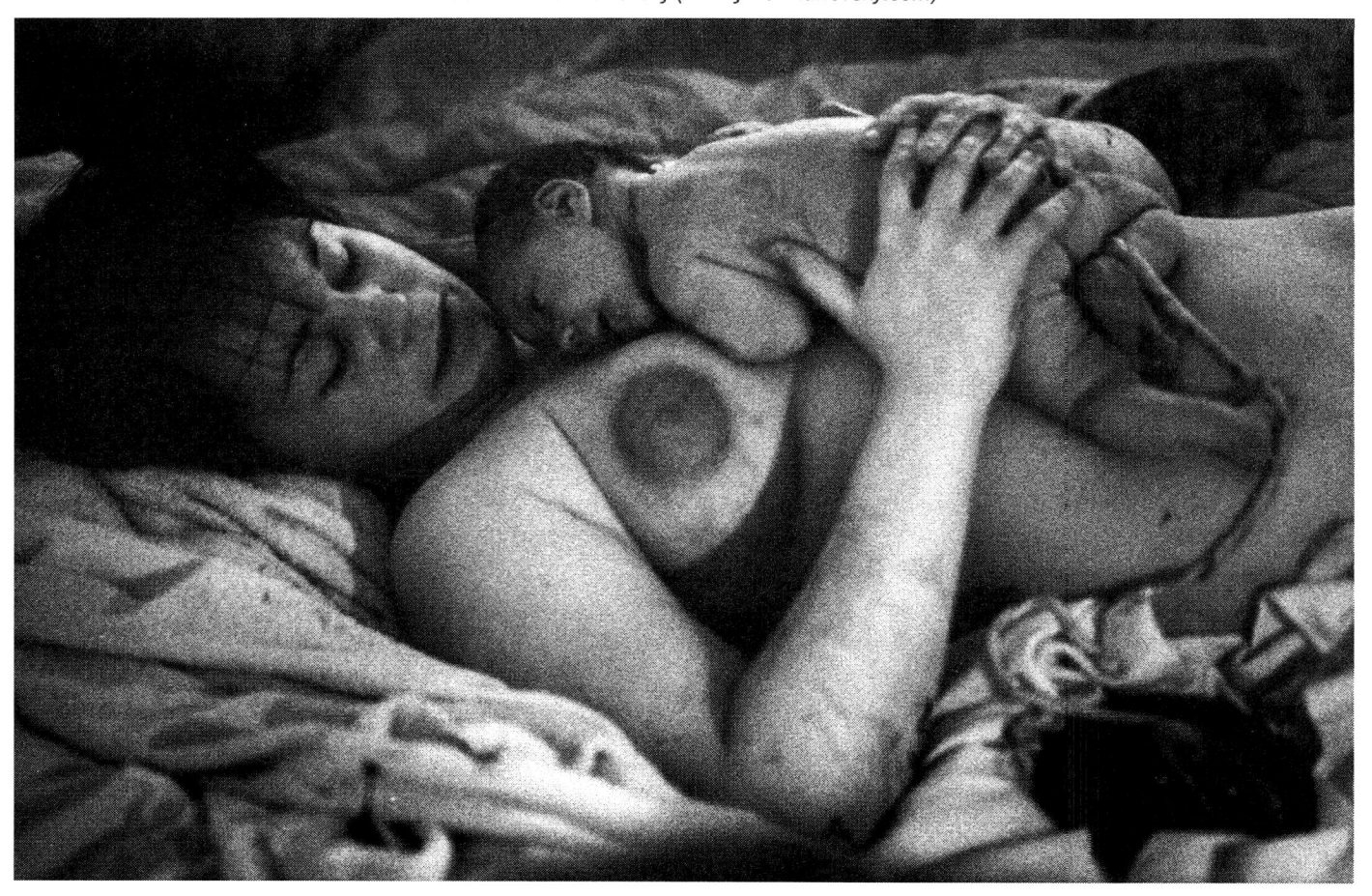

Of course, skin-to-skin contact is important after the birth
Photo © Jill Furmanovsky (www.jillfurmanovsky.com)

Note that no commands are necessary to tell the woman how to push. There is no straining, no fear, no control and no management.

I must mention at this point that one midwife disputed this point with me, saying that women often require instructions, guidance or encouragement during the second stage. (I hate mentioning specific conversations like this, but it is extremely relevant in this case, so I will just hope that the midwife concerned will forgive me for mentioning her anonymously like this.) Anyway, after talking to this midwife for a while it became clear that she'd only ever observed *one* physiological birth, and that one was accidental. It was a case of a woman arriving in active labour and being virtually ready to push on admission. My midwife friend had been about to embark on the usual admission protocols when a more experienced colleague stopped her, saying the mother was fine and she should be left undisturbed.

I think there are many cases in life when we *assume* that some kind of guidance or action is vital to the success of some endeavour, even though we might find Zen-like non-action (i.e. watchful waiting) to be more effective in actual fact. I don't know if I am the only one in the world who has had a row with her partner because of a comment made, which has prompted the response, "Yes, I know! What do you think I'm going to do?!" And am I the only person who's taken the advice of the childcare books on sibling rivalry? Sometimes, as advised, I've just sat and watched while my children squabble—only to find that 99% of the time they resolve their disputes on their own, without any 'help' from me. In fact, I'm often surprised by how harmonious and fair their own approach is and dismayed by the way in which my own well-intended interruptions often just make things much worse.

You may think I'm digressing terribly in mentioning these very different scenarios, but actually I think the principle of 'things going better when you leave well alone' applies *even more* in the case of childbirth because of the brain processes which are taking place. As Michel Odent has pointed out, it's as if a woman 'goes to another planet' during an undisturbed physiological labour and birth. In other words, she appears to switch off from her day-to-day reality and move into an entirely different state of mind. Any kind of speech, however brief, can jolt a woman out of an instinctual frame of mind back to cold reality, which naturally usually disturbs birth more than it facilitates it.

What, I think, is particularly interesting is that the labouring woman often *doesn't* feel she knows how to give birth. It is only by being left entirely undisturbed that she manages to reconnect with that deep, instinctual knowledge within herself, which typically emerges very suddenly.

Anyway, getting back to our documenting of the physiological processes... After the baby shoots out of the woman's body, hopefully onto something soft or into your hands. The baby will spontaneously take its first breath just a few moments later, sometimes crying as it does so, and sometimes not. Usually, the woman will pick the baby up or take it from you, if you've caught it.

At this point, both mother and child are usually in a state of heightened alertness, provided her birth attendants (including you!) do not disturb her in any way, either by talking, or attempting to communicate non-verbally. She will continue in this state for some time (again, provided she is not disturbed in any way), and will typically instinctively put the baby to her breast...

In many cases, the baby will slowly make its way there on its own, if placed on the mother's abdomen. The baby's suck is very strong and effective because it will have no opiates in its system. Of course, during this first feed the mother will usually be gazing at her new baby and as part of this first examination, she will spontaneously check the baby's gender. (Needless to say, *telling* her the baby's gender would be a disturbance which would stop the birth from being entirely physiological. If this seems extreme at this stage, please bear with me here... As we will see later on, any disturbance changes the hormonal environment and therefore the smooth-running of the physiological processes—and speech is particularly powerful.)

The continued smooth production of hormones then ensures that the placenta is released safely and speedily—probably within two hours of the birth, but often within seconds or minutes of the baby's birth.

The umbilical cord is cut when it stops pulsing or can remain intact until it spontaneously breaks away from the baby's body a few days later—unless it snaps before this!

Suddenly, provided there is no disturbance, the placenta is born too—usually in one smooth, slippery movement. In an undisturbed physiological birth, this happens very soon after the birth of the baby (even one or two seconds later). Breastfeeding also stimulates the production of the hormone (oxytocin) which makes the birth of the placenta possible.

As we've already noted, if the woman was upright (squatting, semi-squatting, or on her hands and knees) at the moment of birth, it's very likely that her vagina, and indeed her entire pelvic floor will be undamaged after all these processes have taken place because the perineum is naturally stretchy and the woman's complete awareness of every sensation will help her to make sure the birth does not cause any injury. This means she'll have no pain after the birth, beyond a little discomfort the first time she passes urine and a bowel motion, as well as the experience of her womb contracting back to its normal size. She will feel completely normal when sitting or walking around. Obviously, this is in stark contrast to the postnatal experience of many women who have analgesia or anaesthesia in whatever form because of side effects or the increased risk of tearing, not to mention the likelihood of a 'cascade of interventions'.

One very interesting aspect of all this, from a midwifery point of view, is that a truly physiological birth usually involves far less mess. When the placenta detaches itself quickly and extremely efficiently (as happens when the woman and baby are completely undisturbed by at the time of the birth and afterwards) there can be virtually no blood loss. (This is something Michel Odent has observed many times.) And, of course, this also has enormous safety implications because an efficient third stage means a much lower chance of any life-threatening PPH.

The reduced blood loss after a true fetus ejection reflex also means that the woman is extremely strong after the birth, which puts her at an enormous advantage.

If this or any other aspect of this description seems unlikely or exaggerated to you, let me finish by saying that I've experienced all these things first-hand so can vouch for their accuracy. I have been repeatedly distressed when listening to woman describe their experience after opting for 'pain relief'. It really does seem a bit of a misnomer...

Even if there is some mess after the birth (faeces or blood), as is likely, both mother and baby will certainly be fully conscious and active during and after a completely physiological birth, and a number of pleasant mind-body states are typical. These include wonder, alertness and euphoria—and it seems, from both the babies' facial expressions and research evidence, that the baby experiences these too. Many midwives have also reported greatly increased job satisfaction when attending physiological births because some of this euphoria seems to rub off on them! Perhaps it's just nice being around people who are clearly happy and fulfilled.

The hormones which the mother and baby will be benefitting from will continue to affect their behaviour not just in the hour or so after birth, but even for a week or so afterwards. Of course, this all means that women have a much easier start to motherhood because they are behaving instinctually at each stage, rather than having to be directed by outsiders or prompted from within.

The impact of natural hormones on the processes really is quite remarkable. A woman who is usually self-conscious about being naked will happily strip off her clothes and get into unusual positions when she's completely involved in her labour. In a similar way, even if she has planned not to breastfeed she is likely to do so after a completely physiological birth. Obviously, the implications are enormous. Michel Odent has remarked that it's as if the woman 'goes to another planet' when the verbal side of her brain is allowed to become inactive.

Another interesting thing about physiological birth is that the baby does not need to be 'caught'. The mother-to-be can simply prepare something soft for her baby to land on and can position herself above it. This means the woman can also be alone, while her midwife (or midwives) wait in the next room, or in the corridor, monitoring by listening and observing through a crack in a door. An alternative, if this prospect makes you nervous would be for only one very unobtrusive and sensitive midwife to stay with the woman giving birth, while another waits outside—if a second needs to be present. Whatever the arrangement, the processes seem to work best when the smallest possible number of people are present. (In Michel Odent's opinion, the more people there are, the longer the labour.) With only one or two other people around (or in an adjoining room), the labouring and birthing woman truly has a feeling of privacy and security (because she knows her attendants are there) so relaxes completely into the birthing process.

Finally, to state the obvious, I hope this description has made it clear that literally *nothing* needs to be done to facilitate the birth of a baby: it all happens without any prompting or facilitating. Although a back-up system is essential for optimality, no help of any kind is needed after most completely physiological births—except clearing up! After all, the baby's reflexes help him or her to adjust to life outside the womb. Coughing, sneezing, rooting and sucking all take place completely spontaneously, when necessary, and the newborn will almost always breathe without assistance. If something does need to be done by an outsider—for example, if the umbilical cord is wrapped around the baby's neck—the mother herself, who is fully conscious and active, often spontaneously does it herself, so true sensitivity is required by midwives.

If you're used to something quite different, I hope this detailed description of birth will provide food for thought.

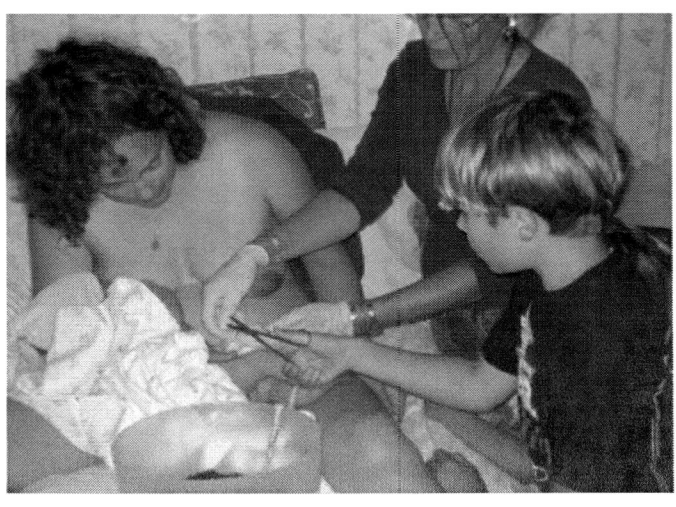

Cutting the cord

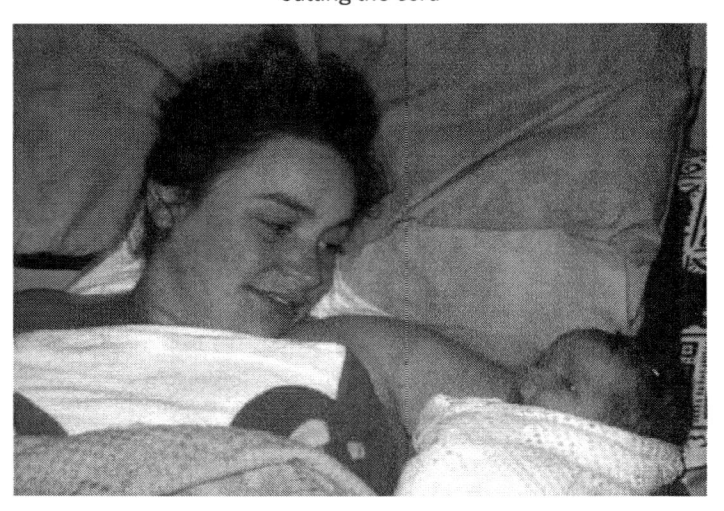

A mother snuggling up with her newborn just after the birth

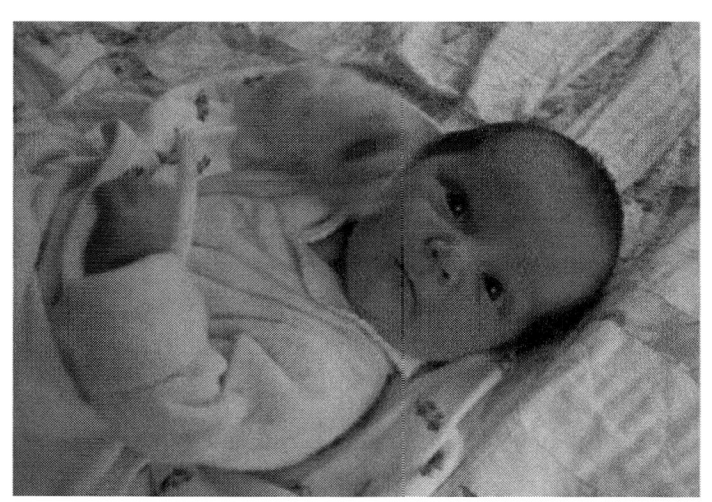

Another alert newborn baby after a physiological birth. Of course, babies who have been born without any drugs in their system are extremely alert and keen to take in all that they find around them—especially people, and in particular their mum!

Of course, babies who have been born without any drugs in their system are extremely alert and keen to take in all that they find around them—especially people

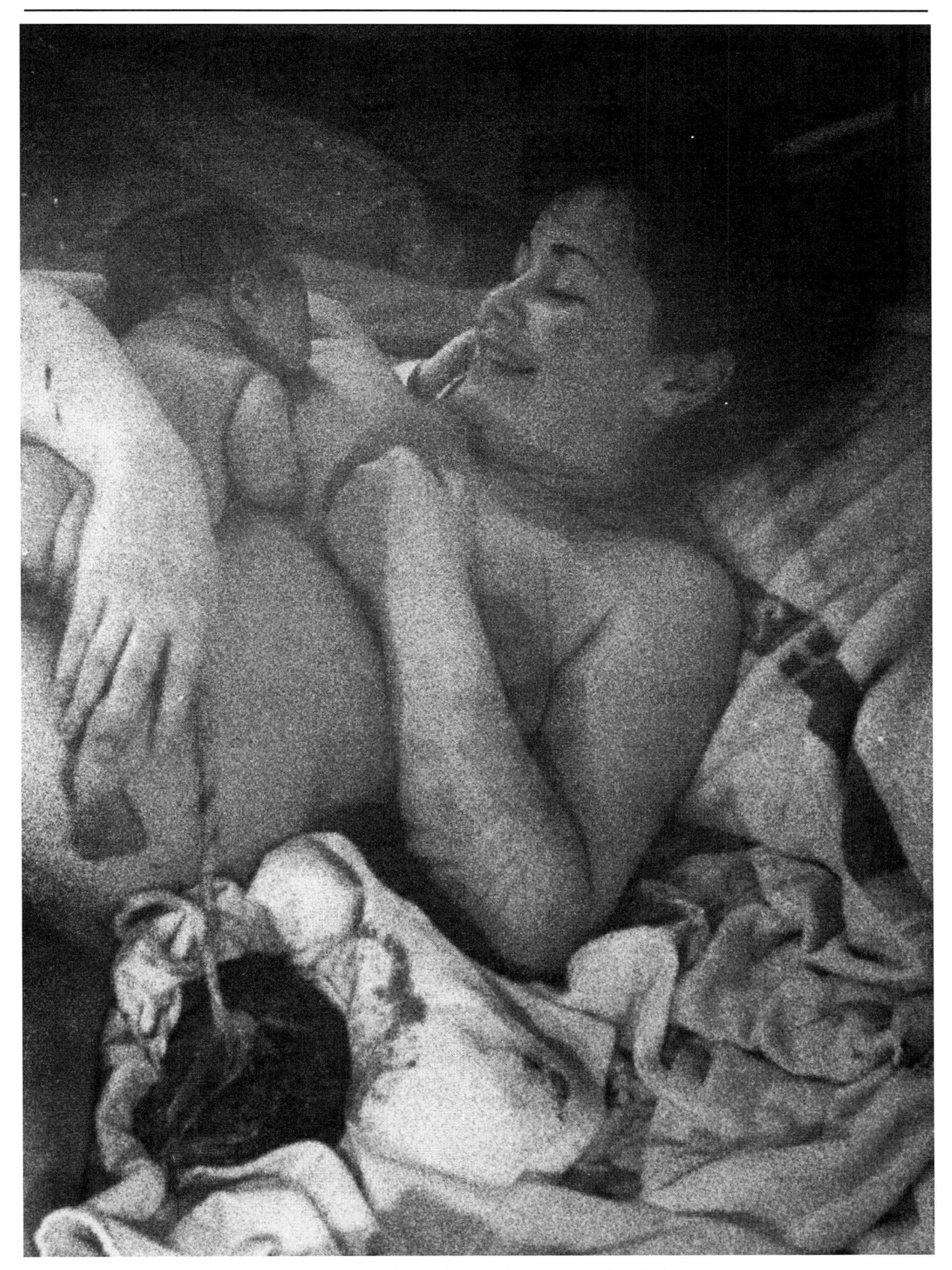

The mother we saw on pp 2 and 26, Nuala OSullivan, bonding with her newborn
Photo © Jill Furmanovsky (www.jillfurmanovsky.com)

Postpartum

After-birth scenarios obviously vary enormously. Mother and baby are usually both very alert for about an hour after the birth. In that time, as we've already noted, the baby usually starts breastfeeding to get the creamy health-sustaining colostrum. Mother and baby—and often the father too—start bonding, as the baby gazes, cuddles up, sucks and eventually drifts off into a contented sleep.

If you are the birth attendant, you will carry out your normal checks at this point (Apgar scores, etc.), If you are making the birth entirely physiological you will avoid any practices which disturb the baby (or mother), such as suctioning (unless necessary to establish the baby's breathing), the administration of Vitamin K (by any means), or the Bart's test. You will also not give any instructions so as to 'facilitate' breastfeeding or mothering behaviour because this should all take place smoothly, triggered simply by the appropriate hormones being naturally produced by the mother's (and baby's) body. Having said all this, you would of course intervene if there were any life-threatening problem.

You will carry out your usual checks on the mother at a time which seems suitable, so as to cause minimal (or zero) disturbance in early bonding. If the baby's father is around, this might be a good time for him to say his first hello—meaning, of course, that the baby need never be separated from his or her parents in the first few hours (or days) of life.

If you're not used to this kind of birth, you may be surprised at this point to find you have an extremely active mother on your hands! She may want your support though while she has her first shower soon after the birth (if she feels messy). And she's sure to appreciate any help you can give her tidying up. (Oh, the joys of being a midwife.)

The baby's extreme alertness may also come as a surprise to you, if you're used to seeing babies born with drugs in their systems. The baby's personal priority at this stage is probably to make use of this alertness to take in as much as possible of his or her new world, outside the womb. He or she will definitely not be worried about having a first wash... so don't worry about arranging this. In fact, so as to facilitate bonding between the mother and newborn, it's best to leave the baby with his or her beautiful newborn aroma, because this can never be restored, once washed off. The baby can simply be cleaned up by wiping with a clean cotton cloth, put in some kind of nappy, and dressed or wrapped appropriately, depending on the weather.

Quite soon after the birth, perhaps after eating and drinking, both mother and baby—although initially in a heightened state of alertness—may well want to sleep. Obviously, they will have been through quite a lot together. Of course, there is no reason why they shouldn't sleep together... As is well reported, mothers who breastfeed are very sensitive to the needs of their babies and—incredibly, but reassuringly—this is true from the very moment of birth. There will also be afterpains postnatally, as the uterus returns to its pre-pregnancy size, and after a physiological birth these may well be *more* painful, because the process is likely to take place more efficiently than after a 'managed' birth.

No doubt, you will also have to complete your usual record-keeping afterwards...

Here a few people explain how it happened for them...

> I was surprised when the placenta shot out from between my legs as I reached down to pick up my new baby. So fast and easy!

> My physiological third stage was surprisingly painful, but very fast. Then suddenly, it was all over.

A midwife's notes:

> 10.24 Baby delivers, brought straight out of water by Georgina and G. Baby cries instantly.
> 10.35 Baby lying in Georgina's arms.
> 10.40 Baby still attached to placenta but cord ceased pulsating now. Georgina has period-like pains and feels the placenta beginning to come. Water temperature increased after the birth (temperature now 37.3 degrees centigrade). Baby feels warm. Baby is lovely pink now.
> 10.50 Baby is feeding from Georgina now.
> 10.55 Placenta membranes delivered spontaneously in the water. Baby still feels okay but has been covered up with a towel now. Cord clamped now and cut by his daddy.
> 11.00 Georgina out of the water. Bleeding minimal, estimated all in all at approx. 100 ml. Perineum observed, no tears at all. Georgina just feels sore and bruised but it all looks healthy and well.
> 11.05 Placenta looks complete. Membranes x 2 present and 3 vessels in cord.

> The placenta had a strange smell and didn't look as I imagined it would.

> I got out of the birthing pool for the 3rd stage and had a small tear, which didn't require stitching.

> There was no need for stitches afterwards.

> It might be of interest to note that although I had what seemed like a lot of blood loss when the placenta was expulsed (without the use of syntometrine), this large loss of blood is considered a good thing in many so-called undeveloped countries (according to Sheila Kitzinger's research) and this seemingly large quantity of blood was followed by very little lochia. On Day 1 I seemed to be soaking pads fairly consistently but from Day 2 onwards I have had very little discharge.

> Postpartum, I just needed 'mini' pads.

> Postnatal problems? I simply didn't have any. I think problems can sometimes be triggered by drugs given in labour, catching infections, unnecessary interventions, etc.

Postnatal problems? I didn't have any

In case you haven't ever had a baby yourself, or need reminding of what it's like, here are a few comments from mothers who did the whole thing entirely physiologically...

> I can't tell you what an amazing feeling it is to hold him, touch him, look at him making funny, suspicious faces and wrinkling his brow. I can see Mum was right when she said romantic love is nothing compared to this feeling of utter astonishment and prostrated adoration of this minute creature. My husband and I both feel it. My husband went home to get a few things and run some errands the next day. "I got home to the empty house and it all seemed so pointless. All I wanted was to be back with the two of you." He is utterly taken by the baby. We haven't needed any name for our son in these timeless days at the hospital, with no one but the three of us, a tiny universe.

> Somehow the house feels entirely different now. We have a home now where we're sheltering somebody infinitely precious. Before it was just a post-college pad for two of us to hang out in and amuse ourselves. Now it all has a point.

> I was a bit confused after the birth for a while. I almost felt like I'd failed because it wasn't totally enjoyable. I kept having to remind myself of what I'd achieved, which wasn't hard—I just had to look at my baby and I knew I'd done something wonderful! Being just me and my husband at the birth made it very special and intimate, we didn't need anyone else. After the birth it was all very peaceful and beautiful.

> Babies are such a wonderful way to start people!

> Mum left on Sunday. That afternoon we took him for the first walk of his life, in Regents' Park. All the other parents with children looked calm and collected. We got hot around the collar trying to put the pram together with him in it.

> My partner and I rowed horribly in the first weeks after our baby was born, partly because she was so incredibly interested in everything all the time and so disinterested in sleep! We constantly criticised each other's attempts to care for her and I felt tremendously alone and unloved. Fortunately, things eventually settled down and our second baby was incredibly easy and obliging, although also clearly as bright as a button.

> I really threw myself into the childrearing and I remember at least one person said to me "What about you? You've got to give some time to yourself" and I remember saying "This is me. This is important." Not to say, there were times when I didn't get exhausted.

Words from a mother of six, expecting her seventh child:

> If there was one piece of advice I'd give to new mothers, it'd be this... Forget about the idea of having routines! Just try to meet your baby's needs and go with the flow.

Such a wonderful way to start people

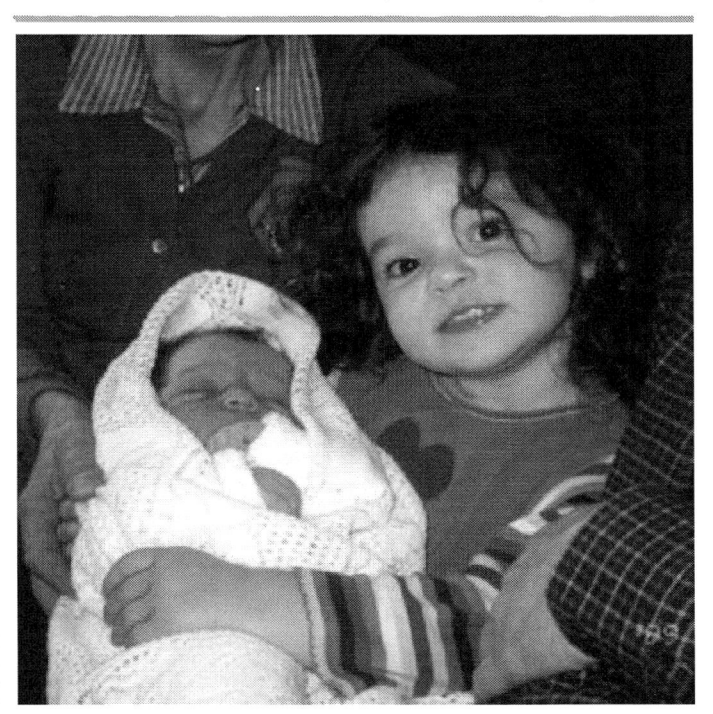

A little girl who's delighted to be involved

There's nothing quite like having a new baby in the house!

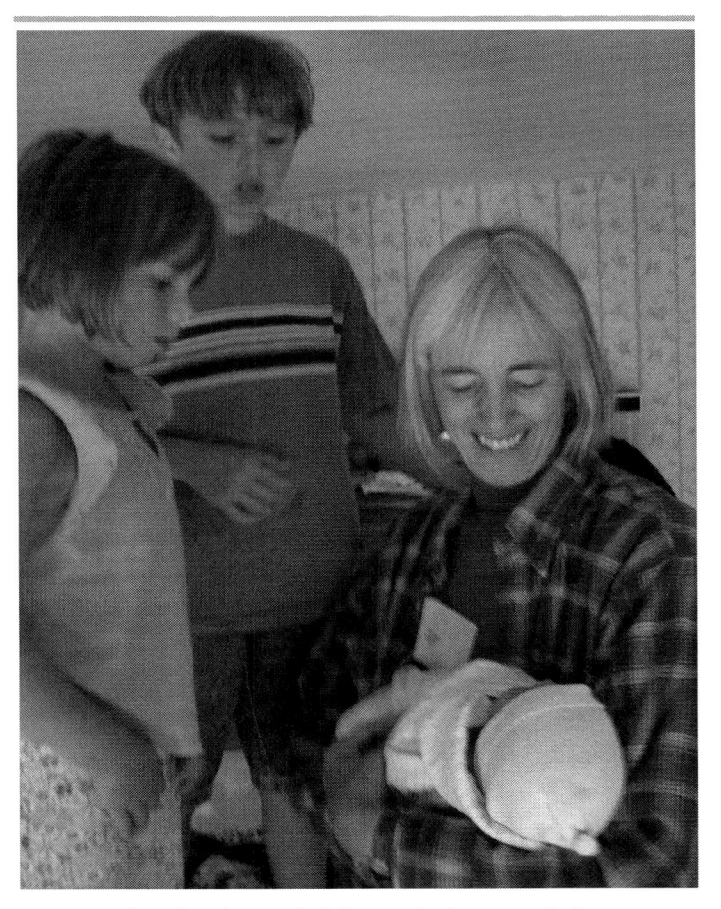

Grandmother and siblings enjoying a new baby

BIRTHFRAMES

I shall now present the first of a few 'birthframes'. These birth stories and are intended to help you visualise real life scenarios and see where my own personal views have come from. Incidentally, I've created the word 'birthframe' to refer to any true account of a birth experience, part of it, or even only part of the labour or pregnancy—or it may cover more than one birth. The word 'birthframe' reminds me of 'window frame', through which you can get a glimpse into someone else's world, and 'frame of reference', which helps put other things in perspective.

Here's my own first birth story...

Birthframe 1

I didn't meet the man who seemed to be my life partner until the age of 36. We decided we'd like three children, so went to our local Family Planning Clinic for advice. "Have them as quickly as you can!" they said, with an air of alarm. This wasn't quite what we'd been expecting, so we went away rather bemused.

By the time we decided to stop using contraception, I was 37 and we were living in Sri Lanka. I started taking folic acid, ate even more healthily than usual and read any pregnancy books I could get hold of. I got pregnant immediately, but then miscarried after falling out of a boat—a freak wave appeared as I was being helped out. Although I was upset, the very next month I was delighted to find I had conceived again.

It soon became clear that the obstetrician I initially registered with intended to intervene in all kinds of ways. As a result I gradually realised I felt strongly about doing things naturally. I didn't find an obstetrician who would support me until I was 30 weeks' pregnant. Not only did this man agree to my birth plan, he also suggested he could ask for permission for me not to be moved to the delivery room for the birth. This would mean I could avoid the things I didn't like about that room. (Was I taking this 'natural' thing too far, I wondered?)

I worked full-time right up until the day I went into labour. That morning, which was already four days past my due date, I felt as if I was fighting off a migraine. This was unusual, so a sympathetic boss sent me home. I had what I thought must be a show in the afternoon and started experiencing some mild contractions for a few hours. That morning I'd at last got my old electronic piano working, so I spent the early part of my labour playing through my old piano music. At around 8.30pm my partner got home, then at 11.30pm he took me along to the hospital. There, my contractions soon stopped, only to restart gradually a couple of hours later.

After a difficult 'posterior labour' and 'face-to-pubis' delivery I gave birth at 1.20 the next afternoon in a supported semi-squatting position. Strangely, the first downpour of the Sri Lankan monsoon season that year came a couple of hours after my baby's birth.

There were some extremely bad moments, but somehow I managed to get through them. This was due to luck as well as effort, if you like to call it that. I had asked for an epidural at one point. I was told I could only have one if I transferred to the local (more modern) hospital, which I didn't want to do. I was offered pethidine, but I refused that too, remembering that it would weaken my baby's suck—and I was very keen to breastfeed. I also asked for gas and air, but that wasn't usually available and the obstetrician and nurse couldn't get the cylinders working. Luck and judgment, I suppose.

Through the OK moments and the dire my partner, Phil, had supported me by massaging my back. I'd screened out the many people who wanted to ogle me by turning away from them and leaning over a wickerwork chair in a corner. Michel tells me I would have had a much easier time if they hadn't been there because I was clearly constantly being disturbed. I did at least have the periodic support of my obstetrician, who popped in every now and then until close to the birth, when he stayed until after the third stage. A few weeks after the birth he wrote to me saying: "I am enormously glad that I had the courage to take you on and it was a pleasure looking after you... Looking back, I think it was a good effort on the part of the staff and even myself. It was the first time, and I am sure many of the girls there would not have even dreamt that anyone would want to have a baby the way you did. They unanimously agree they will do it again."

I made sure my wishes about the birth and afterwards were respected by reiterating them to each new midwife who arrived, miming whenever I thought they didn't understand enough English. And I stopped the 'commanded pushing' when it came by telling the midwife to be quiet. (When she ignored me, I appealed to the obstetrician, reminding him of my birth plan. He then told the midwife she did need to be quiet. This was just as well because I later learned that commanded pushing is can cause transverse arrest in face-to-pubis births.)

Anyway, it did all go smoothly (and noisily) and Anjula, our new daughter, was delightful—very, very alert and interested in everything. To my surprise and relief, I spontaneously found myself achieving what I thought was impossible—I breastfed her immediately. (My mother hadn't been able to.) The placenta came out about 20 minutes after the birth and although I felt faint for a couple of hours due to low blood pressure, the pain was completely gone.

Later that day, I walked across the courtyard to another, airier room for a couple of days' cosseting. While I was there, the nurse-midwives did a wonderful job of teaching me how to bathe my baby and change her nappy. Looking back, it was fortunate that they completely ignored all feeding issues. Despite ongoing feelings of nervousness (worrying that something would soon go wrong), I had no problem establishing breastfeeding and had no postnatal problems, beyond a few mild afterpains. Penny Stanway's book *Breast is Best* and La Leche League's *The Womanly Art of Breastfeeding* were all I needed, along with the hormones which my body automatically produced after an optimal birth.

In the end I breastfed Anjula for almost two years, by which time I was over five months' pregnant with No. 2.

Here's what happened the second time I gave birth...

Birthframe 2

I look back on my second child's birth with a great feeling of peace, happiness and even wonder. Nina-Jay was born on 15 December at 11.30 in the evening, just two hours after I experienced the first contraction; the placenta came out painlessly with another contraction, a few moments later. Her Apgar score was 10 and she weighed in at a healthy 7lb (3.2kg). There was no problem with blood loss and no need for any stitching—I only had a little superficial tearing, which healed in a couple of days. I started breastfeeding Nina-Jay moments after she was born and we continued—with breaks!—until she was nearly two years old, with no problems.

In the three weeks before the evening of her birth I had experienced numerous painless or low-pain contractions. The contractions which started at 9.30pm on her 'birth day', while I was doing the washing up, came on very suddenly. They were much stronger than any I had felt in the days and weeks before... In fact, they were completely absorbing. I was immediately on my hands and knees on the kitchen floor.

Fortunately, Michel Odent, my birth attendant, was already in the house when these contractions started so there was no problem about it being such a short labour. Just before I'd started doing the washing up, he and I had sat at the kitchen table after an enormous dinner, talking about my life and all my problems and I realise that something in me had relaxed during that conversation. I'd been worried about the future but Michel had somehow reassured me that things would work out OK. I didn't know why, but I did somehow believe him. The evening before I had telephoned him, thinking I was in labour, and had had to apologise when he arrived since my contractions had stopped. He decided to stay at our place that night and in the morning said he would like to come to dinner again later that day and again stay overnight. (We were living in Reading, a long way from his home in London.) I must say, I wasn't keen when he said this because I had visions of cooking for him and apologising for the next two weeks—but it turned out that he was right to return so soon. When he arrived at around 4pm, I was fast asleep, having had a huge lunchtime curry. My husband was at home that day because of a quirk in his timetable, so I hadn't needed to worry about looking after 2-year-old Anjula.

With these sudden overwhelmingly powerful contractions, I soon felt the need to stagger upstairs to the bathroom and to start some sonorous groaning. Michel, hearing the noise, emerged from the room we'd assigned him—next door to the bathroom—and asked if he could please check the baby's heartbeat and position. His brief examination reassured him that conditions were ideal for me to labour undisturbed. Firstly, palpation of my 'bump' had told him I had a full bag of waters. Of course, this meant there was little danger of the umbilical cord prolapsing or becoming compressed. Secondly, he established that the position of my baby was fine (LOA). (However, Michel later told me his 'treatment'—i.e. to leave me to labour undisturbed—would not have been different if she had turned out to be posterior too. He was just reassured to find that conditions were optimal.)

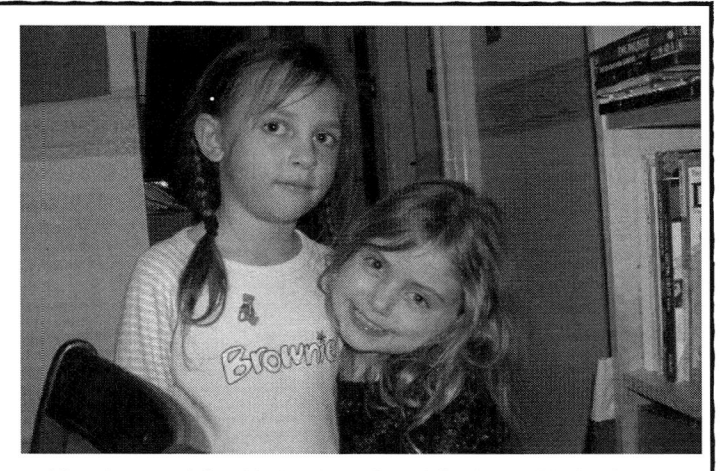

Nina-Jay, aged 6, with the little sister I finally decided to have

He said he has found that women with 'posterior' babies find better positions for turning the baby if left alone, undisturbed. During this check Michel also confirmed with a Pinard that the fetal heartbeat was strong.

Watching me discretely, Michel was then reassured to see that on my return to the bathroom I was spontaneously labouring in favourable positions—leaning forward, either standing, on my hands and knees, or on my knees in front of the toilet when I was throwing up! He knew this would mean avoiding compressing the vena cava, which is of course important for the baby's oxygen supply. So he left me to labour alone, in peace, while he waited and listened from the room next door. He even waited outside while I delivered both the baby and the placenta.

My partner, strong and sensitive, was there to help me during that brief two-hour period. I felt totally alone, though, and regretted not having arranged for a woman to attend me. Also, as each contraction ripped into me I fully understood why some women choose pain relief or a caesarean—but I knew I must not even mention any of these thoughts out loud. A few contractions into my labour I said to Phil, "Two children are enough! We really don't need to have a third one, you know." Wisely ignoring my comment, he ran up and down the stairs fetching things for me—candles for candlelight, something to tie my hair back... [By the way, an arrow like this one will show you when something continues on to the next page.] ▶

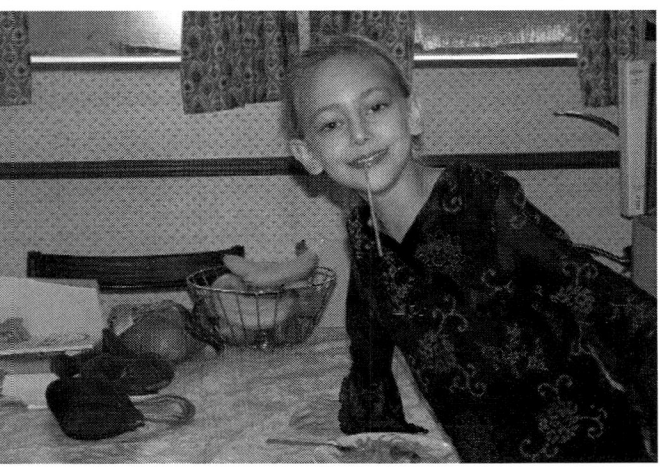

Anjula, aged 8, eating spaghetti

Meanwhile, Michel Odent continued to keep watch from the next room, without making himself seen. He knew from long experience that the best support would be to leave me completely undisturbed, with a feeling of being unobserved. The sounds I made would be enough to tell him that all was going well. Of course, he administered no drugs and insisted on no routines. Nature had her own routines in mind...

Then, within two hours of feeling that first contraction, I gave birth. Moments before, Anjula had woken up so Phil had had to go and console her. Suddenly, having been sitting on the toilet for a few minutes, straining to do a non-existent 'poo', I arose and stood firm and erect, yet somehow also in a semi-squat since my knees were slightly flexed. Between my feet, bundled up in a large ball, was the plastic sheet I'd been 'relocating' around the house in a preoccupied manner for the few days before I went into labour. So much strength was coursing through my body, I didn't need anyone's help or support.

I thought about various things I'd read. I thought of Eskimos—Inuit—supporting their wives from behind and pushing down on the 'bump' so as to help the baby and I focused in on my own baby within me. Then I thought, "Baby, be born!"—calm, joyful words which passed through my head quite spontaneously. Then suddenly, I gave two wonderful strong, clear, purposeful pushes. The ring of fire I then felt made me consciously realise my new baby's head must have crowned. I momentarily felt worried I would tear.

Then—thinking, "Oh, I don't care if I rip in two"—I flicked my hips forward. Reaching down to feel what was going on I was shocked to feel a head. "Michel!" I shouted, anxious that I should be giving birth without his help.

Knowing it would be dangerous to disturb me at this point, he ignored me and carried on simply silently watching through the crack in the door.

There was a moment's pause, then again I flicked my hips forward. In a sudden gush my baby was born and, confused, I felt another gush seconds later.

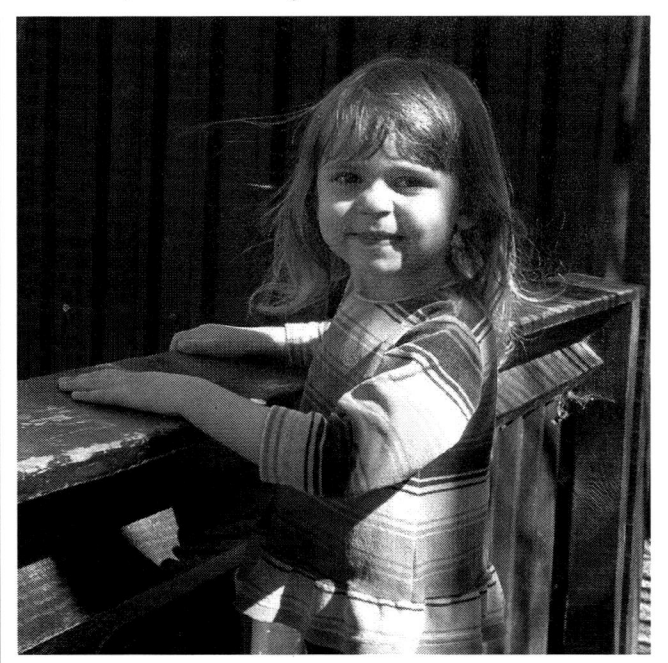

Nina-Jay, born by fetus ejection reflex, aged 3

I looked down, transfixed for what must have been only a few seconds, admiring my new baby's features. Suddenly she let out a cry and saying, "Don't cry," I took her up in my arms and instinctively put her to my breast.

I calmly, joyfully thought, "Baby, be born!"

There was none of the hesitation I'd expected to feel. Having read about so many problem situations, I had wondered whether breastfeeding would be so easy the second time around. My new baby sucked as if for the thousandth time, not the first, and her life was begun. As I looked down it dawned on me that the second gush had been the placenta... It was all so fast! Beautifully alert, my baby was gazing quizzically into my eyes as she breastfed.

Michel came in at this point and was reassured to see the placenta lying by my side, born and whole, a sign that all was properly finished and safe. My partner was sad to have missed the birth and my 2-year-old daughter who'd just woken up looked amazed at her mother holding a new sister in her arms.

It was wonderful not having someone else 'catch' the baby for me. It was also wonderful being able to discover her sex myself and pick her up for the first time without anyone observing or 'checking' on me. The most wonderful aspect of this birth, though, was the feeling of strength I had. I felt so strong, both physically and mentally. I didn't need anyone to support me as I suddenly stood up, swung round, raised my arms in the air, elbows bent, feet planted firmly on the floor some distance apart, knees flexed. I certainly didn't need anyone to tell me I was fully dilated. Somewhere deep inside, I knew it was time to push. The feeling of pushing—two long, clear, happy pushes—was very positive and also completely painless. The ring of fire which I immediately became aware of at the end of these pushes was also not painful or 'weak-feeling'. There was never any need to 'pant' or control my breathing—I just felt poised, focused, very alert and decisive. And I was strong physically in the sense that I had no problems with low blood pressure and no feelings of weakness after the birth. This had been a truly authentic fetus ejection reflex. And, with so little disturbance I had really entered that other-worldly state of mind which Michel calls 'going to another planet'.

After everyone had come in and Michel eventually cut the cord, I passed the baby to Phil, climbed over the side of the bath without any assistance and had a shower. Michel just hovered in the background to make sure that I was OK. It was really wonderful feeling so strong and capable. Of course, I also felt that I had given my baby the best possible start in life by giving her an undisturbed, undrugged birth. She was a very contented baby.

As the hours passed after the birth, there was just one worry left in my mind. What on earth could I say to the neighbours about all the noise I'd made? With my one-day-old strapped to my front in a Wilkinet carrier, I ventured out. The neighbour on one side chatted for a few moments before realising with astonishment that the 'bump' on my front was actually now a baby. The neighbours the other side—two single women—were calm and friendly. Apparently, they'd been at a party the night before. So that was the end of that.

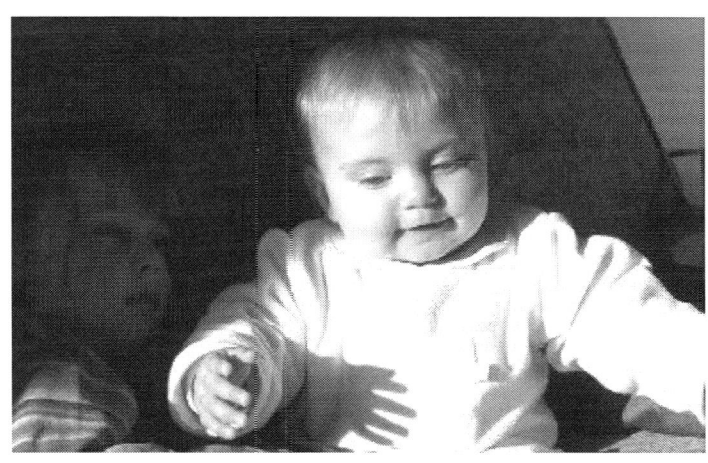

Jumeira at 9 months old (with Nina-Jay on the left!)

Birthframe 3

And here's my third birth story... the abridged version.

> By the time I conceived our third daughter, I was 43 and still working on this book. Would I be able to give birth naturally all over again? Did those natural processes really work reliably when a body and a baby were left undisturbed? We'd moved to the Middle East, to Oman, some time before but we returned to the UK partly because of my pregnancy. I discovered that not only was home birth illegal in Oman, the hospitals were also extremely interventionist. Anyway, my husband managed to get a job in Birmingham, so I had a lucky escape from my dilemma. I was 30 weeks pregnant when we moved into our new rented house.
>
> Some 10 weeks later I knew I was in labour when a powerful contraction woke me at 3 o'clock one morning. I soon went back to bed and to sleep but gentle contractions kept coming here and there throughout the morning. Between-times I managed to get my two little ones to their playgroup and home again. While they were out I pottered round the house.
>
> When they were home again I sat on the floor, listening to a CD, rocking to and fro, while 2-year-old Nina-Jay and 4-year-old Anjula played in front of me in the living room.
>
> Eventually I phoned my husband at work. As soon as he got home I went up to the bathroom alone. After two hours of labour there (spent mostly kneeling forward in the bath) I shouted downstairs to ask Phil to call the midwives. "Are you sure?" "Yes. Call them now."
>
> Five minutes after the midwives arrived I gave birth standing up, completely unassisted. I'd told the NHS midwives (who I'd never met before) to wait outside and locked the bathroom door so I could give birth in peace.
>
> The placenta came out a few minutes after the birth, just after I'd sat down on the toilet to breastfeed.
>
> As usual, I experienced no problems postnatally. I was up and about immediately after the birth and busy with housework and the usual errands the next day. This time I didn't have the 'problem' of being pregnant again— I found my breasts became too sensitive while I was pregnant—so I breastfed Jumeira for over three years. Seven years' breastfeeding experience in total! My body had served its biological purpose...

The natural norm

The last few accounts, describing my own births, are what I like to call 'the natural norm'. In the light of your own experience you may find this very surprising. Think about it though, please....

Isn't this how human beings should be giving birth. (Yes, I realise I'm pushing the definition of the word 'norm' here, but I mean that physiological birth *should* be the norm, even if it isn't at the moment in most, or even many, parts of the world.)

In our efforts to improve birth experiences for mothers and get babies born quickly, we've moved a long, long way from what should be normal. To make matters worse, whenever births are featured in the media, they are made to look *abnormal*.

Media coverage is particularly unbalanced because editors are looking for unusual things to report. I was reminded of this when I contacted a Features Editor of a well-known women's magazine, when I was researching this book. At the time I was looking for a vaginal breech birth story. The editor initially seemed enthusiastic to pass material on to me, but completely changed her tone when I said I was also interested in any births which had involved life-saving intervention. "Ah no," she said. "You wouldn't be able to have any of that. That's precisely the kind of story *we're* interested in." In other words, it was clear that the magazine's objective was not to accurately portray reality, to present a balanced picture of what childbirth is for most women, or to help women consider what it might be. It was to catch people's interest through the sensational.

Perhaps as a result of our constant media exposure, perhaps because of our fear of failure (or litigation!) and our desire to control things which seem *out of control*, the present-day climate in hospitals is one of worry, habitual intervention and insensitivity to a labouring woman's needs. Or is it oversensitivity to labouring women, who appear to be in an unbearable amount of pain, which must be stopped at all costs? In any case, it's not surprising that many women don't experience 'optimal'.

Of those who do, most feel no need to talk—as Michel has pointed out—precisely because they haven't been traumatised in any way. (See his comments on p130.)

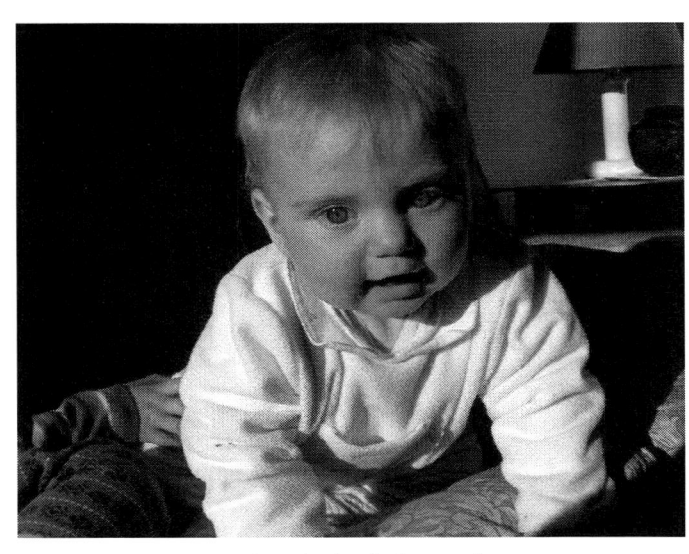

Jumeira having a crawl

When I chanced upon somebody who had given birth naturally, it was usually rather difficult to get an actual account. The women concerned were quite open about their experiences, but they didn't make a 'big deal' of them. This generally meant that if I asked people to write anything down they usually said, "But all I did was... There was nothing special about it." Sometimes my 'potential contributors' did indeed realise there was something special about their experience, but they clearly felt no driving need to talk about it. As a result I had to do quite a bit of hassling to get hold of many of the natural birth stories in this book.

In the end though, after eleven years of perseverance, I managed to obtain contributions from over 200 people. In the version of this book which is for pregnant women (BIRTH: Countdown to Optimal) I feature 100 birthframes and include 180 comments too. I obtained accounts from all kinds of women (and men!), from vastly contrasting walks of life—making it clear that it wasn't just 'hippies' who give birth physiologically!

What was particularly interesting (if not obvious?) was that many of my contributors had a fully physiological birth the *second* time they gave birth. This reminds me of the viewpoint of the !Kung San tribe in Botswana: their ideal is to manage to give birth alone by their third child. Before that they are only 'practising'. Clearly, many women in the developed world do the same. To give you an idea of what I mean, on the right and below are other accounts.

> This time round I was in control the whole time and I knew what was going on, I was more prepared mentally and physically.

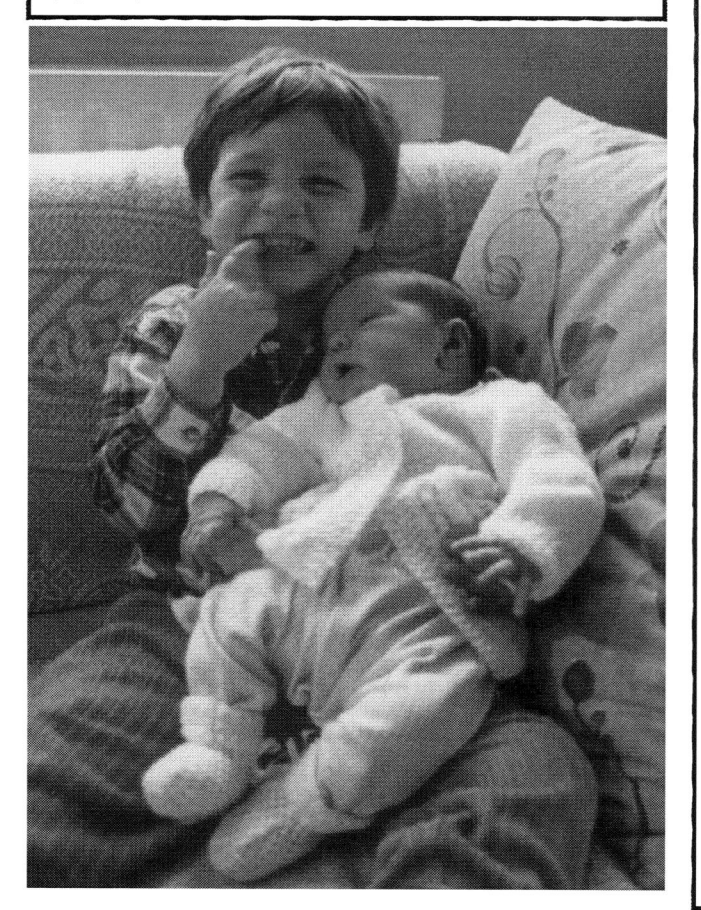

Here is Maria's first son with his physiologically born sister

> After having forceps and a postpartum haemorrhage the first time round, my second birth was totally straightforward with no time for the TENS, birthing pool or gas and air, which I had planned. I stood up for delivery, supported by my partner and pushed the baby out myself, the midwife 'catching' her well. I had no injection [of syntometrine] to speed up the placenta and control the blood loss as it was just not necessary and this third stage was completed in about 20 minutes.

> For my first child I'd planned a water birth but ended up with a four-and-a-half hour labour that was very traumatic. I was rushed into hospital and into a very clinical environment, with bright lights and at least six people standing around me. Jamie was a forceps baby and I ended up having to be stitched. It was almost enough to put me off having any more children. So when I got pregnant again I knew I wanted things to be quite different and I was prepared more. After Arion's birth I felt so empowered that it had gone right the second time.

Birthframe 4

This is the story of a woman full of ideals, who became disillusioned after a bad first initial experience of birth when all kinds of intervention had seemed inappropriate. Would she be able to rediscover her innate, instinctual ability to give birth if left to her own devices?

> I was very frightened about my ability to give birth properly, and questioned all my ideas about home and water birth. I called the Active Birth Centre in London and explained my experiences at the hospital when I had my first baby, Fiohann. I asked if there was anyone I could talk it through with. They gave me a few names, and then suggested Michel Odent. I couldn't believe that I actually had my revered Michel Odent's phone number.
>
> Before I could think about it, I forced myself to phone him. I explained to him what had happened, and although, understandably, he wasn't prepared to comment on the hospital treatment, he did explain that not many midwives had experience of water births, and could panic, thinking the baby would drown. I told him it was a dream of mine that he would deliver our baby, and after hearing when the conception date was, he found that it did fit in with his schedule of international conferences, and that yes he would. I had to pinch myself!
>
> He came around to meet us and I cannot describe what a gentle, intuitive and passionate man he is. He filled me with a quiet confidence and reassurance, and was so different to our doctor, who had originally told me that if I wanted a home birth I would have to find another doctor. Another difference was that he had absolutely no problem with calculating the due date from the conception date: it was a simple nine months later. The community midwife could not cope with anything more than the date of my last period, which I did not know exactly, since I never paid any attention to my cycle. Her date was two weeks before Michel's estimate. The pregnancy went well in that I was fit and healthy, but my partner and I started to have problems and when I was six months pregnant he left home for a month. I felt desperately insecure and cried through most of my pregnancy. Another pregnancy filled with grief, but so different to the first. We went on holiday and decided to try again. ▶

◀ I hired the birthing pool two days before the earliest due date and waited. The midwife got increasingly agitated and by the 21st July was telling me that I would be causing the fetus brain damage because my placenta was past its sell-by date. Michel calmed her by telling her it was due on the 26th, which she could not comprehend. Sure enough, on the 25th, which happily was a Saturday, I went into labour. I called Michel and he promised to be over in a couple of hours.

We filled the pool, put the low music on and had candles ready, and I tried to relax, but found it difficult because of my doubts in myself. Michel arrived and asked me how I was, felt my tummy, and said he would go to sleep in the next room, because I had a few hours to go yet. My partner went to sleep in our bed, and I spent most of the night sitting on the loo having contractions; it felt the most comfortable place to be, looking at the stars through the bathroom roof window, and going back to bed trying to doze before the next one.

Early next morning, things started hotting up and I decided to get into the birthing pool to ease the pains. It did ease them immediately, and as soon as he heard the change in my noises, Michel got up and came in. He can tell where a woman is in her labour by the noises she makes, and just that small change had indicated to him a change in me. I told him I didn't know what to do, asked him what I should be doing, so different from my first birth, and he told me just to listen to my body, just as I had done in the first. I yelled that I didn't know what it was saying, and was very fearful. How different to the first time, with my confidence now in tatters. He calmly created an environment where I would have to listen to myself, by leaving me alone and getting my partner to go and have some breakfast. Our Brazilian au pair was beside herself that I could be moaning and wailing alone with no doctor, and took it into her own hands to go and tell Michel in no uncertain terms to go in to me and induce me! In Brazil, apparently, over 40% of women have caesarean sections because it keeps their passages honeymoon fresh! He handled her sweetly and reassured her.

My body did know what to do after all—I just had to get my doubts out of the way

Things really got going at about 8.30am. I was gnawing on the side of the birthing pool, thinking about the benefits of knives and drugs, half hoping that she wouldn't come out at all, would go back and stay safe inside me.

But that doesn't happen, and finally I got that huge push urge, when all you can do is that colossal push and your whole body is intent on turning itself inside out.

It did know after all what to do, I just had to get my doubts out of the way. Her head came out in the water, just like Fiohann—my son. Michel reached down and checked the umbilical cord was not in the way, and then said that because she was so big, we needed gravity to help us. With her head still between my legs, he lifted my legs, and my partner lifted my torso out of the pool, and I hung from his arms, with Michel ready to catch her.

Two more big pushes and out she slid, our beautiful girl. I flopped to the floor and Michel gave her to me immediately. I held her close and within a few minutes she was nuzzling at my breast ready to suckle, still attached to the umbilical cord.

Right: *Maria with Eowyn and Fiohann*

Michel was delighted at the perfection of it, but said that before she settled into it he would tie off her cord with string rather than the metal clamps because it was more comfortable for the baby. I lay on our bed with our wonderful baby and as she suckled I realised that it would have been no different for Fiohann. If only.

Michel left me to deliver Eowyn's placenta naturally, which came easily shortly afterwards. What I hadn't expected was the sharper pains as my uterus contracted back again, but apparently this is a normal feature of a second childbirth.

I had no tears and was perfectly fit

Michel wrote to our doctor to inform him of the birth and our baby's 'top' scores, knowing that we would be left undisturbed until Monday. Once again, I had no tears and was perfectly fit. The day following Eowyn's birth we had a celebration barbeque, and I walked around Tesco shopping for it, feeling so proud and happy, as if everyone must be able to tell that I had just had a baby! Michel came with his son, and was thrilled to see us so clearly well and happy. It was perfect.

I walked around Tesco shopping, feeling so proud and happy

Our doctor and his doctor wife arrived Monday morning, demanding to know how long she sucked on each breast and making appointments for paediatricians to see her. I had no idea how long on each breast and I declined the paediatrician offer, which they seemed a bit put out about.

Finally they left, leaving the midwives and health visitors to do their checks, etc. and eventually we were left in peace again.

Eowyn is now a very fit and healthy 4-year-old.

Maria Shanahan

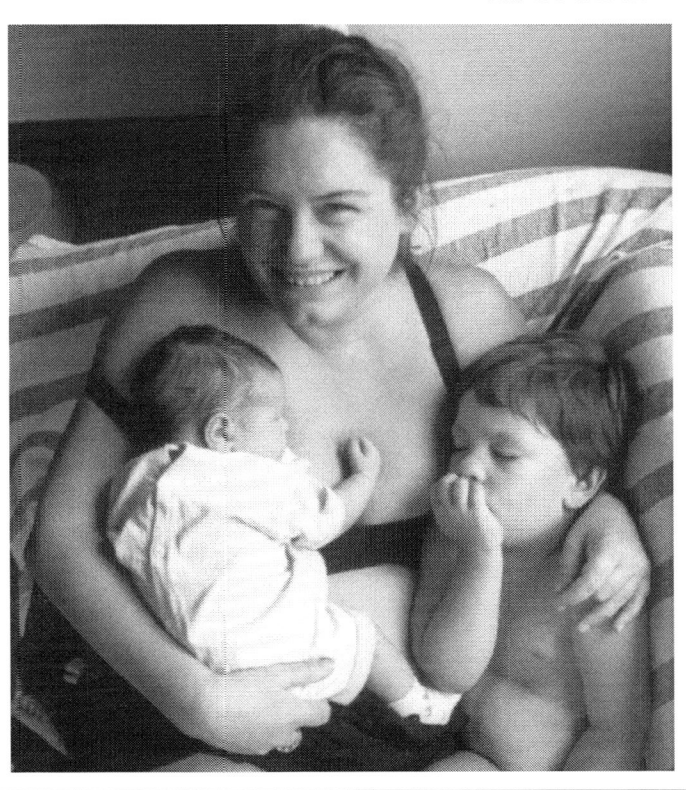

Here's a quick overview of a few more reasons why many women might not experience the 'natural norm':

- Pregnant women may be overly cautious and fearful about childbirth, so request interventions which aren't really needed. (For example, they may ask to have their waters broken if they're overdue.)
- They might feel convinced they can't face the pain of labour, so request pain relief which necessitates other interventions.
- Perhaps they've never met a woman who's had a completely physiological birth and can't imagine it.
- They've met, read about and watched (on television) numerous women who've had interventionist births for various reasons.
- Their care providers may be cautious because of a lack of experience dealing with women who are unmedicated. Mostly, they might fear litigation.
- Pregnant women might be classified as 'high risk' out of over-cautiousness or for the wrong reasons.
- Lack of one-on-one care during labour or birth might mean women are disturbed and lose confidence.
- Pregnant women may not know their midwives well.
- Without good midwifery support, pregnant women are likely to lack confidence in their ability to give birth.

This is Beth Dubois, a mother who experienced a physiological birth for the birth of her first child, despite a history of sexual abuse—and all the psychological baggage that usually entails. Through careful preparation and support from her midwives, she managed to give birth naturally and also breastfeed. Her detailed account is included in BIRTH: Countdown to Optimal, the companion volume to this book, which is for pregnant women.

Birthframe 5

Rachel, a first-time mother, was amazed to find her labour and birth really did happen as Michel had predicted...

I gave birth at home, at age 38, in water without using any drugs. My [identical] twin sister had had a baby the previous year, with the usual story of failed home delivery due to minor complications followed by the cascade of interventions at hospital ending in a caesarean.

I read Michel Odent's *Birth Reborn* and was inspired at the stories of natural birth—the fact that he finally avoided the use of chemical pain relief altogether because it seemed to interfere with the natural pain-relieving processes of the body.

I searched widely for a sympathetic midwife and was so lucky to eventually find one, who visited me at home and helped my confidence. I think state of mind is so important—I also did some hypnosis, or visualisation of the birthing process, which I think helped.

My baby was born after a 9-hour labour. To my amazement, it was like Michel described—I became almost like an animal, or went into another level of consciousness beyond pain. The part I remember as the most difficult was the beginning—moments of fear—then gaining confidence—more moments of fear—reassure-ance once from the midwife—then feeling like a fish in water being thrown about by the contractions and finally roaring as she came out, not with pain (as is so often the stereotype we see of labouring women) but with power.

It left me feeling so proud of my body.

Rachel Urbach

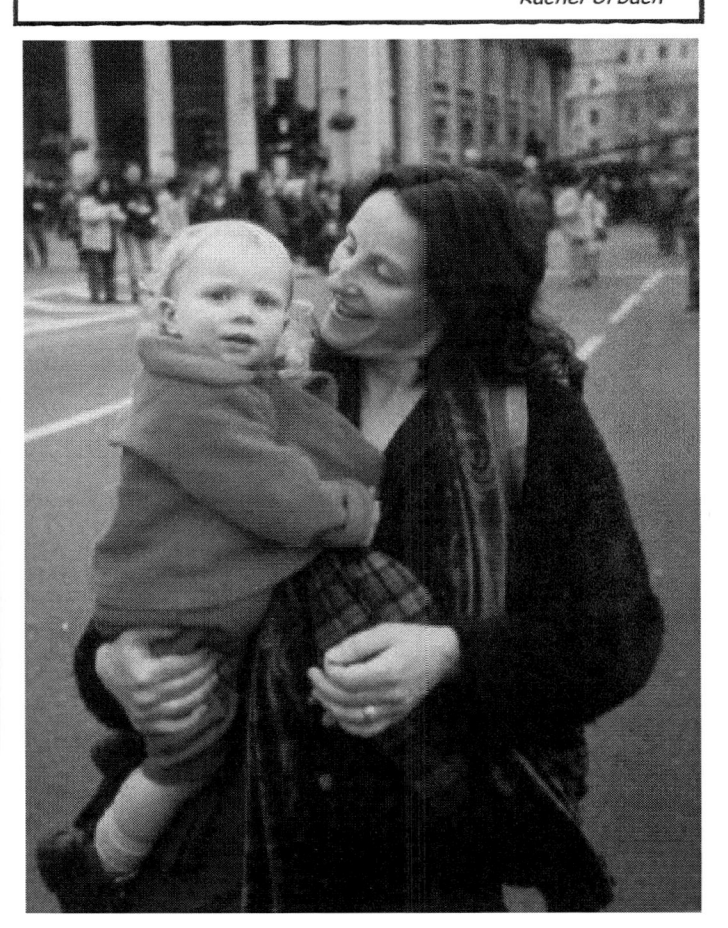

Rachel with her baby, several months after the birth

Life-saving intervention

Birthframe 6

Sometimes, of course, medical intervention is necessary to ensure optimal outcomes. In the next account we see how it made it possible for a couple to have another child against the odds. This is a clear case of medical support being life-saving for both mother and child.

Having had one fairly straightforward birth, it came as a shock when I realised things can go wrong in pregnancy. My second pregnancy was ectopic so at nine weeks I had an emergency operation. Luckily, I did not lose the fallopian tubes but they did end up damaged.

So, in order to have any future children the only option was to go through a lengthy, costly IVF programme. We were extremely lucky to be successful on the first attempt, where I became pregnant with twins. However, fairly early on I developed hyper-stimulation (painful swelling) and one of the twins died by the 10-week scan. (You have a lot of early scans with IVF to detect ectopic pregnancies and check that everything is developing normally.) As I had lost one of the babies I was told to expect some minor bleeding. They also mentioned that bleeding can be a response to all the vaginal scans... So when I had some small bleeds before the 13-week scan I was not surprised, but a little worried. At the 13-week scan I was told I had placenta praevia, which was fairly low down, but was told that for most women by the mid-term scan and certainly by 28 weeks, the placenta moves sideways and away from the cervix, along with the growth of the baby. I continued to get small bleeds and was up and down to the hospital like a yoyo. At the mid-term scan (20 weeks) I was told that I had major placenta praevia, being classed as Grade 4+ (1 being minor and 4+ being serious). This meant that the placenta would not be able to move away from the cervix as it was completely covering the os, and in some places was adhered to the cervix. I was told I would not be able to give birth naturally and would have to have a caesarean.

At 25 weeks I started to have a fairly heavy bleed and was admitted for the duration of my pregnancy. Luckily, I stopped bleeding but had to keep a cannula in just in case I started to haemorrhage. I was allowed home occasionally as long as someone was with me 24 hours a day and I was within 10 minutes of the hospital. This is because I would have to be on the operating table within 20 minutes if I started to haemorrhage, as the worst-case scenario is death of both mother and child. At my 28-week scan the earlier diagnosis was confirmed—there was no way I was getting away with a natural birth.

At the 13-week scan I was told I had placenta praevia, but was told the placenta usually moves sideways, away from the cervix by 28 weeks

I started to have contractions at 32 weeks, which caused problems as I was not allowed to go into labour. (This is because the cervix dilates in labour and this would mean the placenta would rip, causing a major haemorrhage.) After being monitored on the labour ward to see the strength and frequency of contractions I had an emergency caesarean under general anaesthetic. [As you no doubt realise, it was necessary to have a general anaesthetic in this case for the sake of speed. An epidural takes much longer to set up and sometimes doesn't become effective the first time it is administered—which then means needing to try again.]

I'd have to be on the operating table within 20 minutes if I started to bleed

I was extremely poorly after the caesarean because I did end up having a haemorrhage, as well as some sort of reaction to the anaesthetic. My daughter spent a short time on the special baby ward before being whisked into the Neonatal Unit as she was having breathing difficulties. Mother and baby are now both fine—and the 'baby' is now three years old!

In general, I would definitely be on the pro 'natural birth' side of things, wherever possible. My pregnancy was clinical and from the outset not only was it a traumatic experience, I was unable to hold my baby for nearly two weeks after she was born. I was not aware I had had a baby until four hours after the birth.

Caesareans as a birth option are ridiculous. Mothers 'opting' to have an elective caesarean when it is not a necessity are totally nuts! I did not recover properly until four months after the birth. It is major abdominal surgery.

Birthframe 7

In this case, the problem was ongoing nausea and vomiting in pregnancy.

You've probably heard of the drug 'thalidomide', which eventually became known as a teratogen (i.e. harmful to the growing baby). It was originally prescribed to pregnant women in the late 1950s to treat morning sickness, but it eventually became clear that it caused gross deformities when taken within a certain period during the first trimester.

Health care professionals are now more careful about any interventions or prescriptions during the first trimester because the after-effects in pregnancy or during birth are still unknown in most cases, or unconfirmed. However, experimental intervention does sometimes seem necessary or desirable in certain cases, such as the one described in this case...

It was December 2001 and I was delighted to find out that I was expecting our second child, if a little apprehensive following a miscarriage earlier in the year. With our first child I had started feeling sick at about Week 8. This sickness had then rapidly intensified until I was vomiting up to six times a day.

A sympathetic doctor diagnosed hyperemesis and allowed me time off from my full-time teaching job. After three months of this sickness level and some anti-emetic drugs, I gradually felt better and the pregnancy continued uneventfully until the birth of our healthy first son in the May of 1999.

▶

The memories of this were still fresh two and a half years later when we decided to try for our second child. I had not really researched the condition of hyperemesis and naively believed the many comments I had heard about every pregnancy being different and the unlikely event of this level of sickness returning.

In the fifth week of this pregnancy I was understandably anxious when I started to bleed again. After two scans, however, the hospital were able to reassure me as far as they could and told me to come back in Week 8 for a further scan to see if they could detect a heartbeat.

> The vomiting started on the Sunday and by the Monday—which was Christmas Eve—I could hardly get off the sofa... How would I get through the celebrations of Christmas Day?

Then, on the Saturday commencing my sixth week of pregnancy I woke up feeling weak, battered and extremely sick. The vomiting started on the Sunday, and by the Monday—which was Christmas Eve—I could hardly get off the sofa and was wondering how I was going to manage to get through the celebrations of Christmas Day. At first I felt cross with myself and kept repeating that it was only morning sickness, even if it did last all day. But by the following week I was having difficulty keeping even sips of water down and my New Year's Eve was spent lying dehydrated on the sofa until my partner arrived home smelling of wine, which immediately sent me rushing for the toilet again. I could not tolerate the smell of anything and started to sleep on my own. Even the smell of the sheets on my bed would make me retch uncontrollably.

> I was having difficulty keeping even sips of water down and my New Year's Eve was spent lying dehydrated on the sofa

Two days later and despite having a hospital appointment for a scan the following day I felt I could not wait and went to see the doctor. By this stage my partner had to practically carry me in and out of the car. The doctor asked me to give her a urine sample but, as I explained, I couldn't because I had not really had anything properly to drink for days. She took some blood and explained that although it was unlikely, if the results were abnormal, she would contact me the following day. She did contact me the following day and left a message on the answering machine. I never heard it as I had already been admitted to hospital.

My hospital appointment on the next day appeared to go well. I had been having some bleeding and I was reassured to see a healthy heartbeat. After the scan, my partner and I were unclear about whether we should wait again to see a doctor or go straight home. I wanted to go home because of the terrible way that I was feeling, but we waited anyway to have the results of the scan confirmed by a doctor. I was sick again while we were waiting and heard a nurse say, "What's the matter with her?" "Oh, just morning sickness", came the reply.

> I had not known about ketones or that it was possible to be hospitalised for hyperemesis

The doctor confirmed the pleasing results of the scan but said that it was obvious that I was suffering. She explained that high levels of ketones had been found in my urine, that I would need to come into the hospital to have some anti-emetic drugs and a drip, and that I would feel a lot better after about 24 hours. I had not known about the existence of ketones, or that it was possible to be hospitalised for hyperemesis. I also felt frightened as, apart from the birth of my son, I had been lucky enough not to be hospitalised before. Little did I know then this was to be the first of seven hospitalisations and the beginning of six really difficult months for our small family.

The attitudes of the nurses in hospital varied. Some were sympathetic, others appeared to think that you were wasting a valuable bed—despite repeated vomiting and fainting every morning when I was forced to get up to allow the bed to be changed. (I later found out that low blood pressure is one of the symptoms of this condition.) There were other difficult aspects to being in hospital with this condition—for example, sometimes I was placed in wards with women suffering from miscarriages, and I was forced to smell the food at mealtimes.

There were other side effects of the illness that I did not know, or that nobody explained to me. As I previously mentioned, my blood pressure was very low and I passed out daily, which was both unpleasant and frightening. After a few months of the sickness, apart from the weight loss, my skin started to look yellow, I was constantly cold and shivering, my hair started to fall out and I started to vomit small amounts of bile and blood. The latter, I was reassured, was normal and simply caused by small tears in the stomach. It was intensely painful and started to create a fear of being sick any more. I was constantly cajoled in hospital to drink more if I wanted to get better, when every sip made my sore stomach retch. I found the cajoling patronising and felt that it showed a lack of understanding, with the implication that I was not helping myself. I was also given a variety of anti-emetic drugs which did not work for me, and this was echoed by other women that I talked to with this condition. The pattern followed that after being on a drip for two or three days, the ketones would be gone, I would be sent home feeling only marginally better (because of not being dehydrated any more) and within 24 hours I would be back in the same state again. After two or three hospital visits, I was given some ketone sticks with which I could measure the levels of ketones myself at home. For the first four months of the pregnancy I had constant ketones and would only go back to the hospital when I really felt that I could not stand it at home any longer.

I found other women really supportive

Being in hospital did provide the invaluable opportunity to chat with other women suffering from this condition, and we talked about how even the smell of our children and partners would make us retch. I also discovered some Internet sites where other women who had similarly suffered had written their stories and I found this really supportive in the times when I thought I must be going mad.

My son, who was two and a half at the time, appeared to take it all in his stride—that his mummy had simply stopped looking after him and spent the whole time sleeping and being sick. My partner and I had a bedroom in the attic and when he left for work I would be too weak to get out of bed and climb down the ladder, so I simply stayed in bed the whole day, vomiting and retching into a bucket. He would arrive home and I would attempt to get up, but even this effort would send me into more retching and vomiting fits. Without his unceasing sympathetic support I would not have got through this pregnancy.

> I would be too weak to get out of bed and climb down the ladder, so I simply stayed in bed the whole day

We moved house when I was twelve weeks' pregnant as the sale had already gone so far along. Three days later, I was back in hospital again, dehydrated. My partner had a wonderful boss who was supportive whenever he took time off to take me to hospital or to take care of our small son on the days when the nursery had no space. Before the pregnancy, I had been studying and working part-time as a supply teacher. I suspended the study at 20 weeks and, of course, received no pay for the supply teaching as I was only casually employed. That was the financial effect of the hyperemesis.

At about four months, in desperation I started to research the condition and I found one particular study linking the use of antibiotics to curing hyperemesis, so I went to persuade my doctor to give this a try. This was my own doctor, who I had not seen since the start of the pregnancy. She was shocked at my condition and despite having no ketones in my urine, she sent me in an ambulance straight to the hospital. There, after breaking down in tears, they readmitted me and I persuaded a sympathetic doctor to try out the antibiotic theory. He did, but it didn't work and the pain of taking the antibiotics was difficult with such a sore stomach. He suggested, however, that there was one last solution: a high dose of steroids with about a 1 in 5 chance that they would affect the adrenal glands of the baby. I was desperate so immediately agreed to take them.

After about three days, the effect was remarkable. The constant nausea and retching had gone and I was finally able to slowly start living a more normal life again. The high dosage made me agitated and unable to sit still, but this seemed a small price to pay. I was ecstatic and could not stop moving about and eating, after months of enforced starvation.

A follow-up appointment a week later with the obstetrician led to the immediate question as to who had given me these and why. The obstetrician explained that I had to come off them as soon as possible, which has to be done gradually with steroids. This took about five weeks and as the dose started to diminish I could feel the nauseous sensation starting to return and then gradually I started to actually be sick again. After coming off them completely, I ended up in hospital again, but this time for the last time. After about 25 weeks, the sickness was no longer so severe that I needed to be hospitalised, but it did continue 5–6 times daily until the last 6 weeks, when it was just once or twice a day.

The controversy of the steroid treatment led to a close monitoring of the rest of the pregnancy, with numerous growth scans and blood tests, etc. The heart of this controversy appeared to be that this was not a conventional treatment for this condition and I was informed that there was a 1 in 5 chance of the baby's adrenal glands being affected. I did feel that the steroids relieved the symptoms of hyperemesis, but also that the hyperemesis probably reduced in severity on its own by about seven months.

> A follow-up appointment a week later with the obstetrician led to the immediate question as to who had given them to me and why

At almost two weeks' overdue and following an induced birth, I had our second whopping 9lb 8oz son. He is 11 weeks old now and completely gorgeous. When I hold him, I cannot believe how placid and gentle he is, and how lucky I am to have him.

Tina C from the UK

Birthframe 8

Here, we have a clear case of obstetric knowledge being used to ensure an optimal result. Although the woman giving birth used a TENS machine for pain relief, she did manage to avoid all other drugs and interventions while she was in labour. Clearly, both she and her care providers realised the advantages—from the babies' point of view—of minimising interference in the natural, physiological processes.

I found out I was expecting twins when I was only 10 weeks pregnant and was immediately put under the excellent care of Lawrence Impey and his team at the Feto-Maternal Medicine Unit at the John Radcliffe Hospital in Oxford.

Due to the twins being identical—sharing a placenta and monochorionic—I was informed straightaway of the complications that could occur, particularly of the risk of twin-to-twin transfusion syndrome. I was told I would be monitored closely and have regular scans.

Throughout my pregnancy I was healthy and reasonably comfortable until at 32 weeks I developed obstetric cholestasis.

I was given medication to control this [ursodeoxycholic acid] and my pregnancy continued as normal.

At 36 weeks I went into labour and I gave birth to healthy twin boys, weighing 4lb 6oz and 4lb 8oz, with no caesarean, no epidural and only the use of a TENS machine for pain relief.

I was very lucky to receive such outstanding care at the John Radcliffe Hospital. I believe that it was the positive attitude of the medical staff towards vaginal twin births and natural pain relief that enabled me to have such a wonderful natural birth experience.

Jo Siebert

Birthframe 9

Here's an account where medical support became necessary even when the mother and all those around her were hoping for a completely physiological birth. Perhaps it's never possible to know the real reasons for undesired events in our lives. I find it interesting that there is a clue in the following account for what follows even in the first line—in the phrase 'all being well'—the feelings of the mother's *mother* are intriguing...

My daughter had planned, all being well, to give birth at home.

The very strange thing was that months in advance I couldn't see it happening. I never said a word to anyone, but on a few occasions when it was quiet, I sat down and wondered... Why? What could happen? Was my daughter to change her mind? Would something go very wrong? Impossible to tell, I just could not see her home birth a reality. But don't think I was full of fear or negative thoughts, it was more like a fact, a reality that I could not comprehend.

Three weeks before her due date she went into labour. Michel Odent came at 10pm and we all went to rest. At 2am Marisa woke me up, she was fine, she wanted to be by herself, but thought Michel had better know she was still having contractions.

Michel, after listening to the baby, asked if he could do an internal. Marisa had no problems with that. I wondered why, but I didn't ask questions. No words, but Michel looked different, a bit tense. Marisa decided to go back to her room, where her boyfriend was asleep.

At 5am I saw Michel was nervous. I questioned him and his reply was: "Footling breech. I can't wait any longer." I had no time to think, he was pushing us into a taxi. Marisa said she was having contractions every 20 minutes. She looked lovely. What to do?

Michel could not take it any more. You probably know, Sylvie, that for footling breech the policy is elective caesarean. For a breech birth Michel will only accept a home birth if it is quick, between 4 and 5 hours. They can be very quick. Some of these babies are born on the way to hospital. The worst thing to do is touch them when you see the lower part of the body appearing—any stimulation can get them 'stuck', so there are many deaths or brain damaged babies. I suppose you know all this. But quick undisturbed, undiagnosed breech births can go very well.

So I talked to Marisa and she said, "That's fine. Let's go". Baby Ryo was born two hours later by caesarean. To me it was a shock. First time in my family.

Marisa, with her 18 years, took it quite well. She is fine, the baby is adorable, and she had plenty of milk from Day 1. They all sleep together. Even in hospital after a c-section, they were happy for mum and baby to be together all the time.

We will never know what could have happened if we had stayed at home. One of the risks is cord prolapse. With their feet they kick so much that if the membranes rupture, cord prolapse can follow (although not necessarily, of course).

Sometimes, it is a problem to know all this.

Liliana Lammers

The worst thing to do is touch them when you see the body appearing...

Grey areas

In some cases it's not easy for professionals to decide on the best course of action. Different midwives have different approaches and obstetricians may disagree with them. The pregnant woman may also have her own opinion, deduced not from years of training and experience, but from an evening spent researching the Internet. Other women may be better informed, having researched their own situation and medical condition thoroughly over a course of weeks and months, their concentration having been made sharper by their very personal need to 'get things right'. What can be done?

Many professionals are loathe to challenge the protocols within their institution. Others stick their necks out... but why? What could their motivation be? Why do some midwives go so far as to endanger their jobs, their bank balances and even their freedom (in the case of American midwives who go to prison for the sake of their principles)? Why do some midwives support women who seem to be making outrageous requests, which quite frankly come across as demands?

The answer is twofold. Firstly, research is on their side. Isn't it odd that so many protocols fly in the face of research, especially given the NICE guidelines? For example, the protocols in some units stipulate that women need to have EFM for 20 minutes on admission, despite the well-known fact that EFM has not been associated with any improvement in outcomes; the only confirmed outcome of EFM is an increase in the caesarean rate, which is not seen as being a good thing. Secondly, women have the right to make decisions about their own care and the care of their babies. Their only problem is to find professionals (especially midwives) who will agree to support them. After all, most women who make seemingly bold choices as regards their care do so after extensive research and do not want to give birth unassisted. They *want* the support and expertise of midwives who will act in their interests with love and sensitivity.

Birthframe 10

I am a 40-year-old woman who gave birth to twins naturally five months ago in an NHS hospital. It is possible!

I did it with a lot of persistence and research, after several meetings with various midwives, consultants, head and consultant midwives and by finding independent midwives and a consultant who supported me in trying for natural deliveries for our babies. With some luck, a very supportive partner and midwives, and a consultant who went beyond the call of duty by being available for me in the labour ward (though by my request, not in the delivery room) when he was not normally on call, I gave birth to the first twin in a birth pool, and the second on land, without any drugs or intervention at 39 weeks and 2 days. Both babies were well and weighed in at just over and under 6lb. I would like to encourage other expectant twin mums or those with a high risk pregnancy to inform themselves of what the risks associated with their pregnancy are, what the birth options are with their various pros and cons and to persist in trying to lay the conditions and plans for a natural delivery if that is what they want. Giving birth to our babies is one of the most satisfying, joyous and proud experiences I have had.

As we've already seen earlier in this book, in many cases women who are categorised as high risk for some reason or other still manage to avoid intervention, while still ensuring that the care they receive helps to ensure safe outcomes.

Birthframe 11

I first read about Debbie Brindley, a midwife working within the NHS, in *The Complete Book of Pregnancy* (NCT Publishing 2000). Thanks to careful preparation, she managed to arrange a very natural water birth for the birth of her twins. (For her first baby, she'd had a water birth at home.) When I wrote to her to ask her a few questions, I discovered that even during her pregnancy, Debbie really did care about the care she received…

What's your view on the use of ultrasound in pregnancy?

Our unit policy is for regular serial scans. However, it only appears to be safe, doesn't it? Research is not conclusive so I feel it should be used as with all medical intervention and technology—when it's needed and not routinely. Following this philosophy, I chose to have two scans: an anomaly scan at 20 weeks and one further scan at 34 weeks to check presentation (they were both cephalic)—so I could then plan how to manage my labour. Growth was diagnosed clinically on palpation.

But, presumably, the midwives who looked after you while you were pregnant used a Sonicaid to check the fetal heartbeats at each appointment?

Carole, my community midwife, did all my antenatal care (at home—I'm so lucky) and she agreed to listen to the fetal hearts with a Pinard instead of a Sonicaid [which uses ultrasound]. They always had good movements so we were both happy with this.

And how were the fetal heartbeats checked while you were in labour?

I was happy to have the heart rates checked with the Sonicaid, as the Pinard's awkward in labour because the labouring woman may have to lie down for it to be used effectively. I had a 10-minute CTG [cardiotocograph], i.e. electronic fetal monitoring, which the student midwife held on, while the pool was running. Beforehand I had agreed to a short CTG of the second twin when the first had been born but in the event, it turned out there was no time!

I discussed my birth plan with my consultant, who then signed it

Did you make any special requests of your birth attendants for your labour. I mean, did you want them to behave in any particular way?

I wanted as much privacy as I would have had if I'd been at home and I didn't want people 'popping in' or coming for a look. (Not that any of my colleagues would dare!) I believe in needing a quiet, relaxing environment so as to raise endorphins and lower adrenalin. I agreed to Carole's student witnessing, though, as Carole had been so kind to me. Otherwise, I wanted midwives only. I wrote a detailed birth plan and then made an appointment with my extremely supportive consultant to discuss it. (I met him twice in all, once early on in my pregnancy and then at 34 weeks in order to discuss my birth plan.) He agreed with most of it, we discussed one or two points regarding monitoring and physiological third stage and then he signed it. In the birth plan, I requested privacy and he and the paediatric consultant kindly agreed to wait outside in the corridor during the birth. My consultant was there in case I needed any help—even though he wasn't officially on duty. He's a very special man.

They agreed to wait in the corridor

I definitely didn't want to deliver my twins in a large, clinical delivery room

What was the room like where you gave birth in hospital? Did you make any requests about this in advance?

It is common to deliver twins in a 'theatre' delivery room—large and clinical, usually with an IV [intravenous drip], epidural and in the lithotomy position [lying on your back]. I definitely didn't want this, so asked to use the small standard delivery room connected to the pool room. The room was reasonably but not fantastically homely, but at 9cm dilated on admission I didn't care. It was night, so it was dark and warm and it was down the quiet end of the corridor.

Under what circumstances would you have accepted intervention?

I trusted my midwife implicitly and if she had voiced any concerns I would have accepted any interventions necessary. I strongly believe in the importance of a positive birth experience but my babies' welfare was always more important. I wouldn't have accepted any interventions unless I had thought they were for the direct benefit of my twins. I wouldn't have accepted a routine intervention.

I trusted my midwife implicitly

Presumably, you had syntometrine for the third stage—this is pretty much routine, isn't it?

No, I didn't have syntometrine for my third stage. I'd had a physiological third stage with my first baby and had wanted to keep this labour natural too. I discussed this with my midwife and we agreed to have something ready in case I needed it, in which case I would have happily accepted it. Actually, this was syntocinon, rather than syntometrine because it has less side effects because it includes no ergometrine. Syntometrine is a combination of ergometrine (which is rapid-acting) and syntocinon—i.e. oxytocin (which has sustained action). Ergometrine's side effects can be raised blood pressure and vomiting, dizziness, headaches… so syntocinon (oxytocin) alone can help avoid these.

The placenta was expelled within a few minutes and blood loss was minimal

Anyway, I felt if I had strong labour contractions then the chances are that my uterus would effectively expel the placenta. And I had no complications. The placenta was expelled within a few minutes and blood loss was minimal. Of course, having a physiological stage means that the cord can be cut later and I think the transition to extra-uterine life is more gentle with delayed cord-cutting. Cutting the cord later, babies receive their intended extra bonus of blood.

Caesareans: optimal or not? The facts...

Despite the fashion for elective caesareans in some places, amongst certain groups of people, the caesarean certainly doesn't seem to be an optimal choice in cases where it is not medically indicated. In fact, in the light of research it's quite absurd to suggest that the modern caesarean operation represents an ideal. Instead, it is simply an extremely effective and now mostly safe rescue operation for cases where things would otherwise go wrong.

Most midwives would not disagree, but since a few obstetricians still view the caesarean overly positively in cases where a woman could otherwise give birth vaginally, it is worth considering what's 'wrong' with it. The main problem is that it represents a great departure from the natural processes and is less pleasant, less safe and less healthy for both mother and baby, unless of course the operation really is lifesaving. It's possible that being born by caesarean has long-term effects on the psychological development of the baby firstly because of the enormously different hormonal environment present when a woman has this kind of major abdominal surgery, secondly because of the experience itself and thirdly because of the disruption to the normal bonding processes after the operation. The absence of oxytocin (dubbed by a researcher, Niles Newton, 'the hormone of love') is the key concern here and may interfere with the baby's development of the ability to love. Michel Odent has discussed this at length in his book *The Scientification of Love* (Free Association Books 1999). Of course, efforts can be made to counteract this potential problem but the point is that a caesarean birth is not ideal for the baby, unless of course it saves his or her life, or that of his or her mother. It is also not ideal for a mother in terms of minimising damage to her sexual anatomy firstly because damage to the pelvic floor (which includes the muscles around a woman's vagina) usually occurs during pregnancy (particularly when the woman is overweight) and secondly because of the enormously important psychological aspect of arousal, response and orgasm, which may be affected by artificial birth experiences.

Research was actually summarised in 1998 in the *British Medical Journal*. According to this summary, women who have a caesarean (rather than a vaginal birth) open themselves up to all kinds of dangers. In the short term, they have a far greater risk of haemorrhage, infection, ileus, pulmonary embolism and Mendelson's syndrome. Long term health problems faced by caesarean mothers apparently include the formation of adhesions, intestinal obstruction, and bladder injury. Uterine rupture is also a possibility in a subsequent pregnancy, especially if labour is induced or augmented. Research also shows that women who've had caesareans are more likely to have fertility problems, an ectopic pregnancy or a placenta praevia later on. It's also more likely that there will be a need for a hysterectomy, which would also have an obvious impact on fertility. There is even evidence that the health of caesarean mothers' future children may be affected by having an older caesarean-born sibling. Psychological problems, such as postnatal depression, are also more likely for caesarean mothers, especially if the operation was carried out under general anaesthetic, and these psychological problems are likely to affect the mother's ability to bond effectively with her baby (or babies).

Research has also shown a significantly higher death rate for caesarean mothers, but it's impossible to determine how high the risk is. This is partly because it would never be possible to carry out a randomised control trial and partly because the level of risk would depend on the reason for the caesarean and the woman's general level of health. Some writers and researchers claim that a woman having a caesarean is twice as likely to die as a woman giving birth vaginally, and some even say she is 16 times more likely to die. The imprecision of these estimates is obvious if you consider any other risk in life—such as the risk of crossing the road, which is affected by numerous personal and situational factors. The estimates are also absurd in a sense because without the operation any one woman might have died anyway, or her baby might have. For a complete up-to-date review of research relating to the effects of caesareans, see *Pushed* (Da Capo 2007). In conclusion, we can see that in cases where either mother or baby is in serious danger it is obviously best for this life-saving intervention to take place because it is currently the only means we have of dealing with certain obstetric emergencies, so it is indeed 'optimal' in these cases. The risk of the operation then becomes less than the risk of the alternative (i.e. potential death of either the mother or baby). So the small minority of women who really do need to have this operation are best advised to focus on the life-saving properties of the modern c-section than on any negative aspects and to be thankful that they can be helped in a difficult situation. If, on the other hand, any particular woman is likely to be capable of a vaginal birth, my research has certainly led me to conclude it is better for her to take this route.

In other words, the caesarean is a real rescue operation in high risk cases but for low-risk women capable of having a safe vaginal birth (even a VBAC) the evidence shows that it's far from ideal. This is not really surprising, when we think that it constitutes major surgery and a lengthy disruption to the normal mother and baby bonding processes.

THE OPERATION ITSELF

We have already considered vaginal births in great detail, describing their less pleasant aspects as well as the exhilarating moments. Therefore, the equivalent level of detail is provided overleaf for a caesarean birth. This will hopefully give you more of an insight into what women are letting themselves in for when they commit themselves to a date for an elective caesarean, particularly in cases where they could just as easily opt for a vaginal birth. And of course, you may want to share these details with some pregnant women, if you feel this is appropriate in any particular cases.

For the following account, I am indebted to *The Caesarean* (Free Assoc Books 2004), *Obstetrics by Ten Teachers* (Hodder Arnold 2000), *Myles Textbook for Midwives* (Churchill Livingstone 2000) and *Abdominal surgical incisions for caesarean section* (Mathai M, Hofmeyr GJ. Abdominal surgical incisions for caesarean section. *Cochrane Database of Systematic Reviews* 2007, Issue 1. Art. No.: CD004453. DOI:10.1002/14651858. CD004453. pub2). Some details are vague because of the variation in protocols in different hospitals or different countries.

BEFORE THE OPERATION...

- The pregnant woman (or her partner) is required to sign a consent form.
- In some countries outside the UK, in the case of an elective caesarean, the evening before the operation some glycerine suppositories may be given. These will help the woman clear her rectum. The woman's pubic prep is also carried out.
- An antacid may be given so as to prevent the contents of the woman's stomach from becoming acidic.
- Drugs to prevent thrombosis are sometimes given as well as antibiotics, in case infection develops. An intravenous drip (an IV) is inserted for the further administration of drugs.
- In many countries a catheter is installed so that urine can be continually drained from the bladder.
- A blood pressure cuff is placed around the woman's arm.
- Jewellery, nail varnish and make-up are removed, so that small changes in colouring can be observed. Contact lenses are also removed. Teeth are checked so that no loose ones are inadvertently swallowed during the operation!
- The woman is asked to change into a clean operation gown.
- The woman is asked to lie down on her left side and a wedge is placed under her right buttock.
- She is then asked to curl up into the fetal position if an epidural is to be inserted or topped up, or a general anaesthetic is injected via the IV. (In the case of an epidural, she may also be allowed to sit up while this is inserted.)

DURING THE OPERATION...

- The surgeon wears a double layer of plastic gloves and a clear plastic shield around his or her face. This is to protect him or her from exposure to the pregnant woman's bodily fluids.
- The woman is turned onto her back so that her abdomen can be easily accessed. At the same time, the operating table is tilted slightly so that the woman's head is lower than her feet. This is to help establish a level of anaesthesia which will be high enough to make the woman's abdomen numb, but not so high that it will affect her ability to breathe.
- A nurse then paints the skin on the woman's abdomen with an antiseptic solution. Someone on the surgical team will then cover the abdomen with drapes and sterile plastic—leaving exposed only the area which is to be cut. The drapes are put over a bar above the woman's chest so that she cannot see the operation itself... er, except in the reflection of the light above in some cases!
- In one clear motion, the obstetrician then makes a horizontal, crescent-shaped incision, just above the usual site of the pubic hair. In the standard technique, the incision is made deep into the skin, so as to cut through all the superficial layers. In a more recently proposed technique (developed by Michael Stark in the 1990s), which Michel considers to be optimal, the scalpel only sinks one inch into the layer of fat and the so-called lateral tissue underneath is torn apart using two fingers. (Techniques involving tearing, rather than cutting, are generally recommended, where possible.)
- Continuing to use fingers and a thumb, or using a scalpel and tiny forceps (which are like tweezers), or even electrocautery (if the 'Pelosi' technique is used), the obstetrician then tears or cuts deeper into the subcutaneous tissue. He or she then reaches a thick layer of fibrous tissue, called the fascia. After that the mucous membrane called the peritoneum, which is the last layer of the abdominal wall, is opened. This is done either by cutting or tearing in order to gain access to the abdominal cavity—which, of course, contains the uterus.
- After the bladder is pushed away, another peritoneum (which loosely lies over the 'low segment' of the uterus) is cut. The so-called 'low segment' of the uterus is then also cut open using short, careful strokes of a knife.
- The small original cut is then extended to a length of at least 15cm with the use of fingers or blunt-ended scissors.
- If the membranes around the baby are still intact—they may have burst open by this time—they are punctured and opened.
- The obstetrician then places one hand inside the uterus, under the baby's head and exerts pressure on the upper end of the uterus with the other hand so as to push the baby through the incision. (An assistant usually helps with this.)
- In some places, the baby's mouth is immediately suctioned with a small ear syringe and then the shoulders and the rest of the baby are eased out.
- Held up in the air, the baby usually begins to cry. When this happens the new baby is frequently held over the mother (if she is conscious) so that she can see the baby's genitals! The assumption is that her first priority will be to know whether she's got a boy or a girl.
- The cord is clamped and the baby handed over to a nurse holding a warmed towel. Mothers and babies may also have some skin-to-skin contact at this stage because modern caesareans rarely require general anaesthesia.
- There have been reports of some women complaining of pain during the next few stages of the operation, or of having difficulty breathing, although both are probably rare occurrences nowadays. Some women also vomit while their organs are being handled and the damage repaired. If any of these occur in the next stages of the operation, the woman will be immediately sedated.
- The placenta is then pulled out and passed to an attendant, who gives it a thorough check. He or she might be soaked in blood and amniotic fluid by this stage.
- Next, the uterus is sutured (sewn together), either while still inside the abdomen (as advised by *Obstetrics for Ten Teachers*) or after being taken out to rest on the outside of the abdomen.
- The loose peritoneum covering the uterus is sutured closed, or left open for spontaneous healing if the obstetrician considers this to be preferable. Then the fascia (the thick fibrous layer) is brought together with heavy thread stitches because it is this layer which holds all the abdominal organs inside and keeps them from coming through the incision. The subcutaneous tissue (which is mostly fat) is sometimes also closed using loose stitches. The skin, the final layer, is sewn up with silk or synthetic thread, or joined with metal staples.
- A dry dressing is placed over the woman's incision and taped to her skin.
- Finally, the drapes are removed.

46   Optimal Birth: The What, The Why & The How

AFTER THE OPERATION...

- Both the woman and her baby are transferred to the postnatal ward together as soon as possible.
- Wherever she is, the woman's blood pressure and pulse may be recorded every now and then and her temperature noted every two hours or so. Whether or not this is done, and the frequency with which it is done will depend on the woman's apparent condition. If she is talking and alert, no checks may be considered necessary.
- The woman's wound is inspected every 30 minutes to check for blood loss and her lochia is also inspected. If the woman has had a general anaesthetic, she is left in the recovery position until she is fully conscious because she is still at risk of airway obstruction or regurgitation and silent aspiration of her stomach contents.
- Analgesia is prescribed and given. This may take the form of an epidural opioid, rectal analgesia or intramuscular analgesia (i.e. an injection). If the epidural route is chosen, the woman's breathing also needs to be carefully recorded.
- The baby is put on the mother, skin-to-skin if possible. He or she may also be put to the mother's breast in such a way that the mother is disturbed as little as possible.
- Even if the woman feels very hungry, she is only allowed to have fluids at first because there is a small risk of paralytic ileus. The woman still needs to have an intravenous infusion for a while after the operation.
- The woman is helped out of bed and encouraged to walk around as soon as possible so as to reduce the risk of deep vein thrombosis. She is also encouraged to perform breathing exercises. A physiotherapist usually teaches these and may also give chest physiotherapy. Low-dose heparin (an anticoagulant drug) and TED anti-embolism stockings are often prescribed to prevent thrombosis.
- Blood pressure, temperature and pulse continue to be checked periodically. The intravenous infusion continues and the urinary catheter remains in the bladder until the woman can get up and go to the toilet. The wound and lochia are observed hourly.
- When the urinary catheter has been removed, urinary output is monitored carefully because some women have difficulty passing urine at first or emptying the bladder completely.
- A woman is reassured if—as frequently happens after a general anaesthetic—she feels tired and drowsy for hours or even days after the operation. If, as often happens, the woman complains of feelings of detachment and unreality or feels she cannot relate well to her new baby, she is encouraged to talk freely and is again reassured.
- Painkillers are given as often as the woman asks for them. This usually means giving intramuscular opiates for up to 48 hours (i.e. injections) and oral analgesics (tablets) after that. Alternatively, some women have their epidural topped up and some women don't feel they need any painkillers at all.
- The woman is encouraged to rest as much as possible and visitors may be discouraged. Because she is likely to tire quickly, the woman will probably need help looking after her new baby.
- Finally, the woman is not allowed to drive a vehicle or carry other children for six weeks after the operation—or for the length of time determined by the insurance company.

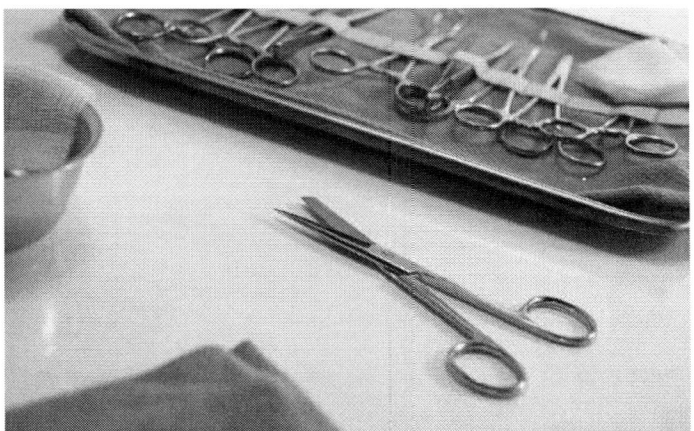

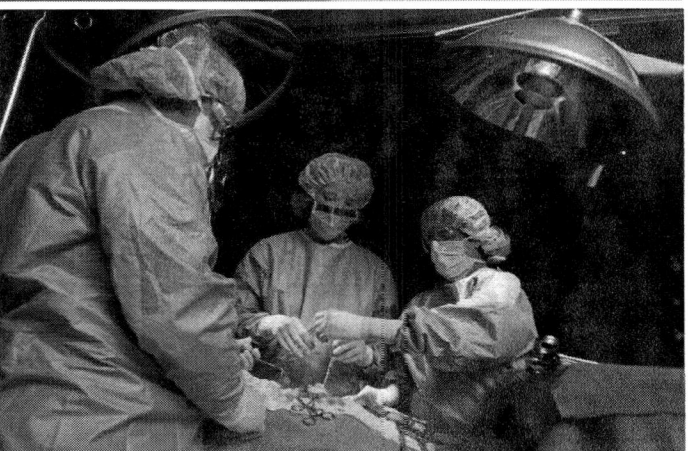

Taking things as they come, or advance hi-tech planning? Intervention or natural physiology? They are very different choices.

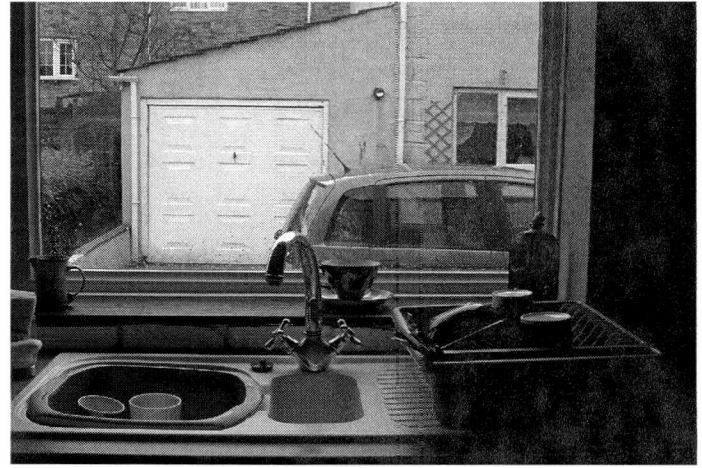

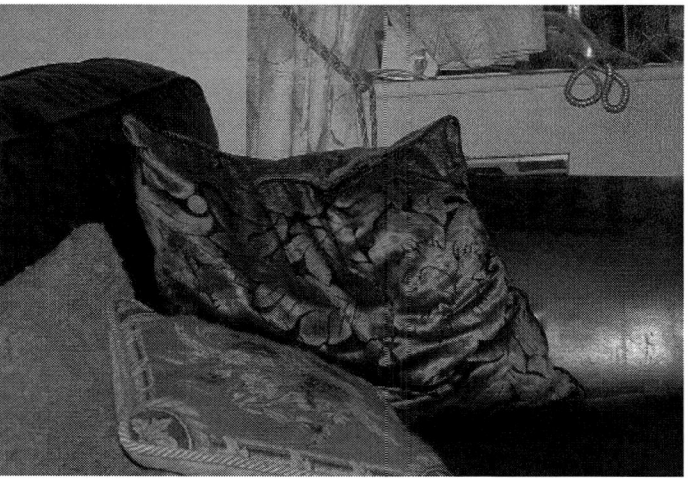

Clearly, a caesarean operation is a complicated surgical procedure, with all kinds of risks, indignities, discomforts and inconveniences. So why on earth has it become fashionable in some quarters to have a caesarean section instead of a vaginal birth?

The fashion

Caesarean rates have been steadily increasing around the world. In England and Wales in 1960 only 2.8% of births were achieved by caesarean section but the figure had risen to 18.0% by 1999—the last year for which figures are currently available. In 2001 in the US, the rate was 22.9% and in the same year in Australia it was 21.9%. In Brazil the overall rate for the country is well above 50% and in private hospitals in big cities such as Sao Paulo and Rio de Janeiro the rate is a staggering 80%.

This modern fashion for caesareans is actually quite easy to understand. Choosing a caesarean section appears to mean choosing to have complete control over a natural process. As one midwife explains...

> The c-section has sadly become part of our culture and an acceptable, if not desirable, way to give birth. Women find the control element of caesareans, particularly elective caesareans, appealing (in my opinion). In our society, generally, women are used to having control of their own bodies and their lives and to give up their body to labour and birth is very frightening to some women. Having 'a date' for their delivery day is another example of control—being able to plan it into their life/husband's holiday leave, etc., as opposed to waiting until the baby is ready.

It's interesting, though, that women who have both elective and emergency caesareans report feeling a *lack* of control when they comment on their own experience, as we shall soon see. In some sense then, the idea that a caesarean gives women control is just a fallacy... Although women might have superficial control in terms of timetables, when it comes to emotions they tend to feel out of their depth. And of course, although the birth itself may be scheduled, post-operative recovery for both mother and baby is highly unpredictable—far less so than with a vaginal birth.

Apart from wanting to control the processes, why else do women actually choose to have a caesarean? One reason is that it appears to mean choosing to blot out pain and discomfort because anaesthesia and painkillers have to be used. It is a fallacy, unfortunately, that no pain will be experienced, mainly because postnatal pain is usually a feature of a caesarean. If physical pain is not experienced (thanks to strong painkillers), often there is emotional pain, so one way or another caesarean mothers seem to get the short straw. Another common reason to have a caesarean is to avoid damaging the sexual organs. Unfortunately, this is also misguided because damage to a woman's pelvic floor usually occurs mainly during pregnancy. The best way to avoid damage to the vagina and perineum is actually to have a completely drug-free, physiological birth because less damage is likely to occur when the woman is aware of all sensation and in control while she's giving birth.

The feeling

What does it actually feel like to have a caesarean?

Birthframe 12

First they put me on the strange, narrow, tipped operating table and increased the anaesthetic drip in my epidural. I was so terrified my teeth were chattering. Two kind young anaesthetists stayed with my husband and me at the head end of the curtain so we wouldn't see me being wrenched open. The operating theatre had one of those strange fly-eye 7-faceted non-glare lamps overhead, lots of monitors checking my heart rate, blood pressure, blood oxygen, etc. They put an oxygen mask on me, to give the baby extra air, they said. When my lower body felt like nothing but lumps of dough, they got to work putting in a catheter and then slicing open the abdominal wall.

"What's happening now?" I asked, because it felt like I was being tugged in all directions. I wondered if the baby were coming out. "Oh, they're pulling apart some of the layers of your muscle wall," the anaesthetist said brightly. "It heals better than when they cut it." I wished I hadn't asked.

Not much later we heard a small cough and a phlegmy squall. "There he is! He's breathing!" I said, and burst into tears. We didn't get to see him right away, because the paediatricians had to check him for any problems related to the meconium and the long labour. We heard him screaming for his life for several minutes. Then they brought him to us wrapped in a blanket. My husband held him and showed him to me. All I could see was a bit of a tiny face in a big white blanket. I didn't know what to do.

(If this ever happens to me again, I will make sure that the curtain is lowered so that I can see the baby lifted out, and have him brought to me right away to be comforted.)

"Can I feed him?" I asked, since I knew that was what you were supposed to do. They said maybe not yet, since I was still swathed in operating sheets to my chest.

"Shall I give him his vitamin K?" asked the midwife. I said no, I didn't want that to be the first thing he ever tasted.

"How much does he weigh?" I asked. Nobody had weighed him yet.

"Would you like me to weigh him for you?" the midwife offered.

I said OK, since I couldn't think of what else to do. So she took him away and I could hear him shrieking in terror as he was made to shiver for the sake of his parents' idle curiosity. I berated myself for being so thoughtless as to allow him to be taken away again so soon. Finally, he was returned to us, still terrified. My husband was led away with the baby to the delivery room. The anaesthetist stayed with me while the doctors finished putting me back together. They lifted me from side to side to wash away the blood and iodine disinfectant that had sloshed onto the table, then they lifted me back onto my wheeled bed, and rolled me back along the corridor to the delivery suite. ▶

◀ Having the caesarean was like getting burgled. Strange burglars, who ransack the house and leave behind the world's most priceless gift, my baby son. But a burglary nonetheless. I was robbed of an experience I'd anticipated my whole life.

Sometimes life forces us to face our worst fears. Perhaps it was necessary for me to go through the caesarean first so that I would be able to appreciate the gift of a normal birth at home. I can't take it for granted. Now over three years later I can say it was a valuable experience. After all, now I've been in an operating theatre and experienced a major operation. Gee whiz. Kind of interesting.

I've experienced all those hospital interventions and I know what it's like. If it's happened to you, I can relate. It is possible to do it another way the second time! From the day after my son's birth, I comforted myself by thinking about what I was going to do differently if I got a chance to try again. The day after I discovered I was pregnant a second time, I started looking for an independent midwife. I really did my homework.

I still regret the terror and pain that my son must have felt being yanked out into bright light by strangers. He is happy and healthy and no one could say, "Here is a child who had a difficult birth." But these things are not visible to the naked eye. Wouldn't it have been so much better for him if I had been able to welcome him to the world in a gentler way? Is that why he cried inconsolably for 36 hours after his birth? They say some babies 'just are' more unsettled than others. How can I help wondering if the caesarean was the cause? Maybe I was the cause of his distress, because I was so upset. Maybe if I hadn't wanted a natural birth so much, I wouldn't have caused him such distress. But I can't be different from who I am. My husband and I were both overjoyed about the baby, nothing could change that. It was a more abstract feeling than after the second, natural birth. After the second one, I felt a physical joy. My whole being was happy. The first time, we were filled with love and wonder for our beautiful son. But my body felt sad.

Nina Klose

After the caesarean I was in a state of shock. Weeping uncontrollably for weeks and months. I became agoraphobic (normally I have to be outside), and couldn't travel in a car because it was far too scary. I was more vulnerable than a cream cake at a Bulimic Congress and the gory nightmares I was having were beyond the fright that most people are required to endure. Worst of all, I thought this was permanent. The good side is that everyone who has this Dark Night of the Soul learns from their experiences and gets stronger, and that's just what happened to me.

Birthframe 13

Post my caesarean with my first baby, I was in pain for a very long time. Even three months after the birth my scar was still nagging and painful by the end of the day or if I went out for a long walk. I remember the horror I felt when the prescription drugs ran out.

After five weeks, a string came out of my scar. The soluble stitches had in fact not dissolved, and my body had had to reject them by sending the length of suture up through the scar and to the surface. I hadn't been warned of this possibility. I was so squeamish and horrified by the whole thing that somehow I managed to ignore this, and didn't even visit the doctor. I think it could have been one of the reasons for the continuing pain. My scar didn't really heal properly and became keloid.

And then it was my daughter's turn. When I became pregnant with her I suddenly realised the downside of an elective caesarean—it makes it much more likely that you'll need one the next time, only this time round you have a heavy child who you're not allowed to pick up.

I really debated whether to go VBAC but was told that I would be allowed only an hour in second stage labour, and effectively as a first timer my chances of an emergency section were considerable. So I booked a maternity nurse and went for it again.

Second time round was incredibly different. After ten days I felt better than I had after three months with my first—I was going up and down stairs, I was off the prescription drugs. My scar healed fine. It made me realise how rough the first time had been, now I had something to compare it with.

Retrospectively I think I'd have done better to go for natural childbirth the first time round: that six weeks after the second child is born when you can't pick up your jealous first child, or put them into the bath, or change them, is really hard. I didn't even think of it when I was making the original decision.

However, it's not the end of the world. My pelvic floor and perineum are intact and my son doesn't seem too traumatised.

Birthframe 14

In case any client of yours happens to be one of the women who needs a caesarean for medical reasons, here's a positive birth story (from *LLL GB News*). It's the story of a woman who was initially in favour of a vaginal birth, who changed her mind after a difficult first labour, which resulted in an emergency caesarean. She describes how she managed to 'optimise' outcomes for an elective caesarean (for her second child), by taking an intelligent, caring and proactive approach.

I feel happy for those mothers who have experienced natural births but concerned that mothers who have experienced other births might feel that their experiences may be seen as somehow less honourable, less heroic. I've had two caesarean deliveries: each time I felt that this birth was an incredibly heroic act. I think all births must be.

The first was performed as an emergency after an incredibly traumatic labour. When my beautiful baby, Tom, emerged he weighed in at almost twelve pounds! After having such a traumatic time, I chose to have my second baby by caesarean. I asked other mothers to share with me their experiences of planned caesareans (through a La Leche League newsletter). ▶

I wanted advice in general and also particularly wanted to know how well breastfeeding had gone for other caesarean mothers, without the hormonal kick-start of going through labour. I was touched and impressed to receive many letters in reply. We are all so busy bringing up young families, with very little time that we can spend writing letters, and yet here were all these La Leche League mothers taking the time and trouble to write long and detailed letters to a complete stranger! It was such a treat to read these handwritten, deeply personal stories and lovely to find that almost all these mothers reported a positive start to breastfeeding.

I've had two caesarean deliveries... each time I felt that this birth was an incredibly heroic act

The day for my elective caesarean arrived and my husband and I arrived at the hospital, as planned, at 7.30am—thanks to one tip I got from a letter to sleep at home the night before. Our hospital's policy is normally to admit a mother the night before for tests and to meet with an anaesthetist, then they simply keep the woman in hospital overnight. The hospital was happy to comply with my request so Tom, our three-year-old, had his granny with him to take him to playgroup and give him lunch afterwards.

After such a traumatic time, I chose to have my second baby by caesarean

I'm writing this account seventeen months later and find I can scarcely remember the hours before Louis' birth. I think I was very excited and also very anxious. When birth begins with labour, one gets swept along in the unfolding experience. Without labour, there is lots of room to reflect on what a truly extraordinary and somehow unbelievable miracle is about to happen—wonderful, but scary. A lovely midwife welcomed me at the door when I arrived back at the hospital, showed me where to put my things and took me down to the operating suite. She joked and chatted with me as the anaesthetist did his work and informed me of what was happening all the way through. She knew I wanted to be well-informed as I'd shown her my birth plan on my visit the night before.

Once prepared, I lay on the operating table, numb from the waist down... well not quite numb, actually, but unable to feel pain. It's a strange sensation, hard to describe. My husband was beside me, dressed up in his little operating theatre hat and clothes.

It was a moment of intense feeling. I was aware that someone was about to cut into my body—OK, I couldn't feel it, but somewhere inside us all must be an instinctive sense that we should not let ourselves be cut. I was aware that of course I was about to meet my baby... Would it be a girl or a boy? Would it look like Tom? Would it be healthy?

I could feel the baby moving about inside me—it had been awake and vigorous all through the preparations. I felt rather pleased that it wasn't being roused from slumber! I also was aware that it would be quite a few weeks before I would begin to feel really recovered from the operation—it's hard to welcome the prospect of weeks of discomfort and limited mobility.

It was a moment of intense feeling... I was aware that someone was about to cut into my body

And I was aware that here I was, about to begin an entirely new phase of my life as mother of two. I also realised that I was lying in exactly the same spot where I had been when Tom was born, exactly three years and two weeks before. Except that this time I was conscious, it wasn't an emergency and the circumstances surrounding the birth were different.

Suddenly, here he was! Our beautiful baby boy, perfect and chubby, and screaming. The midwife wrapped him up straight away and put him on my chest for me to hold while I was being stitched up. Some mothers are able to breastfeed at this point but I was quite happy not to, feeling a bit strange and particularly immobile.

I was aware it would be quite a few weeks before I would begin to feel really recovered from the operation

After a little while, we went through to the recovery room where, as I'd requested, I was able to watch as Louis was washed, checked and weighed (9lb).

Then came the breastfeeding... It's not the easiest thing to breastfeed a baby when lying flat on your back with drips and tubes in the backs of your hands and no movement in your lower body, especially when it's a newborn baby who has never breastfed before. It was agony! I kept taking him off to see if I could improve the positioning but nothing particularly helped. (Breastfeeding continued to often be quite painful for a couple of weeks or so. I have a private theory that some mothers like myself are particularly sensitive to the pressure that the baby's suck exerts on the breast and we interpret it as pain until we get very used to it.)

It's not the easiest thing to breastfeed a baby when lying flat on your back with drips and tubes in the backs of your hands and no movement in your lower body

Louis didn't want to feed for the next 15 hours, although I kept offering him the breast. I was getting anxious. Would the staff insist he should have a bottle of formula? Would my milk take five days to 'come in' the way it had with my first baby? A midwife approached with a bottle of water and I squawked a protest. But she said she only wanted to drip a few drops on my nipple to encourage Louis to latch on. I'd never heard of this before (or since!) but, miraculously, it worked. The milk 'came in' early on Day 3 (and, of course, Louis had the valuable colostrum when he breastfed in the first two days). Maybe there was no delay because I did not start off exhausted after a long labour. Louis grew steadily and has been such a delightful baby. I'm proud of us both.

Of course, it's also necessary to consider the possibility of an *unplanned* caesarean...

Birthframe 15

With so many positive second-birth accounts and so much publicity about the feasibility of a vaginal birth after a caesarean (a VBAC), it is sometimes assumed that it must *always* be possible. However, as the next account illustrates, sometimes a planned VBAC turns out to be another caesarean. This can be extremely disappointing, as the following account illustrates. Here we meet up again with one of the anonymous contributors we've met before, earlier in this book.

For my second pregnancy and birth, I had wonderful, skilled, loving care from a home birth midwife. Labour started naturally, I dilated quickly, and the urge to push came after just a few hours.

I pushed... and pushed... and pushed...

But then I pushed... and pushed... and pushed... and pushed... The three different midwives reached in to try to turn the baby's head to facilitate delivery, to no avail.

After six hours of pushing, as the sun rose, my midwife said my scar just didn't look right, and I walked down the stairs with my midwife and husband, got in the car, and we drove to the hospital in rush hour traffic! (At the time I lived in a western suburb of the nearby city.) I was having immense and powerful pushing contractions, kneeling backward in the car with my midwife helping me.

I was admitted to the hospital, and we all agreed that after the now 7+ hours of pushing, that perhaps an epidural was in order so I could rest a bit. Everyone was very calm and professional. My midwife stayed with me the whole time. I and the baby were both doing fine according to the monitors. They catheterised me to empty my bladder, as I had been unable to urinate much during labour. That was a relief, actually.

In three or so hours, at 3pm, a doctor came in to check me. The baby had not moved down at all, to everyone's great surprise. I had continued to have pushing contractions. I was able to keep that up because I had been so well fed and watered during labour! I was informed that a caesarean would be necessary. I knew they were right, and even my midwife, who was an expert on VBAC births, agreed. I cried. She cried. My husband held me. The nurses were confused, but polite. The anaesthesiologist was kind and professional, as was everyone else.

My midwife sat with me and described to me what was happening step by step. The doctor opened me, looked up and said, "Who did this?" I for some reason thought it was funny he asked, but his voice was dead serious as he repeated, "I mean it, WHO did this? Who did the previous c-section?" I told him, and he kind of snorted angrily. As my daughter's head was exposed and pulled out he said, "WOW, look at the size of that head!" I think he said it just to make me feel better. Her head just looked like a baby head to me! She was beautifully chubby and healthy, (three ounces heavier than my son at 8lb 14oz) and her Apgar score was perfect.

Everyone was kind and professional

I held her after they fiddled with her for a few moments. Of course, I would have preferred to hold her immediately, but it was wonderful to see her. Then my husband held her as they stitched me up.

My recovery was much less painful and traumatic than after the first c-section. There was one nurse who came in and lectured me as I emerged groggy from my anaesthesia. She told me I was lucky I came in when I did and said how dare I try a home birth after a 'failed' first birth. She also said the uterus was so thin when they did the operation I was lucky it hadn't ruptured. I laughed. Did she know I had been in the hospital for over eight hours before the surgery was performed? I didn't actually say anything, I was too groggy. She huffed out.

I cannot describe that feeling of loss— really a physical ache in my vagina

The doctor came in and told me that I had massive scar tissue from the previous surgery, which he had managed to 'clean up'. My bladder had been abnormally adhered to my uterus after the first c-section, which is why I could not urinate during labour. I was catheterised for five days so that the bladder could heal properly. The doctor was amazed that I hadn't had any symptoms from that problem. Neither doctor nor midwife could give any specific reason why I could not deliver vaginally. It was apparently possible that the scar tissue had caused an impediment. My bone structure seemed normal. I dilated normally. My contractions were very strong and coordinated, for hours and hours and hours! She was a baby on the large side of things, but certainly not abnormally large.

I put up with a few annoying staff comments such as "She'll never sleep in a crib if you keep holding her." But as a better-informed second-time mother no procedures were performed or drugs given to my daughter that I did not want. I wish I hadn't had to have any drugs, but I'll take what good things I can.

I cannot describe that feeling of loss—really a physical ache in my vagina, as strange as that sounds. The great expectation of holding the baby there, but then not, again. I don't know what to make of it emotionally. I sometimes don't even want to think of it, the disappointment is still strangely fresh. At least this time, I wasn't pressured into anything, I didn't make decisions out of fear. I had the antenatal care and labour I wanted until the very end. My care was respectful and loving, and I was NOT a particularly 'good' patient! Thank heavens.

I am trying to accept that even when I do everything right, there are some variables that I don't have control over. There is some reason for everything.

At least in this case, both mother and baby were well. Sometimes this may not be the case. Amazingly enough, in these days of high technology and information still approximately 1 in every 100 babies is born dead... and there is still a fairly high maternal mortality rate, which varies from country to country. According to the World Heath Organization, a woman's chance of dying at some point in her life as a result of pregnancy or childbirth can range from 1 in 6 (in Rwanda or Sierra Leone) to 1 in 8,700 (in Canada or Spain). Interestingly—or worryingly—neither the UK or USA statistics are particularly good (1 in 4,600 and 3,500 respectively). Would the rates improve if more women had optimal births?

Are caesareans really necessary?

Dystocia (also called 'failure to progress') and fetal distress are reasons given for a great number of caesareans.

> **Dystocia and fetal distress are reasons given for a great number of caesareans**

While care providers are right to monitor the progress of a woman's labour and her baby's safety, it is essential that they do so without actually causing a labour to become extended or a baby distressed. (We need to remember the association between EFM and the increase in the caesarean rate!) Most of the practices and interventions which are common on labour wards all over the world may well disrupt women's labours and even cause fetal distress. Lack of privacy, interruptions, alienation through the use of machines and impersonal practices, deprivation of food and drink, continuous or constant monitoring... all these are practices which disturb and therefore probably lengthen a woman's labour. An atmosphere of fear and tension, fetal scalp monitors and inappropriate physical positions—such as when the mother lies on her back—are ways which are highly likely to cause fetal distress. It seems the real, psychological and hormonal needs of a labouring woman, not to mention the fetus, are being disregarded in the name of safety. And it all seems to lead to what is diagnosed as dystocia.

One of the emailed conversations I had with Michel while writing this book relates to this problem. I had been wondering how often caesareans might need to be performed, in an ideal world...

Michel, if every woman were to begin labour spontaneously and were to labour undisturbed and unobserved, without pain relief or interventions, what do you imagine the rates of mortality and morbidity, and caesarean might be?

Imagine that the prerequisite to be an obstetrician or a midwife would be to be a mother who has a personal experience of vaginal unmedicated birth. I guess that the caesarean rate would drop below 10% with the same perinatal mortality rates and lower rates of transfer to paediatrics.

Is nature really that inefficient, though? Surely even a 1% caesarean rate would indicate extreme inefficiency in nature...

... or would be a reminder of the laws of natural selection. The huge development of the part of the brain called the neocortex (the brain of the intellect) is a handicap where childbirth is concerned. As long as the neocortex remains active, it tends to inhibit the activity of the primitive brain structures that are supposed to work hard during labour (releasing all the necessary hormones). That is the main reason why a difficult birth is an aspect of human nature. There are other reasons why humans beings are condemned to have difficult births. One is that the fetal head is so large that it has to spiral down in a complex way inside the maternal pelvis. If we add the deep-rooted cultural misunderstanding of birth physiology, one can explain why the rates of caesarean sections are far above 1%.

Can you explain what you mean by 'the deep-rooted cultural misunderstanding of birth physiology'?

I mean a widespread, deep-rooted failure to understand the basic needs of women in labour. Recently, I attended a birth that could be used to illustrate my assumption that the current rates of caesareans would drop dramatically if the basic needs of women in labour were better understood.

Birthframe 16

Here's Michel's account of the birth...

> The woman who gave birth belongs to a family that is familiar with caesarean birth. Her brother, her sister and herself were born by caesarean. When she gave birth for the first time, it was decided after a long trial of labour in hospital that the baby was too big for her and that she needed a caesarean: the baby was 9lb (4kg).
>
> While she was expecting her second baby, she asked me if I would come to her home when the labour started, because she wanted to try to give birth vaginally. My answer was: "Yes, if I'm not in Costa Rica".
>
> The labour started during the night preceding my flight to Costa Rica. I could stay in her home until she was in advanced labour, so that when she arrived at the hospital with Liliana (her doula), she was not far from a point of no return. She eventually gave birth with the help of ventouse to another 9lb baby.
>
> When she was expecting her third baby, she asked me again if I might come to her home when she was in labour. My answer was: "Yes, if I'm not in Italy".
>
> The labour started two days before my flight to Italy. There were ideal conditions of privacy. I was following the progress of labour from another room, through the sound.
>
> Liliana who, as a doula, behaves like a cat, was around, evaluating the progress of labour with her own criteria—postures, sound, breathing patterns, etc.
>
> I did only one vaginal exam. At 12 noon, the father left in order to make some arrangements so that the children could stay in the house of friends. Soon after, there was a series of powerful contractions—a real 'fetus ejection reflex'. At 12.45 the ecstatic mother gave birth to an 11lb (5kg) girl... no drugs, no tears, no episiotomy.

So, as we've said, a caesarean does not seem to be the best way of giving birth unless it really is medically indicated. On the other hand, when caesareans are performed in order to safeguard the well-being of either the labouring woman or the baby, they are to be welcomed.

It is, after all, thanks to the caesarean operation (as well as improved nutrition and sanitation and advances in the fields of antibiotics and anaesthesia, in particular) that childbirth is no longer the potentially life-threatening rite of passage for women that it once was.

With this operation as a safety guard, we can now confidently leave the physiological processes to take place and have an unmedicated vaginal birth, knowing that if we or our baby are in danger, there is a fast and effective operation to rescue us. This represents a new vision of obstetrics, as Michel explains:

My idea is to introduce a sort of futuristic strategy of childbirth which is partly what I have already practised. It is based on having a good understanding of physiology and of the basic needs of human beings in labour—for privacy, a sense of security, etc. If the midwife behaves in a motherly way and disturbs the woman as little as possible, either it works or a caesarean is necessary. This strategy makes it possible to avoid the two main alternatives as much as possible: drugs (which all have side-effects) and difficult interventions by the vaginal route (difficult forceps and so on). If we avoid these alternatives, there are really only two possibilities: a completely undisturbed physiological labour or a caesarean section.

Women just need to find a midwife who will support them in this choice... Could that be you?

OPTIMAL BIRTH—THE WHY

There's some overlap, but let's tease out some reasons...

Reason No. 1:
RESEARCH SUGGESTS IT'S SAFEST TO MINIMISE INTERVENTIONS

If you're finding time to keep up with the latest research, I'm sure you know that many practices associated with modern maternity care are not recommended by research.

As you probably know, a Canadian team of researchers, Enkin et al, did a great deal of work to survey research carried out into the effectiveness of midwifery and obstetric practices a few years ago. Their book, which has been periodically updated and supplemented by CD-ROMs, is *A Guide to Effective Care in Pregnancy and Childbirth* (Oxford University Press 2000). Also see www.cochrane.org.

More recently, the American editor of the revised edition of *Our Bodies, Ourselves* (Touchstone Books 2005), Jennifer Block, researched and wrote *Pushed* (Da Capo 2007). Dr Marsden Wagner, who was formerly Director of Women's and Children's Health at the World Health Organization, also wrote *Born in the USA* (University of California Press 2006). Although both books focus primarily on the situation in the USA, they are packed full of references to practices which are not founded on research, or indeed which fly in the face of recommendations based on research, which are also common in the UK.

Here are a few commonly used interventions which research has shown to be unhelpful or harmful, which cannot be part of an 'optimal birth' scenario:

In pregnancy...
- Assigning a pregnant woman to several care givers
- Using ultrasound routinely to assess fetal growth
- Screening for gestational diabetes

In labour...
- Using EFM as a screening test on admission
- Confining a woman to a bed against her will
- Stopping women from eating and drinking
- Not using one-to-one care or midwifery-led care
- Routinely inserting an IV or heparin lock 'just in case'
- Using artificial oxytocics to augment labour
- Imposing arbitrary time limits

During the birth...
- Insisting on the lithotomy position
- Directing the woman's efforts with commanded pushing
- Imposing arbitrary time limits
- Routinely using episiotomy
- Using forceps or ventouse to speed up 'delivery'

Postnatally...
- Restricting contact between the mother and her baby
- Taking healthy newborns to a separate room or nursery
- Routinely giving babies supplements of water or formula when mothers are breastfeeding
- Restricting visits from younger children to hospital wards

It's easy to see how these practices can adversely affect the safety and success of physiological birth.

Pregnancy
When a woman has no continuity of care in pregnancy, she is unlikely to develop a relaxed, confident relationship with her care provider(s). This will mean she is in danger of succumbing to what Michel Odent has called the 'nocebo effect', i.e. the situation when a woman becomes fearful as a result of care givers' comments or concerns. When various care givers (or even the same one repeatedly) ask the pregnant woman to have ultrasound scans in order to look for abnormalities or check for adequate growth, for example, the implicit message to the pregnant woman is that the caregivers are not actually really *expecting* things to progress normally. Screening for gestational diabetes is problematic simply because the condition is considered non-existent by some researchers, or non-treatable by others. (Other screening tests, e.g. for anaemia, provoke similar levels of controversy, as we shall see later on.)

Labour
As we've already mentioned, although EFM can ostensibly be justified on the grounds that it provides some useful information about a woman (and her fetus) on admission, in research studies it has only ever consistently been associated with a rise in the caesarean rate. It has never been shown to improve maternal or infant morbidity or mortality rates. Partograms have, however, often been used in court cases. They also successfully put a woman in a position where she is subservient to technology and the decisions of her caregivers, which sets the scene for limiting the labouring woman's sense of freedom. Inhibiting a woman's movements and actions by confining her to a bed, stopping her from eating and drinking and inserting an IV or heparin lock also function to make women feel like a patient (who must be ill), as opposed to an empowered woman about to give birth. In any case, research has shown that these procedures serve no useful purpose and in fact that they inhibit the smooth progression of labour. This makes sense when we consider the close relationship between emotions and hormones and the importance of a 'correct' hormonal cocktail if the birthing processes are to proceed smoothly. Of course, imposing arbitrary time limits simply exacerbate any psychological damage done by other procedures (by making the woman feel tense and observed) and artificial oxytocics give the woman higher levels of pain, which is likely to propel her down a cascade of interventions after initially succumbing to some kind of pain relief.

Birth and beyond...
When a woman isn't allowed to move around and give birth in her own time, in a standing position, she will certainly not experience a fetus ejection reflex. Episiotomy has been shown to cause more tears, not fewer, or to make them worse when they do occur and forceps have been found to have lasting effects on babies. The importance of bonding after any kind of birth has been well-publicised so it is tragic if it is inhibited in any way through the procedures listed...

Reason No. 2:
ALL DRUGS FOR PAIN RELIEF HAVE SIDE-EFFECTS

The search for perfect pain relief continues... As yet, no drugs have found which are both effective throughout labour and birth and which also have no side effects. In many cases, side effects are substantial and in cases where they aren't, we must recognise that we may simply not yet know what they are. Here is a little of what we already know:

Gas and air...
- Women are disturbed by the process of self-administering gas and air, so cannot possibly 'go to another planet'.
- Using gas and air probably interferes with a woman's natural ability to produce natural endorphins.
- Experiments into the use of nitrous oxide (50% of gas and air, the other 50% being oxygen), showed it substantially increased the risk of drug dependency in adulthood.

Pethidine
- Women have frequently reported feeling drunk and out of control after having doses of pethidine and even then it has not effectively masked the pain of labour or birth.
- Like any other opiate used in labour, pethidine can cause problems for the woman, such as nausea, vomiting, sedation, itching, hypotension or respiratory depression.
- Pethidine can have dramatic effects on the baby at birth. Since it goes straight through to the baby and is usually still present in the baby's system at birth, it can cause early breathing problems, It can weaken the baby's 'suck' (so has a dramatic effect on breastfeeding), it can affect the fetal heart rate and change neonatal behaviour.
- Research has established a link between the presence of opiates in the baby's body at birth and later drug addiction in adulthood.

Diamorphine
- This drug (which is 100% heroin) is increasingly being used in labour wards, perhaps because it can block out *all* the pain of labour. Interestingly, or worryingly, women are not being told that this drug is actually heroin. Why not?
- It can cause the same problems listed under 'pethidine'.
- The prospect of long-term effects for the baby is worrying.

Epidurals
- Epidurals necessitate continuous EFM because the anaesthetics used cause fetal heart decelerations; this may in turn increase the likelihood of a caesarean.
- They necessitate continuous monitoring of the woman's blood pressure as it may fall to dangerous levels.
- So as to counteract problems with lowering of blood pressure, intravenous fluids have to be used, which can cause excessive swelling of the feet, legs and breasts. Swelling of the breasts can cause infant feeding problems.
- The catheter needed to drain off urine can easily introduce infection into the woman's body.
- Epidurals, when administered to sheep, interfered with mothering behaviour—the ewes rejected their lambs. They may have a similar, but subtler impact on human mothers.
- They may be followed by 6-week-long headaches, temporary or even permanent paralysis.

I seemed to recover so much faster after the birth, not having had pain relief

---

On top of all these possible or definite side-effects, Michel Odent—in his book *Primal Health* (Clairview Books 2002) has documented long-term effects which may occur simply as a result of having certain experiences in what he calls the 'primal period', which runs from conception until the baby's first birthday. Here are a few comments from contributors:

> When I was fully dilated at 3.50pm the midwife took away the gas and air and told me I wouldn't be able to push adequately with it. I found the instant shock of the pain (when the midwife took the gas and air away) to be devastating. I was in so much pain that I could not speak let alone push. My contractions were without respite and the midwife was constantly telling me to relax. It wasn't until 4.40pm that I could actually push effectively.

> I had the epidural, my blood pressure dropped and they moved me around until they found a position the 'baby liked'. I dozed in a stupor. I suddenly had a sharp pain on one side, and then a persistent ache. I could not change position: I was too numb. I was utterly dependent. I called the nurse. Now it was somebody different. I hoped she was kind. I was helpless, and I had to rely on her. I tried to be nice, and as unobtrusive as possible. A good patient.

> I was admitted at 4.45pm and by 7pm I was getting very painful contractions, an epidural was mentioned and after a few more contractions I decided to have it. What wondrous relief except that you are literally numb from the waist down which makes any form of movement amusing. Things then slowed down as expected, so up went the fluid drip and the hormone drip to get things going again.

> The contractions then came stronger and closer together, but, due to the effects of the epidural, all I could feel was pressure on my bowel when they were at their very strongest. I had to be told when to push by the other people in the room.

> After the epidural I could only have ice chips, and I didn't have any because I was too busy screaming and trying to push. I was desperately thirsty, but now was not allowed to have any water because I was being 'prepped'. A few minutes later I was taken into surgery.

> I had an epidural the first time, but didn't the second because there wasn't enough time to get it organised. I was really glad, afterwards, that I hadn't had it. I seemed to recover so much faster after the birth, not having had pain relief while I was in labour.

Reason No. 3:
BABIES ARE BEING DISADVANTAGED, PERHAPS FAR INTO THE FUTURE

The baby's perspective

The baby's perspective is often forgotten when childbirth is under discussion. Years ago, the baby was often regarded as being an insensitive, unfeeling part of the equation of childbirth. Discussion has always taken place as to when a fetus or baby becomes a truly sentient person, with sensations, thoughts and emotions. This debate still continues but research is increasingly providing evidence that our estimate of a person's development of consciousness should be placed earlier, rather than later, perhaps even at a few weeks of gestation… if not before.

Whatever people's conclusions, from the 1920s on, several European psychologists and clinicians researched the effect of birth experiences on human growth and development. Otto Rank's contention in 1923 that adult psychological problems might stem from birth separation anxiety, implying the primacy of the *mother*-infant relationship (over that of the child's relationship with his or her father) was seen (by Freud in particular) as an extreme and unacceptable claim. Today, of course, it is accepted without question, especially as a result the work by Marshall Klaus et al (first published in 1976) on bonding.

Frederick Leboyer, a French obstetrician (born in 1918), certainly felt that a baby was completely sentient at birth and that he or she could be affected by birth experiences. He successfully raised many people's awareness of what he saw as the baby's perspective through his book *Birth Without Violence* (Inner Traditions Bear and Company 2002), which was first published in 1974. To do this, he used a poetic approach, not one based on hard data, and his book spawned a gentle birthing approach which involved subdued lighting and gentle touch, as well as a bath in lukewarm water.

David Chamberlain, a psychotherapist based in North America, also came to believe that birth experiences are crucially important to babies. He came to this conclusion after hypnotising adults and attempting to gain access to their birth experiences, which in many cases he found surprising and important in terms of their later lives. In his book *Babies Remember Birth* (Ballantine Books 1990) he details some of the hypnotherapy sessions he conducted, which seemed to suggest that babies are even sensitive to comments people make at the time of their birth. His research through psychotherapy also led him to conclude that babies became frightened when things go wrong at birth, for example when they have difficulty breathing, when they are suddenly subjected to bright lights or when they are taken away from their mothers. Along with Thomas Verny, he co-founded the Pre and Perinatal Psychology Association.

The idea that babies can be scarred by words and actions at their birth might seem extreme to you, but people in other cultures are more accepting of this idea. Nina Klose, who's done research in Russia comments…

> There's a feeling in natural childbirth circles in Russia that we have a responsibility to our children to try to give them the gift of a natural birth because of the lifelong physical and emotional after-effects of a traumatic birth.

If you're sceptical, imagine for one moment what it must be like to be born under pressure, with artificially-induced contractions (which are stronger and which often compromise the baby's oxygen supply), in an unfamiliar drugged state, with an electrode pierced through your head or suctioned to it. Consider what it must feel like to meet an unresponsive, dopey or merely passive mother, after hearing her lively voice for weeks, and indeed months in the womb. Imagine the reality of having difficulty establishing breathing because of a hurriedly severed umbilical cord or an excess of drugs in your system. Imagine what it must feel like to have unnecessary difficulties with your circulation or with basic temperature regulation. And how must it feel to have something thrust up your nose, or to have something put into your eyes at the moment of birth? Imagine almost immediately being laid on your back so as to be weighed on cold, hard scales… How would you feel as a newborn if you were taken away from your mother so as to be washed and examined? What might you feel when put to your mother's breast only to find that you can't suck because of drugs in your system affecting your instinctual sucking reflex? Do you think you might feel any panic, confusion, sadness, pain or distress? Might you not feel a strange longing for a better birth, which is somehow more sensitive and beautiful?

Some midwives and consultants dismiss the idea that the baby's state of mind at birth is important or their actions or words show a refusal to take it really seriously… This seems strange because interventions or drugs are surely highly likely to affect a baby's feelings and perception of the world. If contractions were artificially accelerated, they were probably more stressful for the baby so he or she is likely to be more tense or tired at birth. If forceps were used, a headache at birth is a probability. If drugs were used for pain relief, the baby is likely to feel drowsy, woozy, sleepy or nauseous and anaesthesia of any kind may well desensitise a baby for up to a month after the birth. Not a very nice way to start life really.

Imagine, for a moment, the alternative: a fresh, alert, happy sort of feeling, with a usefully strong suck; heightened sensitivity to his or her mother's soft, responsive arms, in a room full of kindness, dimmed lights and subdued sounds. Consider the baby's first experience of looking up into his or her mother's eyes, his or her first attempt to suck at your breast—it's likely to be fulfilling if no drugs are affecting the baby's innate ability to suck. Consider the relief at having completed a journey which might perhaps have been a little frightening and physically tiring… Consider this very different transition from life in the womb to life outside it.

When drugs are not used, mothers are clearly attuned to their babies' movements, and right after birth a kind of entrainment may be established to set up behavioural patterns and language. And yet women are still medicated during the birth process, leaving them incapable of responding to the cues of their newborns, while babies—separated from their mothers—are left crying for the expected touch of parental skin. Why are so many midwives not facilitating what should be a very natural path to effective parental care by encouraging the avoidance of drugs and unnecessary interventions? Is it because of a lack of convincing research data?

Hard data

There is quite a bit of hard data to confirm that events before, during and after birth might have long-term effects.

For example, researchers found that obstetric complications (which often result after unnecessary interventions) were associated with a higher incidence of childhood asthma. Children who experienced certain procedures at birth, i.e. caesarean section, vacuum extraction, the use of forceps, or who were literally pulled out by a care provider manually, were particularly at risk. Rates of asthma amongst children who were birthed normally were significantly lower.

Many other studies have shown links between a baby's birth experiences and his or her late experiences or health in life. Michel Odent reports:

> Recently, there has been an accumulation of hard data confirming the lifelong consequences of the antenatal environment and also of the way we are born. In other words, the branch of epidemiology I have called 'primal health research' (since 1986) has developed dramatically. It developed at such a pace that in 1997 we found it necessary to establish and to continuously update a Primal Health Research Data Bank so that everybody can refer to this data.
>
> [See www.wombecology.com and www.birthworks.org/primalhealth]

A lot of hard data have confirmed the lifelong consequences of the antenatal environment and the way we are born

> Today the databank contains hundreds of abstracts of articles published in authoritative scientific and medical journals. All of them show correlations between what happened during the 'primal period' (from conception until the first birthday) and what happens later on in life in terms of health and behaviour. It is not easy to detect such articles because they do not fit into the current classifications. This is the main reason for trying to bring them together.
>
> From an overview of the bank we see immediately that, in all fields of medicine, there have been studies detecting correlations between an adult disease and what happened when the mother was pregnant. It is even possible to conclude that our health is to a great extent shaped in the womb. There are many studies confirming that the emotional states of pregnant women may have lifelong effects on their children. This might lead us to conclude that the first duty of health professionals should be to deal tactfully with the emotional state of pregnant women. This is not easy in the framework of industrialised childbirth, which implies a certain style of antenatal care, constantly focusing on potential problems. Health professionals need to avoid the common mistake of doing more harm than good by interfering with the imagination and belief system of the person they are taking care of.
>
> Through the data provided by primal health research, we are in a position to try to forecast what sort of disaster might be induced by the industrialisation of childbirth [i.e. excessive intervention]. The data indicates there might be more violent young criminals, more teenage suicides, more drug-addicted adults, more anorexic girls, more autistic children... All these conditions have never been as frequent as they are today. We don't know why this is the case. But, for all of them, the Primal Health Research Databank reveals studies detecting risk factors in the period surrounding birth.

Perhaps health professionals should deal tactfully with pregnant women's emotions

Here is some more detail on research reported in the Primal Health Research databank:

- Anorexia nervosa has been found to be more common in girls who have had difficult births, i.e. births where there was clearly a great deal of intervention. Girls were found to have been more at risk for anorexia nervosa after having a cephalhemotoma (which is a marker of a highly traumatic birth) or a vaginal instrumental delivery, i.e. forceps or vacuum. Interestingly, the fact of having had a caesarean birth did not predispose girls to anorexia.

Anorexia nervosa is more common later on after a difficult birth

- Adults who have committed suicide using asphyxiation were usually babies who had breathing difficulties at birth. (This kind of difficulty is more likely when babies have drugs in their system at birth.)
- Adults who have committed suicide by violent mechanical means usually had some kind of mechanical birth trauma caused, for example, by the use of forceps.
- Autism has been associated with various aspects of the period surrounding birth: induction of labour, 'deep forceps' delivery, birth under anaesthesia and resuscitation at birth. Babies born in certain hospitals where induction of labour and the use of a mixture of sedatives, anaesthesia agents and analgesics during labour were routine were particularly at risk.

Autism has been associated with various aspects of 'managed' birth

- A marked increase in the incidence of schizophrenia was shown in adults whose birth showed an excess of complications of both pregnancy and delivery. Although pre-eclampsia (which the mother can perhaps do nothing about) was associated with schizophrenia, other complications would certainly have resulted from inappropriate or excessive interventions during labour and birth.
- One study showed a clear link between left-handedness (which is often associated with behavioural disorders) and complications either during pregnancy or birth. Again, complications at birth might well have been caused or exacerbated by inappropriate or excessive intervention.
- As we have already mentioned, babies born under the influence of nitrous oxide (a component of Entonox, i.e. gas and air) have been found to be more susceptible to amphetamine addiction later in life. The use of opiates or barbiturates (or both), alongside nitrous oxide, has been associated with opiate or other drug addiction (e.g. amphetamines) in offspring later in life. Researchers think that the clear link established could be the result of 'imprinting' during labour. I wonder if there's any link between the widespread use of ecstasy and cocaine in nightclubs and the way the same young people were born.

As if this weren't all enough, there's one other enormous area of possible repercussions to consider...

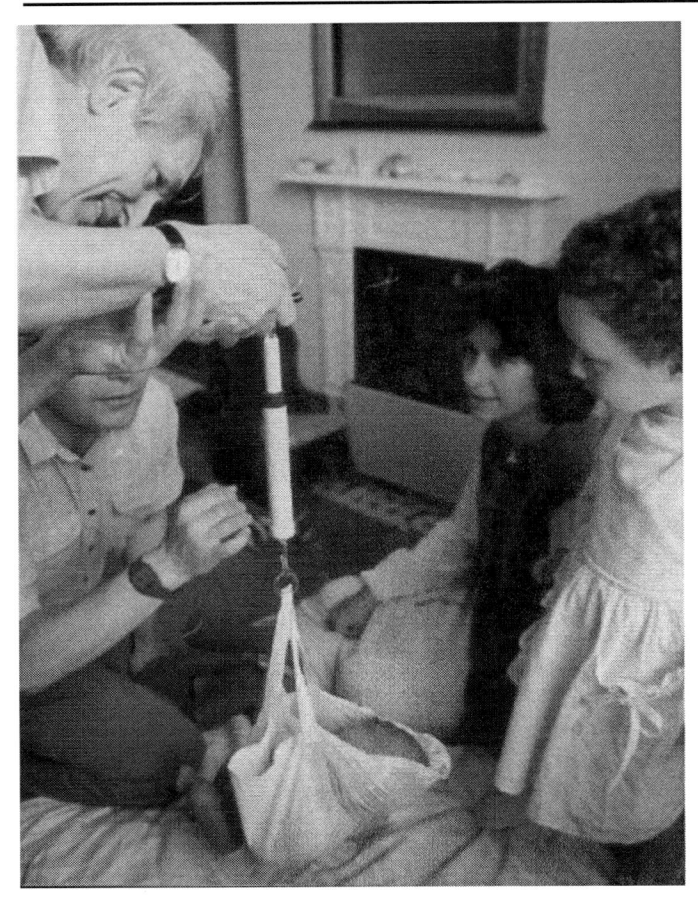

How can you make everything more personal and caring? Here Michel Odent is weighing Liliana's baby after the birth

What about a baby's capacity to love?

It's possible that a person's capacity to love may develop around the time of birth. Michel Odent has argued that this is the case in his book *The Scientification of Love* (Free Association Books 1999). All his hypotheses are backed up by research data, drawn from a wide range of sources. He is of the opinion that even a baby's lifelong capacity to love might be affected by an interventionist birth involving drugs and alienating procedures which disrupt the natural production of hormones in both mother and baby. It's easy to understand how. In a fully undisturbed labour, a woman produces various hormones which may 'imprint' on the baby's mind as he or she is being born. These hormones—oxytocin and prolactin, in particular—produce loving, mothering behaviour in the mother, and they may well also prepare the newborn for a new loving relationship and for relationships in the future. Makes sense somehow.

If these ideas seem extreme, at least allow them to stay at the back of your mind for a while. I remember my own reaction when my obstetrician in Sri Lanka wrote some comments in a letter to me after the birth of my first daughter. "For a long time," he wrote, "and this is no exaggeration, I have wondered if violence at birth contributes to making a violent society." I must admit, it seemed an almost ridiculous notion to me at the time. But the more I think about it and the more I study the research data, the more I feel inclined to think a link may not be so outlandish after all.

What impact do drugs have on babies?

If you are about to interrupt me to say that babies born in the developing world don't always grow up to be gentle and peace-loving, do note that these countries may be the places where most intervention and disturbance is going on. I only learned this through living in Sri Lanka and Oman and through extensive travel elsewhere. In Sri Lanka, in a very rural place called Ella—a tiny mountain hamlet seven hours by train from Kandy—I was astonished to hear from the landlady of our guest house that all women in Ella travel to their local hospital to give birth. (Apparently, it was only eight miles away.) Gradually, I realised that in highly undeveloped places technology and 'Western' ideas are sometimes almost worshipped as gods.

In other places, hygiene may be poor due to lack of resources, climate and lack of training, and these factors may all lead to difficult births. Traditional superstitions also sustain practices which increase the level of risk and the subsequent necessity for intervention. Creating a lot of noise to scare off evil spirits after the birth, before the placenta is born, is an example of this because any disturbance to the mother at this time can dramatically increase the risk of haemorrhage and consequent maternal death. Another example would be stopping the newborn from breastfeeding for a few days because of superstitions associated with the early 'milk', colostrum; obviously this might result in failure to breastfeed at all. All these problems occur in places where female circumcision is very common (e.g. Africa or the Middle East), which makes birth an even more difficult and dangerous undertaking. Very early marriage (from the age of 12) also results in girls giving birth before their bodies are physically ready and subsequent trauma and disadvantages to the babies.

It would be good if researchers could continue to study any links between birth and later behaviour or health more systematically over the next few decades and beyond. Links which have already been established suggest it's well worth discouraging women from using drugs or interventions during childbirth unless they are absolutely necessary.

Whatever our views on the possible long-term side-effects of interventions during labour and birth, we can only be sure that we have minimised any possible long-term effects if we allow babies the smoothest possible introduction to this world, involving an absolute minimum of drugs or unnecessary interventions, and no insensitive comments around the time of the birth.

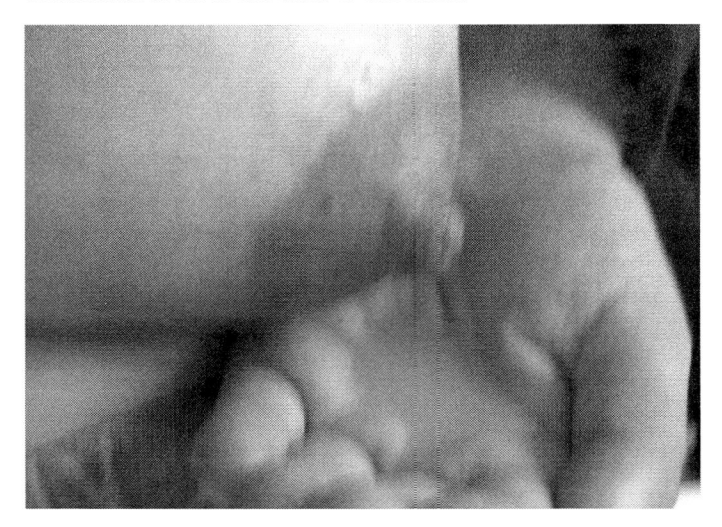

Milk's come in... But is baby able to suck?... or does he have drugs in his system which make it impossible?

Reason No. 4:
WOMEN END UP FEELING DISEMPOWERED, UPSET AND DEPRESSED

Negative emotions postnatally...

Visiting many baby groups in different places has confirmed my early impression that many mothers experience early motherhood as negative and disempowering. Women typically sit around, barely talking to each other or only exchanging superficial information and comments, in an apparent effort to display an ability to cope, despite behaviour which suggests difficulties. Of course, this lack of openness could be attributed to tiredness or a kind of identity crisis after passing into the uncharted territory of motherhood. Certain information and statistics, however, confirm the notion there might be deeper reasons.

A survey commissioned by *Mother & Baby magazine* in 2002, which collated the responses from 3,000 women, turned up some interesting information. Apparently, 86% of the women who responded reported that they were in pain after giving birth for an average of 24 days; almost a third of these said they were in 'considerable pain'. Women who've had optimal births have reported minimal postnatal pain.

According to MIND, the leading UK mental health charity (see www.mind.org.uk) new mothers *usually* get the 'baby blues' for two to four days after the birth. MIND reports that doctors usually put this down to hormonal changes or to 'the experience of being in hospital'. Negative feelings after giving birth—which are said to include feeling emotional, difficulties sleeping and loss of appetite, anxiety, sadness, as well as feelings of guilt and inadequacy—are apparently so common, they are considered normal. Have we as a culture come to terms with the lack of empowerment which results when women don't experience the natural endorphins produced in a physiological birth? When women don't experience the usual postnatal hormones—particularly oxytocin (which is also the hormone of orgasms) and prolactin (which induces relaxation and mothering feelings)—are women plunged into unnatural depression?

The long-term effects of a failure to experience the natural endorphins and hormones of birth and breastfeeding are difficult to estimate, but one cannot help but wonder why 31 million anti-depressants were prescribed in the UK in 2006, many of them no doubt to adult women of childbearing age... Apart from the many women who go to their GPs complaining of general depression, the Royal College of Psychiatrists reports that 1 in 10 women are diagnosed with full-blown postnatal depression. This apparently leaves them feeling depressed, irritable, tired, sleepless, not hungry, unable to enjoy anything (including sex), unable to cope, guilty and anxious.

How many women who don't ever get to their doctors also experience feelings of disempowerment, sadness and depression? How many women go into hospital to give birth feeling optimistic and possibly even excited, but later come out feeling angry, disillusioned and even betrayed? In that survey conducted by *Mother & Baby magazine* over 81% of respondents admitted being frightened during their labour and 53% said that childbirth had been 'far more shocking' than they'd expected. 57% felt their antenatal classes had not revealed the truth about the experience of giving birth in the UK today. That was in 2002. Has the situation changed since then? Are these women representative of all women in the UK? What *is* the truth, which women found so shocking?

Judging from many birth stories I've read (some of them published, others sent to me while I was researching birth), I also conclude that a great number of women feel regrets about some of the interventions they have while they are in labour or giving birth. The simple, but uncomfortable, truth is that many of them are felt to have been unnecess-ary, perhaps done for convenience or control, not safety.

Birthframe 17

I am coming to terms with my anger and bitterness. They eat at me and paralyse my body, while those I am angry and bitter at go blissfully about their work. I believe that the people I entrusted with my care believed that they were doing their best, that they were doing their job. I also believe that in the circumstances under which it was performed my caesarean was necessary. I also certainly believe that those circumstances were, for the most part, caused by my caretakers and were completely preventable. I was caught up in a system that has it all WRONG.

When I realise how much fear I carried with me throughout the pregnancy, how many things I did because of fear, and how little REAL information I got, it makes me heartsick. I had a cascade of interventions leading, finally, to the caesarean. When my baby was taken out, he showed absolutely no signs of the postmaturity that I was threatened with along with insinuations that I was an irresponsible ignoramus for simply wanting to let him come when he was ready. I was so tense and/or terrified for the last three weeks of my pregnancy, it's no wonder that my body would not allow the baby to come. My body knew that babies should not be born where it is not safe. No mammal will give birth in a dangerous place.

I am free to seek expert opinions, but no one else has our interests at heart like I do. I am now a doubter, never taking any statement at face value and now, I trust myself more. I may never learn to trust myself completely, as I have been taught from my earliest moments, like most of us, that the authorities know best. At least I know now that I am worthy of trust.

I have learned that just because a doctor or organisation of doctors says something or holds a belief it does not mean that it has a root in hard science. I have also learned that when something has been discounted as 'never scientifically proven', it may simply mean that no one has yet bothered to do, or been able to get funding for, the research. I have learned that Science doesn't have all the answers. I have learned that most statistics can be cleverly twisted to anyone's end. I have learned that people are lied to by people who have been lied to themselves, ad infinitum, until they really believe the lie to be true. I have given up the naive belief that a woman practitioner or midwife, because she is a woman, will be a sympathetic and knowledgeable advocate.

An unsatisfactory first birth experience often leads a mother to research and campaign for a better birth for a second birth. This perhaps explains the trend for requests for natural birth after an interventionist first experience. And in many cases, women do find that a different midwife (or consultant) will take a surprisingly different approach...

Birthframe 18

I had my first child, Sophie, in January 1985 but what influenced my expectations and hopes was a TV programme I'd watched about four years before. The programme had Miriam Stoppard as its hostess and the subject was Michel Odent and his work in Pithiviers, France as a natural childbirth pioneer. It inspired me to read books about the subject (home births, natural birth— by Sheila Kitzinger and Michel Odent)—and my enthusiasm grew. When I first became pregnant I sought out a doctor who was sympathetic and experienced, who would attend me at home.

The labour started on Saturday morning. The first sign was a little gush of amniotic fluid—but no pain. The doctor examined me, and assessed that I was not dilated at all. He seemed a bit put out that this was happening on a Saturday—he had to visit his sick wife in hospital. I tried the usual tricks to bring the labour on—taking castor oil and scrubbing floors. The doctor said at 3.30pm that we had better go to hospital as some hours had elapsed since the waters had leaked; he said that there was a risk of infection and that the baby could become blind if that happened.

We went to the hospital very disappointed and frightened. The house doctor at the hospital read the letter of introduction from my 'home birth doctor' (who had to go to visit his wife). He looked and acted very disdainfully towards me—that I'd hoped for a home birth and now here I was needing professional help after all. I was wired up to a machine to measure contractions... there were none. I'd heard about the method called sweeping the cervix, whereby the doctor uses his fingers to manipulate the cervix into loosening and maybe rupturing the membranes. I wanted to try this first before resorting to drugs. It was done very painfully and some contractions started.

Over the hours, I was put on an oxytocin drip—the contractions were not strong enough and the baby had to be delivered within 12 hours, according to the hospital's rule, because of the risk of infection. I had the water sac broken so that a monitor could be attached to the baby's head. This was very upsetting and painful. I felt raped. So much water came out—I realised that before it was only a leak and was not as dangerous for infection as the full waters emptying. Then I was persuaded to have an epidural because they wanted to increase the oxytocin to speed things up. The baby's pulse was now dropping so low they were worried, so they phoned their top doctor who advised a caesarean. The epidural was wearing off now and I could feel the baby low down in the canal, almost ready to come out. They still went ahead with a general anaesthetic and I woke up to see my husband showing my lovely baby wrapped up tight in a shawl. She was born at 12.30am on Sunday, nine hours after I went to the hospital.

I was so happy to have a lovely baby that I soon forgot about my ordeal. On Sophie's first birthday I relived the humiliating, disappointing and painful time of her birth. I duly wrote a letter to the hospital. I complained about my treatment. I did receive a reply and I was invited to meet the doctors at the hospital for a talk/discussion. I did not go in the end as I felt that I would be out of my depth at the meeting—and it would be me against them. I had already been through a lot of grief with Sophie's health since she was 8 months old. A doctor at the hospital had told me she had a heart murmur. She was also taking a paediatric steroid in tablet form to try to combat the low blood count they had discovered she had because of a rare blood disease called Diamond Blackfan anaemia. I had enough battles to win ahead of me.

I discovered that a suggested allergy to wheat could be her problem. We discovered that in fact her blood count went up when she didn't eat wheat or other wheat gluten products. It took me three years to finally wean her off steroids. She's now a healthy young lady, though.

My second daughter, Kate, was born in February 1988. I made contact with Michel Odent, who was living in London then. I wanted to try again for a home birth and he agreed to help and support me.

The first sign of labour was a gush of amniotic fluid, as before...

The first sign of labour was a gush of amniotic fluid, as before. This was at 8.30pm. The real labour pains came at 10.30pm. Kate was born on my bed at 2.30am after four hours of labour. It was painful and I was glad to be on my own in the dark of my bedroom. My husband and Michel Odent were there but kept out of the way and didn't interfere.

At the last moment Michel Odent came over and helped, while my husband supported me under the arms as I gave birth in a supported squat position. She weighed 7lb 2oz. I held Kate immediately and put her to my breast. About half an hour later the afterbirth was expelled naturally.

I was in shock for the first half hour after Kate's birth and was shivering—but that is apparently normal—so we turned on the electric fan heater. Kate did not cry when she was born. She lay on my thighs—skin-to-skin—for a long time, contentedly looking around in the half light. I breastfed Kate exclusively (no solids) until she was 6-8 months old. I didn't have my first period until she was 18 months old and carried on feeding her until two months before my third child was born, when she was 2 years 4 months.

My son Adam was born in August 1990. I had put on more weight with this pregnancy than before. He was overdue by a week or so. We had visitors—relatives—staying in our home at the time. The night that the guests went to spend one night away my labour started at 10.30pm. It was a long and hard labour—six hours. The second stage only really started when I forced myself to get up into a squatting position. Michel Odent, who had been outside the room listening to the progress of my labour, came in as I was starting to push. He helped to deliver Adam's shoulders. He later said that his shoulders were broad—he was a bigger baby than the others: 8lb 4oz. I recovered quickly again and breastfed him until my second son (my fourth child) Jake was born in October '92.

Jake was four weeks' overdue. My labour started at 8.30pm and he was born at 10.30pm. I wanted to try a water birth so I was in my extra large bath with lots of lavender oil when the midwife arrived at 9.30pm. (Michel Odent was not in the country at the time.) She didn't think that I was in real labour as I seemed so calm in the water. When I got out of the bath to call her from my bedroom she was surprised. Jake was born on the floor of the bathroom, my husband again helping to support me in a squat position.

I had no tears, he didn't look overdue and weighed 7lb 14oz. I breastfed him till he was over 3. I felt very emotional when I tried to stop. He was my last baby. He's now 9!

Christina from the UK

Although it's possible to write off the ease of Christina's second, third and fourth births (putting it down to 'luck'), it's equally plausible to suggest that the behaviour of her caregivers may have had an influence on the types of labours and births she experienced. The behaviour of professionals is a critical element in any scenario because midwives and obstetricians (not to mention GPs) can obviously do a great deal to influence how a woman feels about herself and, critically, whether or not she feels like a patient or a powerful woman, giving birth. Clearly, the first time Christina thought she was going into labour she very quickly felt disempowered and fearful. The disempowerment which many women feel during their labours often occurs gradually and unexpectedly, as happened with Christina.

There are many cases where the approach taken to caring for a woman is open to discussion or even dispute. Although each of Christina's first two labours began in exactly the same way, the care provided was entirely different. Christina herself certainly felt that the intervention in her first labour was inappropriate and unhelpful. (This is why I didn't include her surname or the real names of her children, although she did supply these to me.)

Here's a list of interventions which some professionals might consider to have been unhelpful and inappropriate:

1. **The internal examination** Bearing in mind that the main risk was of an infection developing, this may have been inadvisable because it increased that risk. Christina could have checked herself for infection by taking her own temperature every hour.

2. **Transferring Christina to hospital** Again, a hospital is a place which is full of germs, so it could be argued that she would be safer from the risk of infection at home, where her body was at least used to the germs around. In addition, given the way most people associate hospitals with illness and emergencies, quite apart from the fact that it was an unfamiliar place, it's likely that transferring Christina to hospital made her fearful and tense. Since this would have prompted her body to produce adrenaline (which normally inhibits the production of oxytocin, the hormone needed for contractions to continue) it's not surprising that her labour stopped on admission to hospital. The doctor's negative behaviour towards Christina—she said 'He looked and acted very disdainfully towards me'—would have contributed towards Christina's anxiety.

3. **EFM** Wiring a woman up to a machine which produces a computer readout—and usually thereby immobilising her too—is a very effective way of making a normal person immediately feel like a 'patient'. Since routine use of EFM on admission to hospital has only ever been associated with a rise in the caesarean rate in all research studies (with no improvement in outcomes), there are more arguments against its use than for it.

4. **Sweeping the cervix** This would again have increased Christina's risk of infection. As an artificial method for inducing (or augmenting) labour contractions it also carries with it all the risks and disadvantages of induction, i.e. it often starts off what many have called 'the cascade of interventions'. This is simply because it is unlikely to be completely effective, so further interventions (to augment labour further) are highly likely to be necessary.

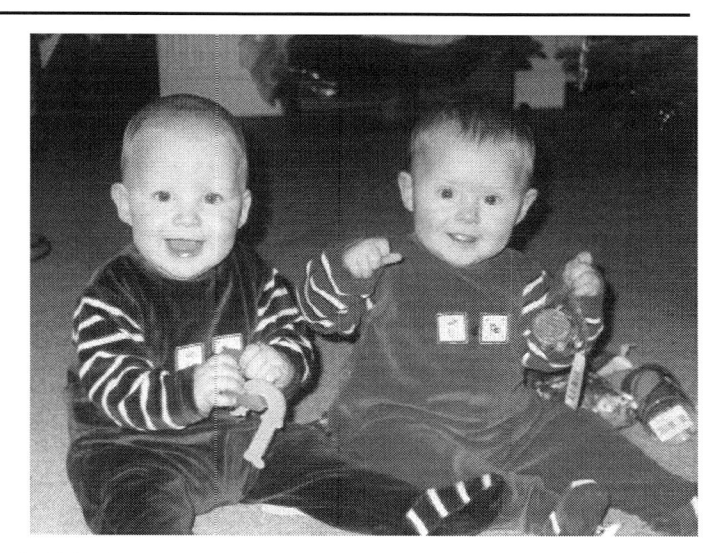

Debbie Brindley's twins Faye and Joe when they were 8 months old [see Birthframe 11]

Do some midwives intervene out of fear? What if the woman refuses treatment?

5. **Syntocinon** Putting Christina on a drip must have confirmed her feeling of being a 'patient' because it implied that she was in need of artificial treatment. In other words, whether or not it was necessary, putting Christina on a drip must have communicated to her nonverbally that her bodily functions were ineffective. This would have accentuated any fear she felt, along with her feeling of disempowerment. In addition, the drip will have increased her risk of developing an infection.

6. **Imposing a time limit** Protocols vary widely, being based on different views. In any case, since the risk was related to an infection developing, checking for this—rather than imposing an arbitrary limit—may have given Christina the extra time she needed to be able to give birth vaginally.

7. **Continuous monitoring throughout labour and birth** Of course, this—as opposed to intermittent, discrete monitoring—became necessary after the initial interventions because they *increased* the level of risk. The use of artificial oxytocics to augment labour makes monitoring particularly necessary because of the unpredictability of effects on any particular woman.

8. **The caesarean** If a different approach had been taken—either because of a different professional attitude or because of the 'patient' actually *refusing* treatment—the caesarean might not have been necessary. Giving a woman a c-section for the birth of her first baby increases her risk of infertility (so may mean she can have no more children); it also inevitably makes any subsequent pregnancy, labour and birth higher risk because if a vaginal birth is countenanced it would necessarily be a VBAC, rather than a straightforward second birth. Given Christina's comments about her feelings on her first daughter's birthday, it's clear that performing a caesarean on a woman the first time she goes into labour may also change the psychological landscape if she gets pregnant again afterwards.

But do you really want an empowered woman?

A woman who felt empowered by the processes going on around her might well have refused any, or even all, of these interventions. This would have been a particular 'risk' if she had been well-informed. Is this really want you want, as a professional?

Firstly, it's important to say that having empowered women around, giving birth, isn't such a bad thing. If you know that the woman you are caring for is having a 'real' experience of childbirth which is likely to result in less pain for her and her baby overall, surely you would be happy? If you know that the woman's choices, even if a little inconvenient are in line with research and are likely to ensure safer outcomes for both herself and her baby, surely again you can't feel bad about those choices?

Secondly, it must be said that the role of a midwife should really be to support a woman in her choices. When I asked an experienced midwife if she felt it was irresponsible for a woman to refuse treatment she replied:

> It's not exactly irresponsible as I do not believe woman will put their babies at risk. I think they know their bodies and we have to work with them and support them if they go against medical or NICE guidance and not threaten them or bully them into doing what they feel is not right for them or their unborn child. Most women are sensible and some make decisions that the medical and some of the midwifery profession don't agree with but it is the midwives' role to support and give care whatever the choices are that the woman makes. However, it is important that the midwife explains any potential risk in a reassuring, accurate and professional way.

As a researcher who has been impressed by the complexity of the natural processes, I personally feel that refusing interventions in cases where there is a choice is in no way irresponsible. In fact, it is the opposite because it is respecting something which is enormously complex and easily disturbed. (We'll come back to this point very soon.)

As an author who has read material from literally hundreds of women, and interviewed many more, I feel sure that refusing pain relief or treatments to apparently ease pain is also wise because it means that women are likely to experience less pain overall, if postnatal pain is also taken into account. Physical and emotional damage caused by episiotomies, forceps bruising and damage, caesareans, catheterisation and disappearing babies (who are whisked away 'for observation' or treatment), can last for years. When breastfeeding proves to be difficult or even impossible because of drug use or disturbance of hormones during the intrapartum period I can't see that the pain relief used provides any overall advantage. (The woman may have saved five hours' worth of pain in order to create six weeks' worth.) We need to remember the advantages for women of full alertness, privacy and dignity, as well as a naturally balanced hormonal scenario, as they meet their new babies.

As a mother who has asserted herself—even when feeling extremely disempowered!—I have experienced first-hand the empowerment that results from an entirely optimal, i.e. physiological birth.

Refusing interventions when there is a choice is respecting a process which is enormously complex and easily disturbed

Birthframe 19

You see, I had a problem similar to Christina's…

> At 38 weeks in my second pregnancy I had a leak of something and I also had the flu. Naturally, I phoned my doctor because I wanted to be checked out. He said it was probably amniotic fluid and that I should go to hospital immediately. I asked him what would be done there. Firstly, he said, a few cells would be scraped from around my cervix to confirm whether or not the leak had been amniotic fluid. After that, I would probably be induced because I was, after all, at 'term'.
>
> Knowing that an internal examination would increase my risk of infection (which is the main danger after a leak of amniotic fluid) I said I would rather not go in. The doctor repeated his instruction to me five times and five times I refused! (A letter followed in the post the next day suggesting he wanted to strike me off his list but a well-considered reply from me managed to persuade him against this.)
>
> That afternoon and evening I searched through my pregnancy books. I also phoned an independent midwife as well as Michel himself, who happened to be at home. (Most of the time Michel is travelling round the world lecturing at conferences or setting up research projects. I was lucky that my due date occurred in his Christmas holidays.)
>
> Both the midwife and Michel said the leak could well have been urine—I did, after all have a bad cough so it could have been 'stress incontinence'—or it could have been a leak of hindwaters, which would 'heal' up. I was told one option was to keep taking my temperature to check it didn't rise dangerously and indicate an infection. Both Michel and the midwife agreed my risk of infection would increase if I went into hospital and had an internal examination.
>
> **I refused to be admitted to hospital**
>
> Two and a half weeks later, after recovering from the flu and after attending my Master's graduation ceremony—looking extremely large!—I had a very straightforward two-hour labour. Nina-Jay, my second daughter, was—and still is!—beautiful and very healthy.

When intervention is inappropriate, it's as if midwives (or obstetricians) are intervening out of fear and a desire to control. Or is it just that they're intervening because they want to get women through their births—this 'awful experience'—as fast as possible, with as little (visible) pain as possible? Whatever the reasons for *inappropriate* intervention, unhelpful interference in birthing processes (which are very delicate) often results in more problems and more risk. This is particularly the case when artificial hormones or interventions are used for induction and augmentation of labour, and when drugs are used for pain relief (either analgesia or anaesthesia) because further interventions later become necessary, and of course, more pain may well be experienced postnatally as a result. In any case, these interventions disturb what's going on already…

Reason No. 5:
THE NATURAL PROCESSES ARE SIMPLY TOO EASILY DISTURBED

It's very easy to underestimate the complexity of the physiological processes. I've already been through each stage of pregnancy, labour and birth but I haven't yet described the hormonal landscape while all these processes are taking place. It's quite incredible...

The hormonal cocktail of pregnancy

The first hormone noticed in pregnancy tests is, of course, human chorionic gonadotropin (hCG). Progesterone, which is initially produced by the ovaries (stimulated to do so by hCG) and later by the placenta, will already have prepared the womb for pregnancy by stimulating the uterine lining to thicken (so that the fertilised egg can implant itself).

Progesterone also has the important functions of stopping the uterine muscles from contracting, thus allowing the fetus to grow undisturbed, and of stopping lactation from beginning until after the birth. It also protects the placenta by fighting off unwanted cells and strengthens the mucous plug, thereby preventing infection.

Fetal growth and maternal breast development, is supported by another hormone called human placental lactogen (HPL) and this hormone also has the important job of ensuring that the mother doesn't absorb too much glucose. Oestrogen, a group of hormones, is also vital and is thought to trigger the maturation of fetal lungs, kidneys, liver and adrenal glands, the production of prolactin, which prepares the woman for breastfeeding, and to regulate bone density in the fetus—amongst other things.

Other hormones—calcitonin, thyroxine, insulin, relaxin, cortisol and erythropoietin also play their key roles. Oxytocin has a key role in pregnancy too, although is 'drowned out' by progesterone until the woman goes into labour. However, as well as stimulating the mammary glands to produce milk, it enhances nutrient absorption and helps the woman conserve her energy by making her sleepy!

The hormonally-triggered switchover to 'instinctual'

According to research, since the hormones of birth are produced mainly in the 'middle' brain (sometimes called the 'mammalian' brain or limbic system), an important switchover needs to take place sometime in the early stages of labour. Instead of being controlled by the neocortex (which makes us rational beings), as is normally the case, the woman must suddenly surrender control to this more primitive part of the brain. Hormones which she spontaneously produces will allow her to effect this important switchover.

Interestingly, these hormones (which allow a woman to experience labour as positive and even enjoyable) also trigger appropriate mothering behaviour after the baby is born, so they have two important purposes. What's more, beta-endorphins, which are produced during pregnancy, begin to be produced at much higher levels, along with CRH (another hormone produced in stressful situations) at this stage. Rising levels of beta-endorphins now and during labour, which peak at birth and subside one to three days after the birth, help the mother to cope with pain and perhaps even experience it as positive. And they also help her to get into an appropriate instinctual state of mind...

The hormones of labour and birth

Despite all we that we know about birth, it is still not known precisely what triggers the onset of labour, but both oestrogen and progesterone are thought to play a part, perhaps because of their changing ratios. Of course, oestrogen is the main hormone which prepares the uterus for the contractions of labour and both hormones also serve the important function of activating the woman's natural opiate-producing mechanisms which operate in the brain and the spinal cord.

Produced in the hypothalamus and released into the bloodstream in a pulsatile manner, oxytocin is associated with positive emotions and sensations. Often called 'the hormone of love', it is produced during orgasm, birth itself, breastfeeding and also in social situations such as eating with other people. (Interestingly, perhaps, the baby produces this hormone as well as the birthing woman and even the placenta, so he or she is swimming in oxytocin-flavoured amniotic fluid! Because of this strange fetal hormonal production at the onset of labour some researchers have suggested that the baby may be responsible for triggering the onset of labour.) Wherever it comes from (i.e. baby, mother or placenta), while oxytocin is thought to be the main initiator of rhythmic contractions, some researchers have hypothesized that prostaglandins assume this same role later on in labour. Interestingly, oxtytocin has been shown to relieve pain in pregnant rats and mice.

Oxytocin is responsible not only for the contractions which open up the labouring woman's cervix, but also for those which push the baby down and out of her body and for the contractions which make her uterus contract back to its pre-pregnancy size postpartum. Intriguingly, though, and something interesting occurs just before the moment of birth in the case of a woman who has been completely undisturbed while in labour. Catecholamines—the fight-or-flight hormones adrenaline and noradrenaline, along with dopamine—are produced alongside oxytocin. (These hormones are usually antagonistic, but they aren't when they are produced spontaneously and smoothly in labour.) Instead of stimulating the body to fight or flee (as they usually do), just seconds before the birth these hormones activate what some researchers (particularly Michel Odent) have called the 'fetus ejection reflex'. From the labouring woman's point of view, there is a rush of energy which makes her want to stand up and perhaps also grab hold of something. (Any birth attendants, including a much-loved midwife, might be abused or shouted at around this time! Frequently, the woman expresses intense fear, anger or resentment.) And then she flicks her hips forward and gives birth! The intense, highly efficient contractions stimulated by the high levels of oxytocin combine with these catecholamines to produce the perfect cocktail for birth. As for the baby, the sudden surge of catecholamines (especially noradrenaline) has a beneficial effect because it protects him or her from the effects of oxygen deprivation, helps metabolistic processes and temperature regulation and improves respiration—which will come in handy outside the womb, in the big wide world.

The newborn helps the mother...

Hormonal production shortly after the birth

Postpartum uterine contractions are made possible because the newborn baby helps the mother to continue producing oxytocin. His or her stroking, licking or sucking actions, alongside skin-to-skin and eye contact, trigger a loving response in the mother, which results in continued hormonal production. Most importantly, perhaps, all this pleasant 'bonding' which facilitates efficient uterine contraction has a safety function because it prevents a woman from suffering from a postpartum haemorrhage. (On this point, though, it's important to remember the role of catecholamines. While they were useful at the point of birth, their usefulness disappears straight afterwards. If levels do not drop—which is likely to occur if the new mother feels cold—oxytocin production will be inhibited, which will obviously increase the risk of PPH. When they do drop, although it's positive in terms of safety, the mother typically feels shaky or cold.

Research has found that oxytocin levels in the mother peak when the placenta is born and then subside over the next hour. Levels of oxytocin in the newborn baby peak around 30 minutes after the birth, but are still high for at least four days after the birth. This generally means that both mother and newborn baby enjoy the pleasant effects of oxytocin in the first hour after the birth and afterwards.

High catecholamine levels at the moment of birth also cause extreme alertness in the baby. Levels typically remain high for around 12 hours, then subside so a much-needed rest is possible.

Noradrenalin, another hormone which is produced spontaneously at this time, is thought to promote mothering behaviour because mice who were bred to be deficient in this didn't care for their young unless they had an artificial injection of the hormone. (It's interesting to note that smell probably also plays a key role in early mothering behaviour. One research study discovered that monkeys who were given caesareans rejected their babies unless the newborns were swabbed with secretions from the mother monkey's vagina.) Prolactin, the main hormone stimulating breast-feeding, also causes mothering behaviour, as well as an increase in appetite (in the mother), suppression of fertility and changes in sleep cycles (which suddenly include more REM sleep), amongst other things. Of course, these changes support the new mother's abrupt shift in lifestyle, which is bound to include a need for a focus on the newborn baby (even in sleep), to the detriment of the mother's own needs.

Finally, it's interesting to note that the beta-endorphins which began rising at the onset of labour continue to play an important role in the mother-infant breastfeeding relationship. With their ability to induce feelings of pleasure and dependency, they usefully help to cement the mother-baby bond. Since they peak approximately 20 minutes after a woman starts breastfeeding at any one time, they continue to enhance the mother-infant relationship long after the birth took place.

Given the extremely high complexity of these processes—which it must be remembered only take place like this in a completely undisturbed labour and birth—it's easy to see how easy it might be to cause a disturbance.

Birthframe 20

In her first labour, Liliana—the doula we met earlier in this book— experienced the effects of having a lot of people watching while she was at the pushing stage. (One doctor and ten students were watching!) This made her decide to avoid hospitals for any future births. With her first birth, the atmosphere of the hospital, the insensitivity of the people, the monitoring—all constituting an atmosphere of feeling very 'observed'—clearly stopped her labour from progressing. The psychological aspect of giving birth is very clear from her three subsequent births. Here, we see how positive birth experiences can be when there is no disturbance from outside.

> When expecting my first child, I registered in a London hospital, as the most natural thing to do... I was born in hospital... and my mother too! It was 1983, I arrived smiling and I was told, after an internal, that I was 8cm. One hour later I found myself in a labour ward, surrounded by ten students, a male doctor and a midwife, and a monstrous fetal monitoring machine was attached to me and sounding very loud. Bright lights, voices everywhere, people coming in and out, my partner at my right... I was soon in a state of shock. Labour almost came to an end. Epidural, episiotomy and a very light and unnecessary forceps followed. "Never again", "Never again", I kept repeating to myself, while holding my baby daughter.

After dinner I rushed into a dark room

> In 1987 I was expecting for the second time. I kept well away from doctors, hospitals and all their machinery. I was feeling wonderful—I knew my baby was well. I wanted to stay at home this time. A friend of mine mentioned Michel Odent... I read a bit about him... "Yes, he will understand me." He did. I had the most beautiful, undisturbed birth one can possibly imagine. Another daughter.
>
> And two years later my son was born. Big boy, 9lb 8oz. Born between lunch and pudding! Literally. I was so lucky to be assisted by Michel Odent again.
>
> I was in labour, but very hungry, to everyone's surprise. I had a big lunch and then, when the cake I had baked that morning was approaching the kitchen table, I stood up suddenly and with an unusually loud voice said, "No pudding. The baby's coming!"—and turning to my partner: "Do the washing up." After this, I rushed into a dark room I had prepared, went on my knees, on the floor, burying my head in pillows.
>
> One and a half hours later I was lying down on the floor, my baby on my chest, both warmly wrapped, the cord not yet cut... and eating the cake! (This child is now 17 and has always had an incredible appetite.)
>
> My fourth child was born at dawn, in a friend's sitting room, at a time when I could only hear the birds singing... and Michel Odent gently sleeping at the other end of the room. It was so magical, sweet, beautiful. My baby girl found the breast in minutes!

It was so magical, sweet, beautiful

Liliana Lammers

Birthframe 21

It's easy from many people's experience to get the impression that home births are always better for optimising birth. As the next account shows, how things are done at home is just as important as where a birth takes place. Disturbing the natural processes by disturbing the woman's sense of security, privacy and confidence can have dramatic consequences whether the woman is at home or in hospital. Of course, as this account illustrates, continuity of care is sometimes crucial.

For the birth of my sixth child, Finn, I had decided on a home delivery for a combination of reasons. The previous five births had been straightforward and progressively quicker and on a practical level it meant not having to worry about where the other children went. The main reason, however, was that by No.6 I had gained the confidence in and awareness of my body and its instincts to want to be left to labour on my own, with as little interference as possible. The birth went beautifully, with the help of some very supportive midwives, who had given me wonderful continuity of care from the start of pregnancy. This is something I'm sure gave me added reassurance and confidence during the birth. Finn is now a very happy and easy-going four-year-old and I am sure that the peaceful atmosphere into which he was born is responsible.

When I discovered I was expecting No.7 (Joseph) I decided to opt for a home delivery again. The pregnancy proceeded uneventfully and despite the baby lying in a slightly awkward posterior position in the last few weeks, everything signalled another hopefully quick and straightforward birth. Ten days overdue, and after a false alarm (contractions caused by the baby turning into an anterior position), labour began at six in the morning. As before, I kept upright and moving, walking around the house and dealing with the contractions as well as the children's demands for breakfast.

By 8am the 'on-call' midwife arrived. On examination I was almost fully dilated and she prepared for the imminent delivery. At this point the 'day shift' community midwives (plus student) arrived to take over. I was surprised, given the stage of labour, that the on-call team didn't stay to see the birth through to delivery. So at transition I had six people—midwives, students and my husband—in the bedroom, all filling in charts and forms or talking in corners and, most disconcertingly, giving each other glances of concern and borderline panic whilst telling me how well I was doing. I paced around them trying to deal with the contractions and not get in their way. Other visitors into the busy bedroom included two of the older children, who were getting ready for school and needed to know where their P.E. kits were. By now, I was beginning to feel the first sensation of pressure from the baby's head and was told by one midwife to push if I wanted to.

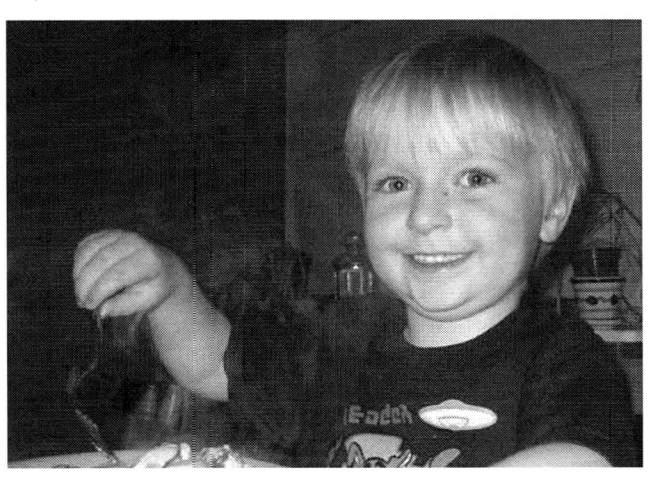

Finn, aged 4

At transition I had six people with me

When, half an hour or so later there was still no sign of the baby's head, an examination revealed that the cervix had swollen, preventing the baby from descending. I was told I would have to allow the swelling to reduce by resisting the pushing urge, possibly for up to two hours. Fighting against my body's overwhelming instinctive urge to push out the baby and the powerful contractions doing exactly that became—after 20 minutes or so of trying—an impossibility. An epidural was suggested to reduce the pushing urge and help with the pain, but this would mean transferring to hospital to have the epidural administered. By now, the pain of resisting pushing was excruciating even with gas and air, which I had gratefully used for the previous 20 minutes. I agreed, and the midwives called an ambulance, which rushed me into hospital. My husband followed the ambulance in our car and just as he arrived to join me in the delivery room Joseph's head was born with a huge contraction over which I had no control. His shoulder then got slightly stuck but with the midwife pushing me into an almost yoga-like position—bringing my feet up towards my shoulders, while I lay on my back—he slipped out and, despite his shock entry into the world, was fine and didn't need any resuscitation.

Other visitors to the busy bedroom included two children getting ready for school asking where their PE kits were

Although the birth was not what I had expected, it worked out for the best. Strangely, the noisiest and busiest part of the delivery was at home. It is possible that being distracted by so much activity at a crucial stage in the labour and losing the control that up to then I had had and had always maintained during previous labours, had an adverse effect. Being told to push before my body was ready may have caused the swelling and the resulting battle with my body, and loss of control over what it was doing led to extreme pain and complications. However, being alone with Joseph in the delivery room after his birth was calm and peaceful. We had a few hours alone—uninterrupted, quiet and warm. I lay back and held him and we were both awake but able to recover from the trauma of the birth and rest together, something I'm sure I would not have been able to do at home with Joseph's brothers and sisters desperate to see and hold him.

Sometimes, hospital births can be peaceful and home births quite chaotic! I think this experience taught me that where the birth takes place is less important than how the mother is treated. Too much well-meaning advice, monitoring, admin, instruction and activity can interfere with the mother's control of the labour and result in more pain and unnecessary intervention, whether it occurs at home or in hospital. Being left to follow her natural instincts and urges in a calm atmosphere can only be beneficial for the mother and child.

Clare O'Ryan

Reason No. 6: INTERVENTION IS AN UNCONTROLLED EXPERIMENT

Experimentation has become the standard approach over the last few centuries, despite the likelihood that any intervention is likely to disturb the physiological processes. Experimental procedures have become routine before research has confirmed they are safe or even helpful. How has this situation developed?

From the birth of time...

Hundreds (and thousands) of years ago interventions were initiated when women or babies were in difficulty. Perhaps it seemed likely the mother was about to die in labour; sometimes the fetus was already known to be dead; sometimes it seemed to be having difficulty getting itself born. Anthropological data (collected by Sheila Kitzinger, Jacqueline Vincent Priya and others) make it clear that other non-life-saving interventions were also common and very culture-specific. They came about as a result of certain beliefs, which were often not based on any facts. These beliefs affected the ways in which birth was facilitated or unintentionally hindered. For example, women may have been isolated or, alternatively, surrounded by people, perhaps given a shock or kept away from all stress and there was often the belief that the pre-milk 'colostrum' was bad for the baby. (Of course, research has now shown us how wonderfully beneficial it is.) Finally, interventions became necessary as a result of the use of pain relief, which usually created problems which then needed to be dealt with.

1800-1900

Intervention was clearly advocated by certain doctors as soon as they started taking over from midwives as the usual birth attendants. One midwife's diary suggests that doctors were already using laudanum for pain relief or anaesthesia. A range of folklore methods had been employed over the centuries, but specific efforts to develop pain relief for labouring women were now being made. It is unclear when opiates began to be used, but they were probably already in use in the early 1800s. Ether (diethyl ether, to be precise) seems to have been first used in January 1847 in Edinburgh, and in April or May of the same year in America.

> In the 1920s in Britain many women died because of haemorrhage or sepsis

By the late 1800s, routine intervention had become commonplace in some American hospitals. For example, at one hospital in Philadelphia it was routine to administer quinine (because it induces uterine contractions), as well as drugs for constipation, sleeplessness and headaches; at the onset of labour women were given an enema and bath, the amniotic sac was ruptured, and at birth forceps were applied; the third stage was helped along by the use of ergot (ostensibly so as to minimise blood loss) with the attendant pressing down on the woman's abdomen.

The 1900s and 1910s

By the early 1900s in both Britain and America, midwives were losing their power, partly because they were becoming associated with uneducated, illiterate women. (First hand experience was seen as being inferior to the institutionalised study of obstetrics, which meant that educated, wealthier women tended to avoid midwives.) In 1902 in the UK the Midwives Act effectively institutionalised a subservient role of midwives to physicians. Up until the 1920s, maternal mortality was still a major problem since 1 in 250 women died in childbirth. According to *Obstetrics by Ten Teachers* (Hodder Arnold 2000), this was because the modern pharmacological treatments for postpartum haemorrhage and sepsis (which killed most women) were unavailable. Research was being conducted in Germany in the early 1910s into new forms of pain relief. The result—a mixture of morphine and scopolamine, which induced a condition known as 'twilight sleep', followed by the use of ether or chloroform—was so exciting to one group of American women that they actively promoted it.

Below: The use of medicines was highly experimental in the past. Here is a photo of the apothecary at the Black Country living museum in Dudley.

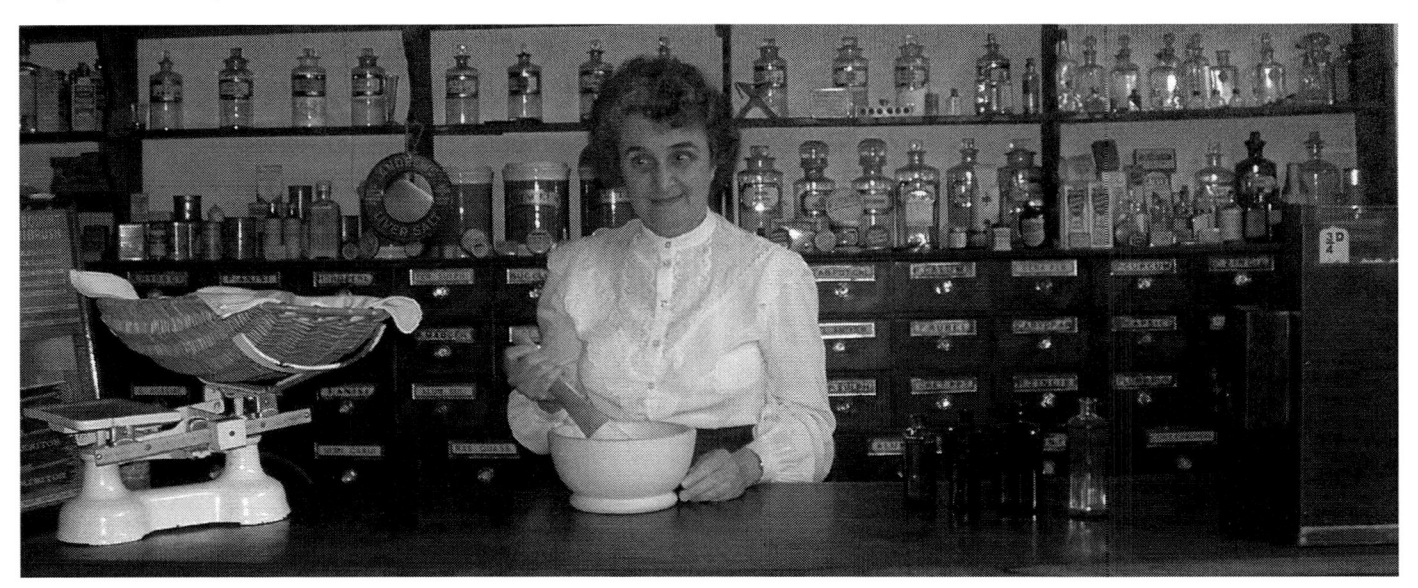

The 1920s and 1930s

In 1920, an American professor of obstetrics, Joseph DeLee—a popular speaker, textbook writer and the inventor or modifier of many obstetric tools—gave a seminal speech to fellow obstetricians, recommending that forceps and episiotomy be routine for every birth, that women should be sedated, that ether should be administered as soon as the fetus entered the birth canal and that ergot or a similar drug should be used to speed up delivery of the placenta. These practices, known as 'prophylactic obstetrics', soon became routine in most US hospitals. From 1928 onwards active steps were taken in the UK to reduce risks through better education, although antenatal care itself was a fairly haphazard process until the 1940s, undertaken only by GPs. In 1937 the antibiotics sulphonamides were discovered and penicillin came soon after. These discoveries quickly reduced the rates of puerperal sepsis.

The 1940s

Before WWII more than 90% of women in the UK gave birth at home under the care of a midwife, and only occasionally with a GP in attendance as well. The increased experimentation with different forms of pain relief from the 1940s onwards meant that hospitalised childbirth became preferable from both a choice and a safety point of view—since more was likely to go wrong when drugs and other interventions were involved. At that time, morphine was widely used, often alongside other drugs. In the US, it was usually used while women were in 'twilight sleep'. In France the morphine was part of a mixture called 'spasmalgine'. In the UK, ether and chloroform were still widely used. It was in this decade that the so-called 'natural childbirth movement' developed in the USA and with it the concept of the husband as 'labour coach'. It was also the time when blood transfusions became safe and when it was discovered that ergometrine could treat and prevent postpartum haemorrhage.

The 1950s

Induction and augmentation of labour now became more of a focus so intramuscular injections of oxytocin became popular, used alongside different painkillers. Since the effects of intramuscular oxytocin were uncontrollable (because nothing can be done after an injection), IV (intravenous) drips soon became common. With a drip in place, if the effect of the oxytocin already administered was too strong and therefore dangerous (i.e. causing too intense and continuous uterine contractions) it was possible to slow down or stop the drip altogether. It was in fact during this decade that IVs became safe because the original rubber tubes—which often caused intense allergic reactions—were replaced by plastic tubes. It was also the time when the vacuum extractor (ventouse) was invented in Sweden. This device appeared to present a good alternative to forceps, which had been in use since the sixteenth century because it seemed to offer less trauma to both mother and baby. Ultrasound scanning was also first adapted for obstetric use in the late 1950s. By the late 1970s and 80s it had become available in most hospitals. Techniques and treatments which we now take for granted (relating to anaesthesiology, antibiotics and blood transfusion) were also further developed.

The 1960s

In the 1960s drips of oxytocin continued to be used widely as a means of inducing and augmenting labour. The main painkiller used was pethidine (a synthetic morphine known as Demerol in the US and Dolosal in France). The caesarean operation, which had until this time been unpopular, suddenly became more appealing to women, thanks to the new use of the 'bikini line' incision (instead of the vertical incision which had been used until then), which was originally proposed by Muro-Kerr in the 1920s. This technique, which was developed in the 1950s, now became widely used, not only because of its increased popularity with women but also because surgically trained obstetricians were now available.

The 1970s

The fast development of electronic fetal monitoring (first invented in 1957) radically changed the atmosphere of delivery rooms. Caesarean rates started to increase dramatically, partly because of this use of electronic fetal monitoring (EFM). Drips of oxytocin and pethidine were still used. The growing public confidence in the technology and pain relief options offered by hospitals resulted in a rapid increase in the number of births taking place in hospital. In the UK between 1960 and 1979 the use of pain relief increased from 25% to 99%. (Thanks to awareness of risks associated with pain management, there has since been a drop in the number of women using analgesics or anaesthesia.)

The 1980s and 1990s

In the 1980s the conventional technique of epidural anaesthesia became available in large departments of obstetrics. So as to facilitate the administration of epidurals, which many women saw as extremely appealing, large well-equipped maternity units were built in the 1990s. Size mattered because it was only economics of scale that made it possible to provide anaesthetists and paediatricians 24 hours a day. Routines and protocols to support the large numbers of interventions now carried out had become commonplace. The injection of an oxytocic agent for the delivery of the placenta had also become routine and women wanting a physiological third stage were often seen as being unusual. Episiotomy was also still routine in many hospitals, although research has now discredited it.

How much takes place now?

In the 21st century there seems to be the implicit assumption that intervention only takes place to save lives. This is far from true since the use of pain relief still constitutes one of the main forms of intervention in modern childbirth and, as we've already mentioned, pain relief usually necessitates other forms of intervention. Here's a brief summary of practices which are still common in some parts of the world, looking at what takes place before any one pregnancy and birth, during it and afterwards. It's necessary to take this broad view because interventions taken at any stage can affect what occurs later on. I've taken an international perspective because we do, of course, live in a very multi-cultural society, with plenty of movement from country to country.

Before the Birth

Many women experience intervention before pregnancy or during pregnancy. This may affect the health of their baby and how successful they can be in giving birth.

Before a woman becomes pregnant numerous old interventions might influence her ability to give birth and her baby's ability to get itself born easily, safely and smoothly. Episiotomies performed in previous labours which have not healed well, old forceps trauma and abortion injuries (especially those inflicted by unqualified surgeons) can all affect a woman's muscular control and comfort when subsequently giving birth. Circumcision (also called 'incision' and 'infibulations') is another practice which constitutes a pre-pregnancy intervention which can affect a woman's subsequent experiences. In the notes accompanying the novel *Possessing the Secret of Joy* (Walker 1993), it is reported that an estimated 90 to 100 million women and girls living today in African, Far Eastern and Middle Eastern countries have been genitally mutilated. The author also states that recent articles in the media have reported on the growing practice of 'female circumcision' in the United States and Europe among immigrants from countries where it is part of the culture. This means a significant number of women are embarking on pregnancy with a compromised physical starting point.

During pregnancy all kinds of screening and diagnostic tests are offered, as well as routine antenatal checks, which I regard as interventions because they must in some way affect either the woman or the baby. They include blood tests, repeated use of ultrasound with a Sonicaid or Doppler machine, maternal serum screening (the alpha-fetoprotein test, the triple screen test or the quad-screen test), ultrasound scans, chorionic villus sampling, nuchal translucency testing and amniocentesis.

There is an enormous amount of what we could call 'psychological intervention'

Psychological interventions might also have an influence either before or during any one particular pregnancy... After all, almost all women are seeing an enormous number of fear-inducing images relating to labour and birth on TV or in magazines and newspapers before they even become pregnant. Perhaps the negative images prevail because they are considered by planners to constitute more exciting viewing than the positive, natural alternatives, which many people wrongly associate with alternative lifestyles or primitive cultures. The prevailing fear of childbirth and tendency to leave responsibility to 'the professionals' mean that many women feel disempowered and incapable of giving birth successfully. A negative mindset is created well before women even begin to actively explore real-life facts and figures, or read about other women's experiences with a view to forming their own opinions. In other words, modern myths about pregnancy and childbirth often replace the reality in people's minds and create a psychological environment of fear and foreboding. (This is even true of midwives, unfortunately.) Antenatal appointments filled with fear-inducing 'routine checks' reinforce this negative mindset in the pregnant woman.

Interventions During Labour and Birth

In Britain, of 3,000 women in the UK who responded to the *Mother and Baby* magazine survey in 2002, 94% used some form of pain relief involving drugs. 24% of these respondents were induced. The caesarean rate varies enormously from 6 or 10% (amongst independent midwives) to 25% in some hospitals. According to the *Mother and Baby* survey, forceps are used in about 1 in 10 births. From my own experience I know that the use of syntometrine in the third stage of labour (to speed up delivery of the placenta) is usually routine.

In the US as many as 60-70% of women in the US have some sort of anaesthesia during birth (according to research conducted in 2005). Intervention of other kinds is also common. 'Listening to Mothers' (Maternity Center Association 2002), a recent US survey apparently carried out with great care, found more than a 99% intervention rate. The caesarean rate is generally reported as being around 25%.

The situation is similar in Australia. Sarah Buckley, a GP and researcher, sourcing her information from a 2001 report from the NCHS [Australian National Center for Health Statistics] reports that in the USA 19.8% of women have their labour induced and 17.9% have an augmentation with synthetic oxytocin (syntocinon or pitocin). She says that according to a 2001 report from the AIHW [Australian Institute of Health and Welfare] 25% of women in Australia have their labour induced and another 20% have an augmentation.

A survey in the UK in 2002 revealed that 94% of women used some kind of pain relief involving drugs

In Israel, according to Wendy Blumfield (author of *Life After Birth,* Element Books 1992), an estimated 30% of first-time mothers and 40% of multiparas opt to give birth without pain relief. (Of course, this means that 60-70% of women do use pain relief.) The induction rates are comparable. Episiotomies were routine for first births up to three years ago. Now they are done according to need. (In other countries, episiotomy is often still routine, but not everywhere.) In Israel, forceps are little used, but together with ventouse, are used in about 4% of births. This figure is increasing because of the increasing use of epidural anaesthesia, which gives women less control over the pushing stage of labour. Caesareans are performed in about 16% of births and are on the rise.

In most other countries—in particular in the developing world—health professionals are highly interventionist and pain relief is widely used. I was surprised to discover this to be true in both Sri Lanka and Oman when I was pregnant with my first and third babies. It seemed odd that so much intervention and so many drugs should be used in cultures which in many ways still seemed in tune with their cultural traditions. The Western model from a few decades ago is being copied, despite growing evidence that it is far from perfect. And I discovered that professionals in these countries often assert the 'need' to use these interventions even when research has clearly shown them to be harmful.

Here are specific practices which I see as interventions...

- **Induction or acceleration of labour by any means**
Both 'natural' and artificial means are sometimes used to induce or speed up labour. Friends, relatives and even care providers might suggest ingesting various substances (e.g. curries or cod liver oil), or they might encourage excessive exercise or laughter. Professionals try to intervene and trigger a woman's labour by administering prostaglandins (by pessary) or pitocin (intravenously); alternatively, they might break a woman's waters (i.e. perform an amniotomy) or 'sweep her membranes'—with or without her consent. When a labouring woman has an IV drip inserted in her arm, it is possible that syntocinon or pitocin may be added to the original glucose mixture to accelerate contractions; again, this might be done without the woman's consent.
- **Prepping** Hospitals and birthing centres always used to 'prepare' women for labour in some way, but now—hopefully—all or most of these routines have disappeared from most institutions. So-called preparation can include asking the woman to put on a hospital gown, shaving off her pubic hair, administering an enema, and setting up a drip ('just in case' it's needed later) or slipping in a heparin lock for the same reason. (A heparin lock is basically a small tube connected to a catheter, which is inserted into a vein in the arm so that an IV can later be quickly inserted.) All these practices constitute interventions because they can disturb the woman (by inhibiting her movements and perhaps by making her fearful) and consequently the processes going on within her.
- **Electronic fetal monitoring (EFM)** This is often part of the routine admission procedures so may be considered a type of 'prepping'. Whether it takes place for 20 minutes when the woman first arrives at hospital or at any other stage of labour or birth, EFM is certainly an intervention which immobilises the labouring woman either completely or partially. EFM may also encourage her to lie down (rather than lean forward, for example) and it's also likely to create a feeling of anxiety.
- **Dietary controls** Women are often told not to eat or drink during labour in case a general anaesthetic is required later. Stopping a woman from following her natural impulses interferes with her natural ability to regulate her intake of food and drink. Appropriate levels of hydration and the absence of ketones (which start being produced when a woman has not eaten for a while) are both important if labour is to progress well. In any case, research has not shown fasting to be helpful even when a general anaesthetic is used.
- **Directed activity** Women are often told to take a bath because it will 'help them relax'. (In fact, it's more likely to slow down contractions, which is unhelpful.) Women may also be encouraged to walk up and down hospital corridors or take a walk in the hospital grounds. Any time a woman is told to do something in this way, an intervention is taking place because the suggestion is likely to distract the woman from tuning in to her instinctual knowledge of how to labour and give birth. The only non-intrusive kind of 'direction' anyone could give a woman would be, "Do whatever you feel like doing." This would simply serve to remind the woman that she can be confident in her own ability to choose appropriate activities and physical positions.

> The nursing staff wanted me to stay on the trolley, to keep an eye on the monitors, but I put the equipment on a little table and got my mother to push them along while I walked up and down 'to the toilet'.

- **Physical constraint** Even when no EFM is used, women are often told to lie down or stop walking around, or their movements are constricted indirectly through the use of some other medical procedure. Even stopping a woman from making noises is a form of intervention because it is a way of stopping a woman from releasing tension in a way which might help the natural processes to progress. Obviously, insisting that a woman give birth with her legs in lithotomy stirrups is also a form of physical constraint and an intervention, because it makes it impossible for a woman to use her natural ability to find a physical position which is helpful for both herself and her baby. Left to her own devices, a woman is likely to want to work with gravity, rather than against it, so will usually spontaneously choose a standing, kneeling or squatting position. Many women who have given birth with their feet in stirrups have complained that it was difficult 'pushing uphill'.
- **Any communication verbal or non-verbal** People often fail to see the role of comments or eye contact in disturbing a woman who is in labour or actually giving birth. Because any comment or communication (including a glance or eye contact) can disturb the woman or distract her, it constitutes an intervention. Giving a woman instructions on how to push her baby out into the world is an obvious form of communicative intervention—but by no means the only one. Merely mentioning within earshot of a labouring woman that something negative or frightening might be necessary is a form of intervention, again because it is a way of disturbing the woman's state of mind as she moves through labour and birth. Negative or frightening possibilities which are often mentioned include breaking a woman's waters, using drugs for pain relief and the so-called 'probable' need for an episiotomy, forceps or a caesarean.

Gas and air is a common intervention

- **The use of analgesia or anaesthesia** The use of any drugs to alleviate pain constitutes an intervention.
- **Techniques for relieving pain** The use of any technique might disturb the normal course of a labour and birth, so must be considered an intervention. This includes breathing exercises, TENS machines, acupuncture, shiatsu, aromatherapy and any other complementary therapy.
- **The use of a fetal scalp electrode** This is often done in order to make the EFM more reliable—which is considered necessary because EFM has been widely reported in research studies to be ineffective.
- **Episiotomy** Obviously, cutting a woman's sexual parts while she is giving birth is an intervention.
- **The use of forceps or ventouse** Large metal 'salad tongs' are used to pull out a baby who appears to have got stuck. In the case of ventouse, a suction pad is attached to the baby's head and he or she is sucked out by a vacuum pump.

After the Birth

Only a few decades ago it was routine practice in hospitals around the world to put babies in a separate nursery from their new mothers, and it still is in some places. Nowadays, a lot of babies spend time in Intensive Care Units (ICUs). If the babies are premature, this intervention may well be life-saving and some full-term babies who are experiencing real difficulties may also need this kind of intensive care. Others who are transferred to ICUs may experience considerable distress unnecessarily. How many babies are affected by this kind of intervention? All premature babies and most multiples are, but in *Immaculate Deception II* (Celestial Arts 1996), Suzanne Arms implies that many singleton babies may also be affected. She writes: "Various studies show that between 15 and 25 percent of full-term, healthy babies born to healthy mothers are also spending days or weeks in intensive care units." Unfortunately, she doesn't refer us to any specific studies but we can at least guess that the percentage is still high in some hospitals around the world. Full-term healthy babies born to healthy mothers may be taken off to the ICU if there are any breathing difficulties at birth or if the mother's (and therefore the baby's) temperature is raised, because this could indicate the presence of an infection. The raised temperature is often the result of the mother using epidural anaesthesia and indicates no problem in the baby but because of the possibility of an infection, babies with a temperature at birth are given what is called a 'septic workup'. This involves repeated blood tests and one or more spinal taps, all of which could be painful and unpleasant for the baby. As with interventions occurring during pregnancy and labour, there is perhaps the tendency amongst health care professionals to over-test in order to be sure that no problems need dealing with. The long-term effects of separating mothers and babies are less of a focus and even humanistic supplementary treatment, such as kangaroo care is not used as widely as we might hope it to be.

Whether or not a baby has started life in an ICU, one other significant intervention which many babies are experiencing is bottle-feeding. Programmed to consider breastmilk their birthright, numerous babies are forced to consume formula made from cows' milk for the first few months of their lives. Despite the fact that almost all women would theoretically be able to breastfeed if they tried, many decide to use formula. The negative experience of friends, relatives and health professionals (who have often not breastfed themselves, or gave up early) as well as the 'scientific' look of formula make many feel they are succumbing to the inevitable. Aggressive promotional advertising by the major formula milk companies was widespread until very recently. Even without it, interventions which take place during labour and birth have an impact on the hormones a new mother does or doesn't produce as she is giving birth and therefore affect whether or not she will spontaneously breastfeed. Fortunately, worldwide awareness of the benefits of breastfeeding is triggering another kind of more positive intervention: various schemes and promotional campaigns are being set up worldwide to encourage mothers to breastfeed, even if they appear to have no desire to do so. This kind of intervention is necessary for mothers who have had a medicated birth because the natural processes have been so badly disturbed that they are unlikely to spontaneously put their newborn babies to their breast.

Finally, writers and researchers such as myself are trying to intervene to create a new awareness of childbirth in the 21st century. Some are angry mothers who have had bad experiences themselves; some are midwives who are disenchanted with practices and outcomes they have witnessed; some are researchers who have uncovered disturbing new data which put old practices into a new perspective.

How much intervention is needed?

How much intervention really is necessary from a health and safety point of view? How much of it is used because protocols are in place, because it is expected or because it impresses the client? How many lives are saved—or endangered—by all this intervention?

Of course, this is the $64 million dollar question. Nobody knows the answer. We have drifted so far away from the normal, undisturbed physiological processes of pregnancy, labour and birth that it's impossible to have a clear answer. We have never really allowed the natural processes to take place on a large scale within the safety net of our modern expertise and technology. Unfortunately, for psychological reasons as well as humanitarian ones, it would be impossible to conduct a randomised control trial.

There are indeed a small number of women who need the help of doctors when they conceive, gestate a baby or give birth. These are the women who—years ago—would have remained childless, who would have had dangerous pregnancies, who would have died in childbirth, or who would have given birth to dead babies. But the great majority of women would probably be better off without so much intervention... don't you think? It seems to me that too many procedures are over-used because of fear, misjudgement or inappropriate protocols. While I was researching this book, I often asked Michel how much intervention had really been necessary, in his opinion, in the case of particular births. We were usually in agreement as to the appropriateness (or otherwise) of intervention. However, all his comments are tempered by his overall view (which also coincides with my own) which he expressed in his book, *Birth and Breastfeeding* (Clairview Books 2007):

> Should the method of the mammals be inefficient in any particular instance, there must always be teams capable of doing epidurals to compensate for the lack of endorphins; to use drips to compensate for a deficiency of hormones from the posterior pituitary; and to perform caesarean sections to rescue babies in distress.

That brings us back to the concept of optimal birth... In other words, perhaps it's time to change the approach typically taken by care providers in modern birthing facilities. Normality, not pathology, must become the new focus. Non-invasive tests utilised to identify the tiny minority of women and babies who really do need intervention should be just that—non-invasive. They should not impinge on a pregnant woman's sense of well-being or undermine her confidence in her ability to give birth. Empowering the great majority of women and supporting them unobtrusively as they labour through a completely physiological birth should be the new aim. Only this shift in focus will enable women and babies to experience safe, life-enhancing births, which—many more people will come to realise—actually result in less pain overall, not more...

Reason No. 7:
OPTIMAL IS MORE BEAUTIFUL...

The dignity and experience of optimal birth

There is a quiet dignity to optimal birth—birth without any unnecessary drugs or interventions—which managed births simply do not appear to have. While the woman is in labour although she may appear to be wild and out of control—difficult *to* control, in fact!—she is certainly not a pathetic creature. Instead, as long as she feels secure and supported (by good, but undisturbing midwifery care—'watchful waiting'), there is a quiet, purposeful strength about her. When both the woman and the newborn baby are fully alert, they enjoy a much more beautiful start to their life together. Is this all not more beautiful than a woman who is drugged?

Here are some comments from a mother who experienced an undisturbed birth, Fiona Lucy Stoppard:

> The world is a wonderful place and there are some beautiful things. Lovely people. Nature. Art. Poetry and music. Writing. Friendships and love. But, basically, what I feel is that at the core of it all—the one real thing, the crux of it all—is pregnancy, labour and birth... and also breastfeeding and bonding. It's like the sun coming out. It really illuminates everything. I'm not saying that if a woman chooses not to have children, she can't have a wonderful life and do a lot—I don't mean that. But it's just that it's like everything else is pushed away, all these wonderful things. It's like the core of life. When women give birth without drugs, they're really connecting then. It's so subtle, what's going on, and drugs just spoil it. It's like some wonderful beautiful flower that's incredibly delicate and beautiful. It just can't be a production line. A production line's for making bread, for very practical things. This is just the absolute... it all needs to be treated with the greatest of care.
>
> I know there are all sorts of different things happening during pregnancy and labour. It would be wonderful if midwives could just look at a pregnant woman and know exactly what was going on and know just how to deal with it. But so often they say, "Oh, something's not right, we'd better induce you"—and maybe that might not have been the right thing at all. I know there are times when it is true the case is "Quick! Hospital! Get the baby out." Great, that's wonderful—you've got a beautiful baby, if that had to happen. But if the woman is healthy and it's a healthy pregnancy then you have to let the baby have the best possible experience. And it's not just the experience at the time, because it affects the future of the mother and the child.

It was actually too much to eat a mango

> I recently talked with a man who has been an anaesthesiologist for over 30 years at a medical centre in the USA. He has been at many, many births administering anaesthesia and has never seen a woman birth without medication. When I briefly described my experience, I could tell he just had no context for it. I think it's so totally different to see a woman birthing in an environment where she feels comfortable, has whatever support she needs, and is not medicated. He probably cannot even imagine the power that moves in the uninterfered-with birthing woman.

Birthframe 22

Lucy Stoppard's account beautifully captures the memory of 'going to another planet'... the process which allows women to tune into their instinctual knowledge of how to give birth. (See pp 24-28 for more on this.)

> My waters broke very, very early in the morning and then she wasn't born until after midnight. The labour was all that day—all morning, afternoon and evening—and she was born after midnight. So it was less than 24 hours. It was very slow for a long time. I phoned Michel and he said "Oh it's fine. It'll be all right. I'll come along later." I don't think I was having contractions then—only very slight ones. He came to see me, then he went home again. He was able to go backwards and forwards a little bit, although there was one point when he knew it was getting close and he said he'd stay.
>
> I don't know what I can remember of the labour—it was just very hard work. A lot of resting. Very hard work. Completely closed off from the rest of the world. I remember asking David once to get me a mango and he went out and bought me a mango which I didn't finish. It was actually too much to eat a mango because I had to concentrate. I went really deep, deep within. Quite spontaneously.
>
> And I remember that the next morning when I woke up I thought, "Oh, I'm here, back in the world again." I looked out of the window and people were doing normal, everyday things and I felt like saying, "Don't they realise what's just happened here?!"
>
> *Fiona Lucy Stoppard*

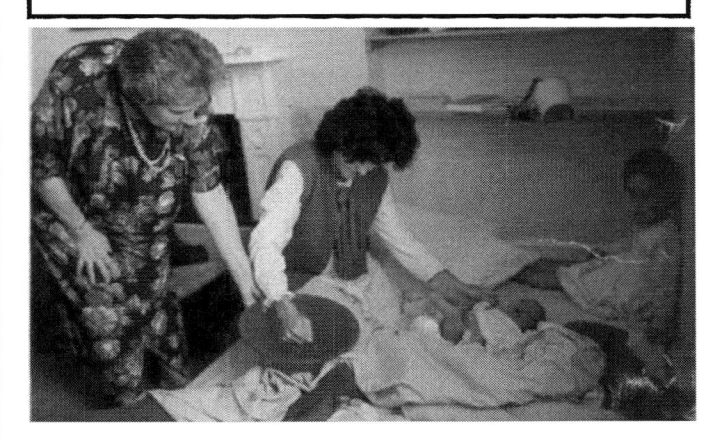

Liliana Lammers bathing her newborn baby [see Birthframe 9]

Birthframe 23

Here is an account to give us a little intuitive insight into the reasons for avoiding the alternatives to normal, physiological birth if at all possible. This account came in very late on while I was writing this book, with this note:

Dear Sylvie,

At last I have managed to find the report and your address at the same time! I am so sorry to have taken so long—I am really ashamed of myself! I do hope this will be of some use to you. I hadn't read it for some time and it really brought tears to my eyes. Rosie's birth really was a magical experience and I so much wish I could have repeated it.

Pauline

I sat down to write about the wonder of Rosie's birth at home, but felt it all started over two years ago with Sean's birth in hospital, which affected both myself and my family so much that we were determined our next baby's introduction to our world would be a happier and easier event. So, firstly, I am writing about the birth of Sean Henry on 17 October 1986.

> Sean's birth in hospital affected both myself and my family so much that we were determined our next baby's introduction to our world would be a happier and easier event

I attended our excellent NCT antenatal classes which helped me to look forward with excitement to my baby's arrival, instead of with the fear of childbirth which I'd always held. I had hoped for a natural and gentle birth but due to slightly raised blood pressure following a family crisis, at 36 weeks I found myself on the local hospital baby extraction line. Although I instinctively and intellectually felt that all the intervention was unnecessary, and indeed dangerous, and that the baby was the best judge of when he would be 'better out than in' (the antenatal ward catchphrase), I did not have the confidence to totally resist the daily pressure from the doctors during my two weeks on the ward. Being told I was killing my baby did not help the situation—or my blood pressure!—although some of the midwives were very kind and supportive and were obviously concerned at the number of inductions being performed. However, I did have the knowledge and courage to decline their frequent offers to break my waters (at 1cm dilation) and 'pop' me down to the theatre for a nice convenient planned caesarean.

Unfortunately, due to the constant harassment and worry, my blood pressure rose even higher and I finally agreed to prostaglandin pessaries and had seven inserted over seven days. Sean still showed no sign of budging, which simply meant that he was not ready for the outside world. (All my other tests on urine and placenta, etc were perfectly normal.) I was then a Failed Induction and subjected to the full panoply of modern obstetrics: waters broken, numerous drips (including oxytocin), gas and air, and meptid. I didn't really know what was going on during 15 hours of labour, except that everything stopped at one point—not surprising with that cocktail of drugs which made me quite unable to stray from the bed.

The resultant birth was a 'normal delivery' with a bullying, insensitive midwife who took Sean away immediately (despite my written and oral requests to the contrary) and returned him to me clean and swaddled, so that I couldn't even get to see or touch his fingers. I didn't have a chance to put him to the breast for four hours, despite frequent requests for help, and Sean and I had great difficulty with feeding for ages afterwards. He was sleepy for a few days due to the drugs he received through me, and I was in such a state trying to fend off the bottles from the night staff, it is amazing we ever got the hang of breastfeeding! Needless to say, it took me nearly a year to get over the trauma of those three weeks, so when Mike and I found we were expecting another baby, we realised that we could not risk the same things happening again, especially as I would have to be on top form to cope with a baby and our extremely boisterous 2-year-old.

The reactions of the medical profession to my request for a home birth could take me through several paragraphs. Suffice to say, it made everyone very twitchy. Tactics used to dissuade me ranged from coercion to disbelief ("There is no such thing as a home birth in this country") and from the usual threats ("What if something should go wrong?") to the sudden discovery of a problem with my antibodies which meant the baby should be checked by a paediatrician at birth!... none of which, of course, were valid.

I pursued every avenue imaginable and pestered all sorts of people in my determination to ensure that this time my baby and I would not start off our relationship emotionally battered. Time was running out when I read an article in *The Independent* about Michel Odent. It appeared that he had attended some home births, so I attempted to contact him via his publisher. A few days later I answered the phone to a gentle French accent—I couldn't believe my luck. Much to our amazement, Michel was willing to attend our baby's birth if possible (he refused to use the word 'deliver'). From then on we just hoped that baby would have the good sense to be born out of rush hour times as we knew that, with Michel, we would be able to truly get to know our new baby during that very sensitive period immediately after the birth and she would be treated with gentleness and respect.

I wake up on 9 October feeling that this would be a good day to have a baby—the sun is shining and I feel well and reasonably energetic for a change. Baby due today, though, so I'm sure nothing will happen. Cathy and daughter Emily (aged 2) are coming to have lunch and spend the afternoon with us.

> I would not start emotionally battered

Around mid morning I feel very mild period-type pains but I had them Friday night so I take no notice. About 1.30pm I have to stop for a moment through the quickening—I couldn't really describe it as a pain—but manage to prepare a simple lunch quite easily. We sit down to lunch about 2pm and I finally tell Cathy that I am having 'pains' but think it is probably a false alarm. About an hour later Mike comes in from painting the gates outside to have lunch and I tell him about the 'pains'. He says he'll finish the gates but I tell him I'd rather he didn't risk welcoming our baby into the world covered in black gloss. It then registers that something might really be happening so he looks a bit panicky and rushes about in confusion.

4.00pm: I still can't be convinced I'm definitely in labour as I'm not really in pain and I don't want to call Michel unless I'm sure, so we start writing down times. Contractions seem to be about 3 minutes apart. Mike gets electric fires and polythene sheets (the only special equipment needed) and looks agitated. I keep laughing because I can't believe this is the real thing. Everything is so normal and Sean is rushing about terrorising Emily, as usual.

4.40pm: Mike decides it's time to call Michel—he's getting worried about being 'in charge', I think. Luck is with us and he is at home and says he will be right over. Cathy sits reading a book with Sean and Emily and I join in, but have to stop suddenly to lean on the back of the chair. Emily asks, "What's Auntie Pauline doing?" "Having a baby, darling". We both can't stop laughing, which is a bit tricky during a contraction. My own sensitive little angel hasn't noticed a thing!

5.30pm: Cathy gets tea for the children as Mike is not capable in present state of agitation. I go upstairs to change but keep getting delayed by a contraction. It's cool and peaceful upstairs and contractions seem stronger.

5.40pm: Mike is looking out of the window and announces Michel's arrival with great relief. I greet him with a smile then wish I hadn't as he tells me I don't look like a woman in labour. We show him our list of times of contractions but he isn't interested. (Michel told us that he can tell if labour is normal and how it is progressing simply by listening to the noises an uninhibited woman makes, and I remember clearly how I could not stop myself from making different noises as labour got stronger.)

5.50pm: I go upstairs with Michel and he checks baby's heart and my blood pressure as I tell him it has been raised... in fact to the same level as when I was admitted with Sean. It's now the lowest it's been for two weeks.

> We show Michel our list of times but he isn't interested—he says he can tell how labour is progressing simply by listening to me

6.00pm: Children having tea with Cathy. Michel joins them to chat to Cathy and asks about their bedtime. (He had previously told us that it is best not to have anyone else around for the birth as the number of people present is directly proportional to the length of labour, and the longer the labour the more likely complications occur.) Mike orders pizzas for himself and Michel due to vivid recollection of no food or drink for 12 hours before Sean's birth, and we feel it will be a long night.

6.45pm: Cathy and Emily leave. Mike takes Sean up to bed—skips the bath today! Pizzas arrive.

7.00pm: Sean asleep in record time. Contractions getting stronger now. I try out the newly acquired bean bag but it radiates heat back at me so I kneel in front of the sofa with my head on my arms, leaning on the seat, swaying my hips through contractions. I had intended to wear my 'Singapore happy coat' for the birth but don't feel like moving now! It is incredible how the contractions have taken off now it is quiet and there are no distractions. Mike has organised our birthing music—Irish harp and Clannad, which is very soothing.

> Michel had told us the number of people present is directly proportional to the length of the labour—the longer the labour, the more likely it is for complications to occur

7.15pm: Contractions stronger so I start moaning through them. Mike and Michel chomping away on pizzas at the other end of the room. Mike comes over to see how I am and reminds me to 'breathe', which I had forgotten! He gets me a pillow to lean on which is lovely and cool. I ask him to hurry and finish his pizza as I'm in pain!

7.25pm: Making a lot of noise now as contractions really hurt, and I'm worried about coping for hours like this. I hear Mike make a move to get up but Michel whispers that I am best left 'in my own world'. Any outside interference will delay things.

7.30pm: Mike now joins me. He is very calm and reassuring and I hold him through contractions.

> Michel comes upstairs and tells Mike to get the electric fire on at the bathroom door—this must be IT!

7.45pm: I feel I want to go to the toilet. I remember this feeling before Sean was born but don't allow myself to possibly imagine baby is coming as I couldn't bear the disappointment if it's a false alarm. Mike helps me upstairs between contractions. I sit on toilet and feel very constipated and confused. Waters break. Maybe baby is coming... I put my hand down thinking I might feel the head and find blood on my hand. Michel comes upstairs and tells Mike to get the electric fires on at the bathroom door—we have a very small bathroom!—so we know this must be IT. Mike helps me off the toilet and they pull my clothes off and Michel tells him to hold me from behind in the supported squat. I feel my uterus push and a burning sensation and give a little cry as (at 7.55pm) baby's head is born. Then my uterus pushes again. Mike and I are still standing in suspended animation as Michel tells us to look down at our baby daughter lying in his hands! We can't believe she has arrived so quickly and easily. Michel hands her to me and I cradle our beautiful daughter in my arms, her lovely virgin skin touching mine. The wonder and joy of that moment, to be holding my newborn babe so close and feeling her perfect little body next to mine, I can never describe. I kept saying to Mike, "We've got a little girl!" and his face was alight with happiness.

> I can never describe the wonder and joy of that moment, holding my newborn babe so close and feeling her perfect little body next to mine

I sat in the bathroom amidst the goo and mess for about 30 minutes while Michel and Mike sorted things out. I was blissfully unaware of what was going on, having eyes only for my baby. I remember Michel tying the cord after about 10 minutes and Mike cut it and found it quite tough! Then Mike took Rose Eleanor while I went to lie on the bed.

About 9pm Michel felt my stomach and said the placenta had separated. He massaged my stomach and the placenta came away with a contraction. Mike was trying to clear up the bathroom and was pleased the birth hadn't been on a carpet! Michel left about 10pm, and we sat in bed marvelling at our new baby daughter. She was very alert and never cried, although she gave the occasional whimper. We had the lights very low for her all the time. She didn't want to suck immediately after the birth but kept nuzzling my breast and looking around. Mike opened a bottle of champagne but I didn't like to drink more than a glass so I contented myself with two packets of Mintolas! We sat and caressed our little miracle and talked over and over about her birth, we were both so excited. About 2am I thought we should get some sleep and maybe Rose Eleanor was tired, so we all snuggled up in our bed. It was incredible that Sean had slept through all this but at 5am he woke and came into our bed. His little face was a picture when he heard Rosie stirring and he laughed and said, "Baby sister!"—he was so happy to see her.

Pauline Farrance

The father's tale...

> I have always opted for nature's way but this had never extended to having a baby—I preferred to abdicate responsibility to the medics

◀ Whenever there was a choice I have always opted for nature's way in areas such as food, environment and general health. However, this had never extended to having a baby and I preferred to abdicate the responsibility to the medical profession, who appeared more than willing to take over.

I attended the NCT classes and that's when doubts began to creep in, especially as I learned of all the medical hardware, paraphernalia and drugs that were deemed essential nowadays for giving birth. I began to realise that the medical profession was perhaps, after all, just as horrified as I at having the responsibility for the birth.

However, we went ahead with the hospital birth of our firstborn as it was decided by a hospital screening process that Pauline's blood pressure was outside the norm, for which she was immediately admitted. Sean was eventually extracted in a very workmanlike manner, some two and a half weeks of protestations, seven pessaries, two gas tanks, two doses of chemicals, ten yards of graph paper, one cup of tea and 15 hours of narcotic trance later. It would be an understatement to say it was a very traumatic time for all of us and I was disappointed at not experiencing the joy one has heard about as the father in attendance at the birth of his first child. It was more a sense of overwhelming relief that the whole episode was over with and all three parties (physically) healthy and alive.

Sixteen months later we found we were expecting our second baby and this time we were determined from the outset that this baby would be born at home so that we could have more control and responsibility. Our GP reluctantly agreed to cover the birth but opposition grew from all quarters of the medical profession and eventually no doctor would agree to cover the birth at home. This again I would attribute to their horror at having the responsibility for the birth. However, in desperation and clutching at any possible straw, Pauline managed to meet Michel Odent, who agreed to be present at the birth, if he was available.

The day of the birth thankfully arrived on a Sunday. Although we had read every possible piece of literature on the subject, I was filled with dread and my heart began to palpitate. I thought I might possibly have to deliver the baby myself if Michel was held up in the traffic... I began to race around looking for textbooks, plastic sheets and the bucket. (The requirement for the bucket had somehow lodged in my mind from the NCT course.)

I was greatly relieved when a French-registered Renault pulled up outside and the calming presence of Michel entered the house. I had by this time got my act together and put on some soothing music. Later, we turned the lights down very low and Michel told me to let Pauline get into her own world, and we chatted casually as we ate the enormous home delivery pizzas while Pauline got on with the business of having a baby, leaning on the sofa with her head in a pillow. For some reason I was convinced it would be a long night and I was building up my reserves of energy in anticipation!

Minutes after finishing the pizzas we were all in our tiny bathroom with me holding Pauline in the supported squat and Michel holding a beautiful baby girl in his hands. She gave what seemed to be an obligatory whimper to let us know she was OK and settled blissfully into her mother's arms and there they stayed for about half an hour. I was totally dumbstruck by the ease and beauty of the birth and just gazed in disbelief. After coming down to Earth, I began clearing up operations and gave thanks for lino tiles instead of carpet in the bathroom, but wished I had not eaten the pizza!

> I was totally dumbstruck by the ease and beauty of the birth and just gazed in disbelief... but I wished I hadn't eaten the pizza!

Michel's presence was quite unobtrusive throughout his visit, but it was his confidence and experience in allowing nature to take its course without any unnecessary interference which made the birth such a trouble-free and memorable event, and gave us so much joy and confidence during the weeks that followed.

Michael White ▶

And afterwards...

◀ We have obviously talked endlessly about the birth and were so happy and grateful that everything had gone so well, but we felt so sad for the vast majority of mothers (and fathers) who are denied the joy of such a precious and unique experience in our so-called civilised society today. It is widely accepted that about 90% of women are able to give birth normally, without complications, so why don't we keep the costly expertise and machinery for those who really need it? Of course, many men and women are happier in the hospital environment, and we would never try and dissuade them from this as the labour will always be prolonged by fear and anxiety. But the present day fear of complications during childbirth is largely unfounded and we should look at the event in perspective as a part of family life.

We were so excited by Rosie's birth that we were on a high for at least a week and had loads of energy to carry us through the sleepless nights, etc. Added benefits of the birth at home include much less disruption and confusion for older brothers and sisters, and it meant so much to my parents to be able to hold their second grandchild so soon after she was born—a privilege not allowed after Sean's birth. In addition, the baby will not succumb to any of the infections which abound in hospital.

To put it all in a nutshell, three days after Rosie's birth we were feeling a little down because we had enjoyed the birth so much. We wanted the clock to turn back to Sunday so that we could do it all again!

Pauline Farrance and Michael White

OPTIMAL BIRTH—THE HOW

Of course I would not presume to tell you how to care for women during pregnancy, labour, birth and afterwards... Having said that, I would like to present some notes and opinions (not all my own), based on both research and experience and informed by current midwifery protocols. I would also like to ask you to consider a few issues. These are some of the issues which could make an enormous difference to any one individual woman's experience of childbirth.

A few questions to contemplate...

Since we all operate under assumptions, which limit what we do in our lives, I think it's a good idea at times to consider questions which challenge these assumptions. Sometimes—as any life coach will tell you—problems can be opportunities.

TRAINING

1. What should midwifery training ideally include?
2. Do you think anything was missing from your training?
3. To what extent did your training focus on pathology?
4. How much time was spent talking about pain relief and concomitant safety issues?
5. To what extent did you focus on the study of normality?
6. How much did you study ways of facilitating birth?
7. How many drug-free births were you required to attend?
8. How many undisturbed physiological births did you see?

EXPERIENCE

1. Is your experience of being a midwife generally a good one or could you improve your professional lifestyle?
2. Has any experience ever influenced your practice?
3. Has any experience in your career ever saddened you?
4. Has any experience in your career ever inspired you?
5. To what extent does previous experience inspire or limit the decisions you make?
6. How do you try to communicate your experience with more newly-qualified midwives?
7. Are you open-minded about having new experiences?
8. Do you ever try and tap into the experience of colleagues or other professionals you meet at conferences, etc.?
9. Do you ever try to learn from non-professionals?

RESEARCH

1. How much do you trust the conclusions of researchers?
2. To what extent do you keep up with the latest research?
3. Where do you go to access research on any given topic?
4. What are the quickest ways of accessing research?
5. What are the most effective ways?
6. How can you evaluate the validity of research studies?
7. How would you go about conducting your own research?
8. In which cases has research changed or influenced clinical practice?

THE LAW

1. Are there any references to the law in any midwifery rules or guidelines you are required to follow?
2. Does a fear of litigation influence the way you practise?
3. Do you know anyone who's been sued?
4. How much are you influenced by insurance?
5. What would you do if a client threatened to sue you?
6. Have you ever refused to support a woman, explaining to her that you're afraid she might sue you afterwards?
7. Do you ever explain or discuss legal issues with clients?
8. Are there any laws you think should be changed?

POWER

1. Do you feel that power has shifted at all between midwives, obstetricians, GPs during your own career?
2. Have there ever been cases where you have been frustrated by any professional hierarchies?
3. How much power do you feel you have within your own working context?
4. To what extent do you think a pregnant woman should determine the course of her own care?
5. How do you feel about a doula influencing decisions which a labouring woman may be making about her care?
6. Is there a dialogue between you and obstetricians?
7. To what extent are you informed or controlled by the NMC (Nursing & Midwifery Council) or by NICE guidelines?
8. To what extent is there a dialogue between you and the local Head of Midwifery and/or Supervisor of Midwives?
9. To what extent do you communicate with local GPs?
10. To what extent do you exchange ideas and information with pregnant women?

PROTOCOLS

1. How do you think protocols are established?
2. Are protocols always in line with research findings?
3. How often do protocols change?
4. How long have specific protocols been in place at your particular place of work?
5. Who influences changes made to protocols?
6. How much power do you personally feel you have?
7. How much power can a group of midwives exert?
8. Do protocols serve the needs of pregnant women?
9. Do protocols ever serve the financial needs of an institution, or any other interests?
10. Do protocols ever focus primarily on midwives' needs?
11. Do protocols ever help you to exert authority over a labouring woman?
12. Which protocols do you like?
13. Which protocols would you really like to change?
14. Are there any protocols which need to be changed for the sake of safety or to ensure better outcomes?
15. To what extent are protocols observed?
16. When is it possible to get permission not to follow protocol and what's the procedure for doing this?

OPTIMALITY

1. How should a midwife ideally behave?
2. How much monitoring do you need to do, in your opinion, in order to ensure safest outcomes?
3. Are there any procedures which you or colleagues normally carry out which interfere with optimality?

A few comments from women on caregivers...

My GP was aware from the start that I again planned a home birth. The consultant at the hospital told me that I could not have antenatal shared care at the hospital if I was planning to have the baby at home and pressurised me into agreeing to come to the hospital for the birth. The midwife afterwards told me not to worry—that shared antenatal care with delivery at home if all was well, or at the hospital if not, was fine.

We moved when I was 5 weeks pregnant, and the first thing I did was find a midwife who would deliver my baby at home. At first I approached the NHS, and spoke to my GP, who I shan't name, because although he read me the riot act and said officially a home birth would be endangering my life and that of the baby, he, unofficially, was glad I wanted a home birth, and said he would support me. I was well chuffed. Next, I went to see a midwife who is also pro-home birth. But as soon as she heard of my previous caesarean she declined her services. I didn't want to press my case because I wanted to make sure my midwife was 100% on my side. I understand the NHS are obliged to attend a home labour, but my faith in the system had been totally shattered. And I didn't want to be hauled from home to hospital in labour under any spurious pretext. So I hired an independent midwife.

I booked with community midwives who are generally supportive of home birth but when my history of a PPH [postpartum haemorrhage] was revealed (by me, voluntarily) I was told that a home birth would be out of the question. I was made to feel that my body was at fault for pouring out a life threatening amount of blood after giving birth—the truth, however, was that mismanagement had caused the heavy blood loss. I soon booked with independent midwives who had the confidence in my body which I had and I gave birth to a second daughter at home in under three hours.

At each check-up at the hospital it became apparent that none of the midwives had any experience of delivering twins and after further research through TAMBA, NCT and general reading it was clear that a first-time mother having a drug-free natural delivery was quite rare. I was told that my babies were cephalic [head down, i.e. not breech] so a caesarean wasn't absolutely necessary but was told to 'keep my options open'. Even my NCT class teacher (who was wonderful) said a natural delivery was, of course, possible but she wasn't sure whether it was realistic. The only positive response was from the consultant himself who, in an evening talk at the hospital, made it 'loud and clear' that he believes it is every woman's right to have a consultant present in a birth of this kind. However, he also said it is more likely there won't be one, so whoever is there is likely to have had little, if any, experience of delivering twins; therefore he said it would be safer to have a caesarean. He was the most amazing man I have ever met. After the talk, when I told him how important it was to me to at least try for a natural delivery, he wrote on my notes to inform him when I was in labour and he would come in. He gave me his holiday dates which I somehow managed to avoid and he stuck to his word and came in on his 'day off' and delivered my daughters. I know I couldn't have done it without him!

I feel that a woman who does not revere childbirth has no place being a midwife

Elaine visited my house throughout the pregnancy for tests, and listened to baby's heartbeat through her wooden midwife's trumpet [Pinard]. We got to know her, and she us, and it was a gentle and caring relationship. By the time I was in labour, my trust in Elaine was complete.

I felt very confident in my ability as a woman to give birth and this decision also let me feel in control of who was to be present during the labour and birth. I was not prepared to let into my home any midwives that I felt didn't respect my rights as a pregnant woman whilst giving birth. This for me was very significant emotionally as I believe that a midwife who does not revere childbirth and show consideration for the labouring woman have no place in being a midwife. As long as there is no danger to the mother or child, the midwife should be led by the labouring woman. If this does not happen it can seriously undermine a woman's confidence in her abilities within herself to give birth, which I think is evident with my first birthing experience.

The birth of my first child felt very institutionalized and governed by hospital policy. The midwife was definitely in control of the entire situation with me as her charge. My second birth was a truly wonderful experience that was influenced by an extremely intuitive midwife who encouraged me to do what felt to be right for me. These experiences have made me highly aware of the dynamics between the birthing mother and the midwife whose main purpose is to provide support for the mother and her partner in labour and who needs to understand both the physical processes and the emotional needs of the mother. I feel that this relationship is one of the most important factors during labour and birth.

Basically, the midwives made themselves invisible. I certainly hardly heard them discussing anything. I do remember hearing them ask Simon to bring clothes and nappies—I couldn't believe I was giving birth already!

Whenever I asked the midwife for guidance about what I was supposed to be doing or how far she thought I was dilated she just told me I was doing really well, coping remarkably well and asked me to feel what my body was telling me to do and to follow that.

Michel was great. He was very calm.

Julie [the midwife] hadn't even got her gloves dirty. She had done nothing fantastically.

THE ANTENATAL PERIOD

Again, let's go back to basics.

What's the purpose of antenatal care?

After consulting various textbooks and professionals, I managed to determine that, generally speaking, you and other health care practitioners are aiming to:
- Confirm a woman's pregnancy and estimate when she is likely to give birth
- Assess any possible risks, based on her previous medical hsitory, age or current circumstances
- Encourage the pregnant woman to take folic acid supplements in the first trimester
- Talk about diet, i.e. encourage the pregnant woman to eat healthily and avoid certain foods
- Confirm the woman's blood group in case a blood transfusion is needed later, and establish whether or not she is Rhesus negative, in which case you will probably recommend a few additional procedures
- Offer the pregnant woman various checks to look for abnormalities and subsequently, if any are found or suspected, offer an abortion
- Offer the woman ultrasound scans to monitor her baby's size and positioning in the womb, to check for multiples and to check the position of the placenta and any fibroids
- Screen for rubella immunity, sexually transmitted diseases, diabetes and gestational diabetes, as well as genetic disorders (if there is a family history)
- Track the woman's blood pressure and urine in case hypertension develops or protein appears in the urine, so as to detect pre-eclampsia and ward off eclampsia
- Track the baby's positioning and the quantity of amniotic fluid, as well as fetal growth, through ongoing manual 'palpation' or the use of repeated ultrasound scans

What are the potential problems?

There are a few, it seems...
- Pregnant women are very emotional, suggestible beings
- Pregnancy, labour and birth does not proceed in a mechanical way, but is affected by psychological factors—because hormones are sensitive to emotions
- One intervention tends to lead to another
- Women often come to appointments wanting to ask numerous questions and leave feeling that they've had no opportunity to ask them
- Pregnant women often feel undermined by caregivers' use of technical terms (either intentionally or unwittingly) ... or even belittled by caregivers' use of 'babyish' terms, when they already know the proper terms
- There are often disagreements between women and midwives about approaches to care
- There can be serious personality mismatches
- Women often 'shop around' for suitable caregivers, so midwives sometimes feel defensive
- While some women want to avoid any intervention, other women come hoping for every possible form of intervention so that they can avoid as much pain as possible and 'control' what seems an unpredictable and scary process

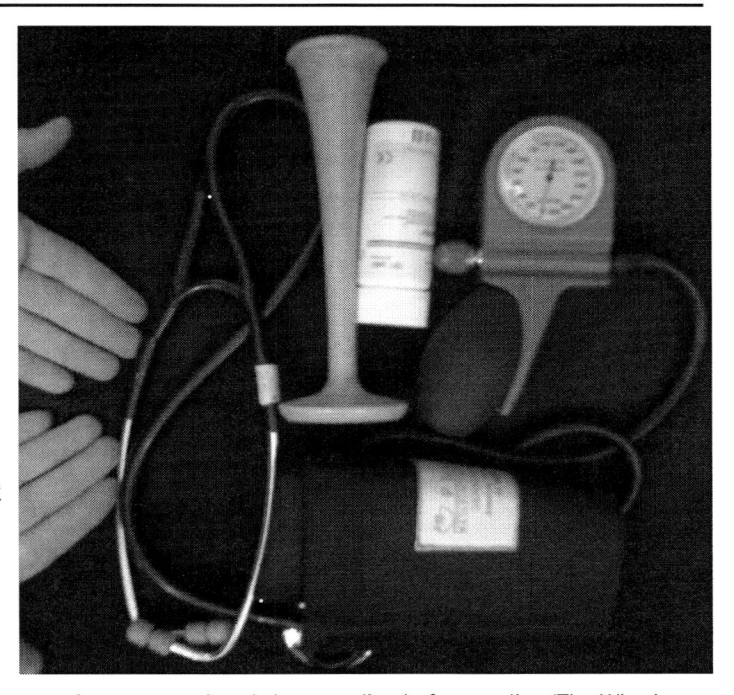

As you may already have realised after reading 'The What', a surprisingly little amount of equipment is needed for optimal antenatal care—but note that hands need to be kept in the picture! Note the presence of the Pinard, instead of a Sonicaid—the aim overall being to absolutely minimise any possible disturbance of the normal physiological processes

What are the potential opportunities?

This could be the source of some professional satisfaction:
- You have the opportunity to get to know a range of different kinds of women
- You may be able to take a 'whole person' approach to any problems by paying attention in a different way, or trying new approaches
- Some women may push you to extend your normal practice by making requests which are new to you
- You can experiment with different ways of communicating with women
- Potentially, you have the power to exert a great deal of influence over any individual woman and the choices she makes as she progresses through her pregnancy, labour and birth
- You can prepare women who are afraid and make them end up feeling empowered and profoundly satisfied
- You can act as a mentor or guide as women pass through this key transition in their lives

What are the potential risks?

Of course, risks aren't always negative, but an intrinsic part of life (as is crossing the road). But do any of these potential risks ever limit what you do? (How many traffic accidents would it take to stop you crossing roads?)
- You may lose a client because of your approach
- You may get sued and lose your job altogether
- You may become too popular! (That might cause jealousy.)
- You may have problems with colleagues or superiors
- You may open yourself up to criticism—can you face it?
- You may get promoted and gain power to inspire others
- You may learn new things from different clients
- You may start viewing things differently if you experiment with different approaches...

Birthframe 22

To zoom in on one of the potential problems of antenatal care, here's an account from a contributor who was not happy with her midwife's approach in her first appointment. (In this case, the midwife didn't take up various opportunities, but instead created new problems.) By the way, this appointment took place in the USA but it could have been anywhere...

I had worked for a publishing company that specialised in some parenting and childcare books, and had published several on active birth, breastfeeding, taking part in one's own care, etc, so I felt happily enlightened. I went to my first antenatal check-up thinking I would know what questions to ask, that I would be an informed patient. I was relieved to see that the head of the 'normal OB' department was a woman, a Certified Nurse Midwife. That sounded proper and competent. Hoping to ask lots of questions, I actually could not get a word in edgewise.

The usual first questions: age, marital status; blood pressure taken, weighed, measured, the pelvic exam. She listened to my heart, then with a shocked look, she said, "Did you know you have a heart murmur?!" "Well, no," I said. "I have had regular medical care my whole life and no one has ever found any heart irregularities." She looked at me in disbelief. I was wondering what the hell she was talking about and was afraid that it might hurt the baby. Later on, another practitioner told me that it is very common for women to develop a mild heart murmur in pregnancy, and it isn't anything to worry about.

Then we had the following conversation.
Midwife: Was this a planned pregnancy?
Me: (ready to laugh and joke about our spontaneity) Well, ha, not exactly, but...
Midwife: What birth control were you using?
Me: Uh, condoms.
Midwife: Did the condom break?
Me: Uh, no ... We were not using one.
Midwife: Well, why not?! Surely you knew what could happen!

I had no response. I was shocked, I think. I just looked at her. I was wondering what about me had given her the impression that I was so young and ignorant, or unworthy of respect. I had come straight from work, was dressed and groomed respectably, she knew I was married. I had no idea. She told me that she had something that could make the pregnancy "more real for people like you". I thought: People Like Me? Exactly what category was that? Middle Class Working Married People in Their Mid-Twenties Who Dare to Be Happy When They are Pregnant? I had a feeling instead I had been put in the Irresponsible Idiots category, which was distinctly shameful. Suddenly, I was 6 years old, caught drawing on the walls.

She wheeled a machine on a little cart into the room and told me to lie down. I was uneasy and didn't like the situation at all any more, but I was also not going to stand up for myself. I had to be a good patient. I was not a troublemaker. The machine was a brand new portable ultrasound, which she had been "wanting to try out". So I was instructed to look at the little screen, to see the baby, to make it 'real' for me.

I went to my first check-up thinking I would know what questions to ask

She didn't know anything about me, hadn't asked me anything about myself or my feelings, yet she seemed certain that I was in denial and this experience wasn't sinking in for me. Looking at the nondescript image on a small greyish-green screen, I thought that my changing body and swelling, tender uterus, my nausea and cravings, were certainly more real than anything she had shown me.

I then got a lecture about nutrition, even though she didn't seem even vaguely interested in my personal diet or knowledge of the topic, and was sent on my way with an order to make my next appointment at the front desk on my way out. The whole thing took about 20 minutes and this was my 'long, personal, initial interview'.

I was suddenly not so excited about this pregnancy and felt ashamed of myself for letting her do those things

I was on the verge of tears all the way back to work. I was suddenly not so excited about this pregnancy and felt ashamed of myself, both for letting her use ultrasound on me and my baby for no good reason (even though I didn't know at the time that there were any risks associated with it) and for being so 'irresponsible' as to get pregnant without 'trying'. I tried to remember why I had been so cheerful on my way in.

Some guidelines for constructive, collaborative communication...

Based on my experience of teaching adults in companies for around twenty years, here are a few pointers...
- Ask women about situations or symptoms, don't *tell* them. In other words, never say, "I expect you're feeling..."
- Ask plenty of open questions, e.g. "How are you feeling?" "How have things been?" "Do you have any preferences?"
- Talk about positives, not just negatives, remembering that talking about risks or potential problems can cause fear.
- Never suggest negative outcomes. For example, don't say 'If *you* get, *you* need...' but use distancing language instead. For example, you may need to say, "When *someone* gets pre-eclampsia, *they* must be monitored closely in case..."
- Explain any technical terms you use, without being patronising. Avoid using 'babyish' language, but consider slang with some clients, especially so as to make them laugh! Take your cue on language to use from the client, rather than habit.
- Never put a woman down for asking 'silly' questions. Positively encourage her, remembering the steepness of the learning curve for a first-time mother. Always give a woman an opportunity to add another question...
- Try and draw out any other concerns or questions, remembering that hesitation may mean the client disagrees with you!
- Explain everything you want to do before you do it, and as you're doing it too, giving the woman a chance to refuse.
- Respect a woman's right to choose her own care and encourage her to plan for a positive birthing experience.
- If at all possible, help women to leave each antenatal appointment on a positive note.

The chance to develop even better relationships

As well as taking care over communication, you could actually aim much higher and work to establish an excellent emotional climate through a different approach entirely. (Hear me out, please... it might be fun!)

Since emotions and hormones are inextricably linked, your relationship with clients is perhaps the single most important factor for determining safe outcomes. Your clients will eventually need to be producing oxytocin in your presence (so as to stimulate or sustain contractions), rather than adrenaline, which would be produced in a stressful or frightening environment. How would this be possible if their memories of you in the past were not terribly positive? (By the way, in case you're worried about triggering a pregnant woman's labour by getting her to produce oxytocin in her antenatal appointments, let me hasten to add that you're aiming here to get her producing the amount someone might produce when having dinner with a friend—not the amount which is usual during an earth-shattering orgasm!)

How is it possible to make a woman feel comfortable when a fair amount of your time during each antenatal appointment will be spent performing checks (auscultation, palpation, urine checks, etc.), which carry the implicit message that there is a risk that something may well have gone wrong since the woman's last appointment?

Here are a few ideas, some of which might seem sensible to you, some wacky. Some you may have already tried. Why not try out some more and think of others too?

- **Maternity fashion shows** You could have afternoon sessions (while women wait for their antenatal appointments). Each fashion show could feature maternity wear. Both local and national companies would probably quite easily be persuaded to sponsor the shows.
- **Singalongs** Michel Odent used to have singing sessions with pregnant women and their partners every week. Why not try something similar? (It could even be a karaoke session involving songs from movies your clients request. There could be a sign-up sheet for suggested songs or movies to sing along to or you could provide a selection.)
- **Partner picnics** These would be 'pot-luck' meals (everyone brings a dish of some kind—savoury or sweet, with no forward planning) to take place at lunch- or dinner-time.
- **Foodie fetus lunches** Nutritious food, prepared according to a sign-up list, could be eaten before a teaching session.
- **Morning munch-time** I've suggested this 'term' rather than 'coffee mornings' for the simple reason that I believe pregnant women should avoid drinking too much coffee. However, a coffee-morning-type idea would facilitate informal chatting between staff and pregnant women.
- **Beautiful bump boasts** These would be workshops in which women could express and discuss any feelings they have about their changing self-image. Photos of trendy pregnant celebrities could be used as discussion starters.
- **Fear focus groups** No prizes for guessing these could be groups in which women discuss and explore their fears.
- **World pregnancy workshops** These could be sessions in which women find out (from you) about birthing practices in other countries. Of course, Sheila Kitzinger's book *Ourselves as Mothers* (Doubleday 1992), *Ever Since Eve* (Oxford University Press 1984) and *Birth Traditions and Modern Pregnancy Care* (Element Books 1992) would provide plenty of material.

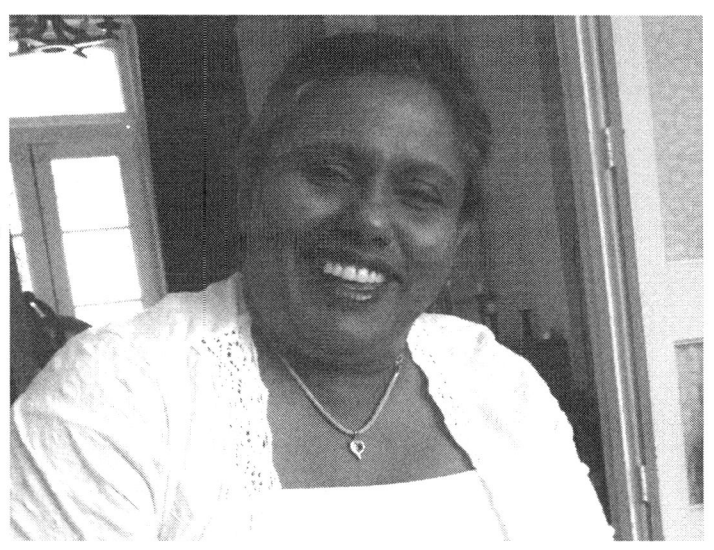

I'm sure your clients already see you as someone who's understanding and supportive... But why not develop your relationship with your clients even more than you do now?

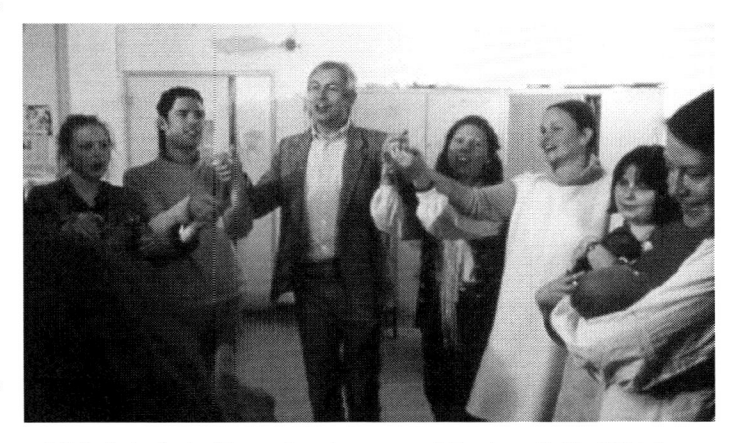

Michel singing with pregnant women at the hospital in Pithiviers, near Paris where he was responsible for around 15,000 births

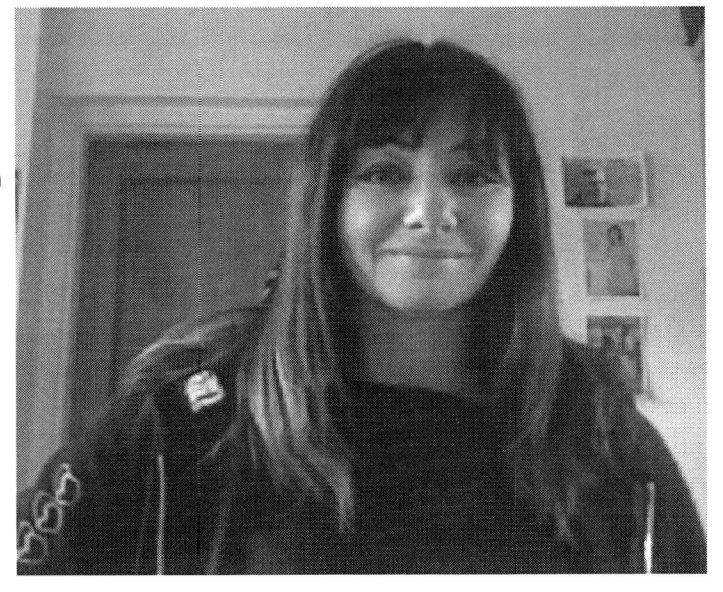

Being a friendly face will in no way diminish your authority. In fact, it's likely to increase it because your clients are likely to open up to you more and put more trust in your judgment—quite simply because you will know your client's situation so well.

The importance of an accurate due date

Given the sense of anticipation most women have about their due date (even though over 95% of births don't take place on it) and given the pressure many women are under once they apparently become 'overdue', obviously it's vital to take this date seriously. When I was pregnant myself I privately felt put out that this calculation was undertaken with only a piece of unimpressive card and that no particular attention was ever paid to the fact that my normal menstrual cycle was 33 days. Despite widespread mentions in the literature that this would mean a strong likelihood of any of my babies being born 5 days after the date the charts indicate, this later date was never fixed as the official due date. Isn't this odd?

In case you would like something to replace a tatty, unimpressive cardboard wheel, here's a reference chart, based—of course—on women who have a 28-day menstrual cycle. In addition, you might consult www.redbabybook.com.

Jan	1	2	3	4	5	6	7	8	9	10	11	12	13	14	15	16	17	18	19	20	21	22	23	24	25	26	27	28	29	30	31
Oct	8	9	10	11	12	13	14	15	16	17	18	19	20	21	22	23	24	25	26	27	28	29	30	31	1	2	3	4	5	6	7
Feb	1	2	3	4	5	6	7	8	9	10	11	12	13	14	15	16	17	18	19	20	21	22	23	24	25	26	27	28			
Nov	8	9	10	11	12	13	14	15	16	17	18	19	20	21	22	23	24	25	26	27	28	29	30	1	2	3	4	5			
March	1	2	3	4	5	6	7	8	9	10	11	12	13	14	15	16	17	18	19	20	21	22	23	24	25	26	27	28	29	30	31
Dec	6	7	8	9	10	11	12	13	14	15	16	17	18	19	20	21	22	23	24	25	26	27	28	29	30	31	1	2	3	4	5
April	1	2	3	4	5	6	7	8	9	10	11	12	13	14	15	16	17	18	19	20	21	22	23	24	25	26	27	28	29	30	
Jan	6	7	8	9	10	11	12	13	14	15	16	17	18	19	20	21	22	23	24	25	26	27	28	29	30	31	1	2	3	4	
May	1	2	3	4	5	6	7	8	9	10	11	12	13	14	15	16	17	18	19	20	21	22	23	24	25	26	27	28	29	30	31
Feb	5	6	7	8	9	10	11	12	13	14	15	16	17	18	19	20	21	22	23	24	25	26	27	28	1	2	3	4	5	6	7
June	1	2	3	4	5	6	7	8	9	10	11	12	13	14	15	16	17	18	19	20	21	22	23	24	25	26	27	28	29	30	
March	8	9	10	11	12	13	14	15	16	17	18	19	20	21	22	23	24	25	26	27	28	29	30	31	1	2	3	4	5	6	
July	1	2	3	4	5	6	7	8	9	10	11	12	13	14	15	16	17	18	19	20	21	22	23	24	25	26	27	28	29	30	31
April	7	8	9	10	11	12	13	14	15	16	17	18	19	20	21	22	23	24	25	26	27	28	29	30	1	2	3	4	5	6	7
Aug	1	2	3	4	5	6	7	8	9	10	11	12	13	14	15	16	17	18	19	20	21	22	23	24	25	26	27	28	29	30	31
May	8	9	10	11	12	13	14	15	16	17	18	19	20	21	22	23	24	25	26	27	28	29	30	31	1	2	3	4	5	6	7
Sept	1	2	3	4	5	6	7	8	9	10	11	12	13	14	15	16	17	18	19	20	21	22	23	24	25	26	27	28	29	30	
June	8	9	10	11	12	13	14	15	16	17	18	19	20	21	22	23	24	25	26	27	28	29	30	1	2	3	4	5	6	7	
Oct	1	2	3	4	5	6	7	8	9	10	11	12	13	14	15	16	17	18	19	20	21	22	23	24	25	26	27	28	29	30	31
July	8	9	10	11	12	13	14	15	16	17	18	19	20	21	22	23	24	25	26	27	28	29	30	31	1	2	3	4	5	6	7
Nov	1	2	3	4	5	6	7	8	9	10	11	12	13	14	15	16	17	18	19	20	21	22	23	24	25	26	27	28	29	30	
Aug	8	9	10	11	12	13	14	15	16	17	18	19	20	21	22	23	24	25	26	27	28	29	30	31	1	2	3	4	5	6	
Dec	1	2	3	4	5	6	7	8	9	10	11	12	13	14	15	16	17	18	19	20	21	22	23	24	25	26	27	28	29	30	31
Sept	7	8	9	10	11	12	13	14	15	16	17	18	19	20	21	22	23	24	25	26	27	28	29	30	1	2	3	4	5	6	7

When I was collecting material for *BIRTH: Countdown to Optimal* I received an alarming number of comments and accounts about problems to do with due dates which were in dispute. So as to avoid confusion or unnecessary anxiety later on in a woman's pregnancy, when you give a client her 'due date'...

- Double-check it's possible for her to have conceived on the date her due date suggests. If her partner was away on business that weekend and only around the weekend after, this might need discussing.
- Double-check the length of her cycle, if she knows what it is, adding on or subtracting dates as necessary.
- Explain that many women experience light bleeding at the time when they would normally have their period in the first and second months of pregnancy.
- Tell your client that very few women actually give birth on their due date.
- Explain that anything from 37 weeks to 41 weeks is considered 'term' (or 42 weeks in some areas).
- Tell her she may later want to read up on prematurity, postmaturity and induction, in case it ever becomes relevant.

The importance of a balanced view

A large number of people (pregnant women, their relatives and even professionals) assume it's necessary to take a very interventionist approach to antenatal care. This is because they feel that non-intervention (as happens in the developing world) results in high mortality and morbidity rates. The feeling of anxiety about outcomes is perhaps exacerbated by the fact that most people nowadays only have one or two children, so a lot of hopes are embodied in each pregnancy. But is this anxiety appropriate? Is it irresponsible to leave nature to take its course? Shouldn't we worry about things going wrong?

Actually, your clients' lifestyles are quite dramatically different from those of women living in developing countries. Your clients have readily available, clean water; they have a good diet; they live in a climate which is less conducive to all kinds of disease (because it's rainy and cold!) and they have quick access to high quality, free healthcare if ever anything should go wrong. What's more, unlike many African women, British women are rarely circumcised, incised or infibulated—i.e. they don't have their genitals ritually damaged in any way—and their healthy diet in childhood means their body grew properly.

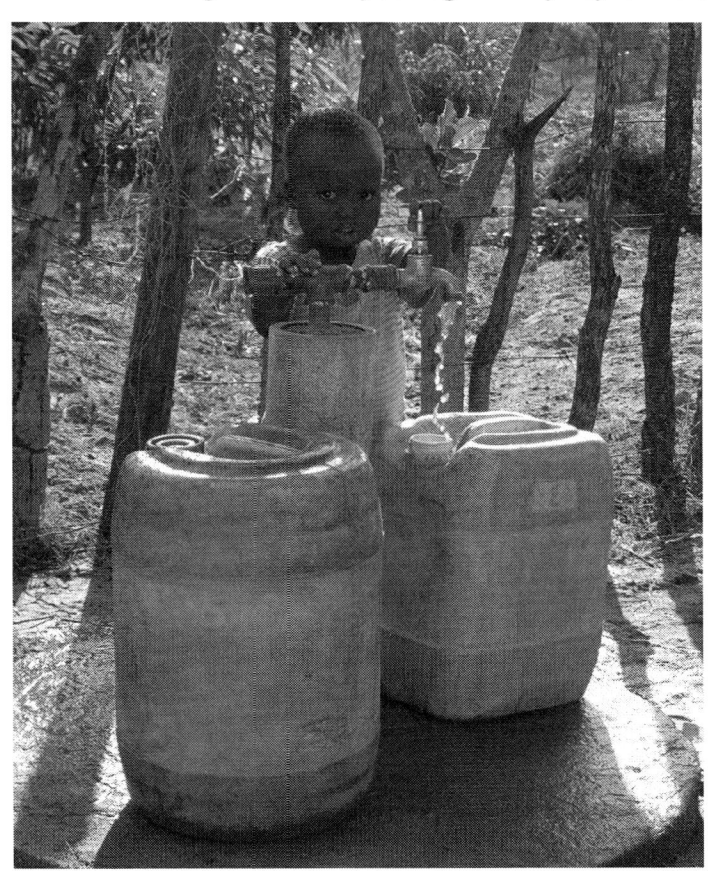

How would you feel about sending a little boy off for water (in South Africa) while attending his mother in labour?

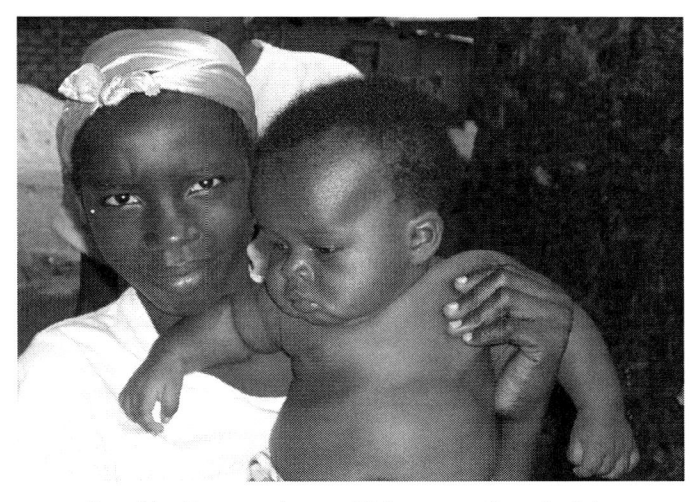

Consider the experience of this woman from Angola. She may or may not be one of the lucky 30% of people who have access to government health care facilities, which were severely damaged during the Civil War up to 2002. Apart from difficulties getting treatment, she and her children will also be in danger of dying from malaria.

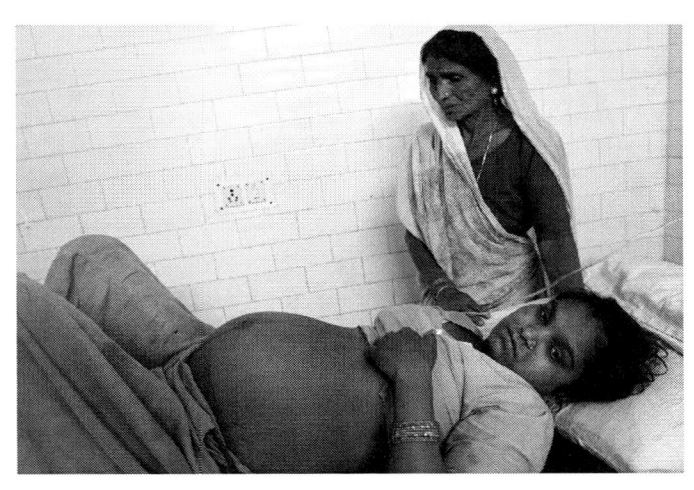

This primie gravida in India started experiencing labour pains at 3am. Her membranes ruptured at 8am. She and her mother reached the 'local' clinic at 1pm. (Many women in India have to travel by bullock cart.) Her condition was by now critical but she was unattended for two hours. (The only doctor present was busy that afternoon with the family planning camp.) Whatever we might say about the situation in Britain, it's quite radically different... [Photo: UNICEF/India/Anita Khemka]

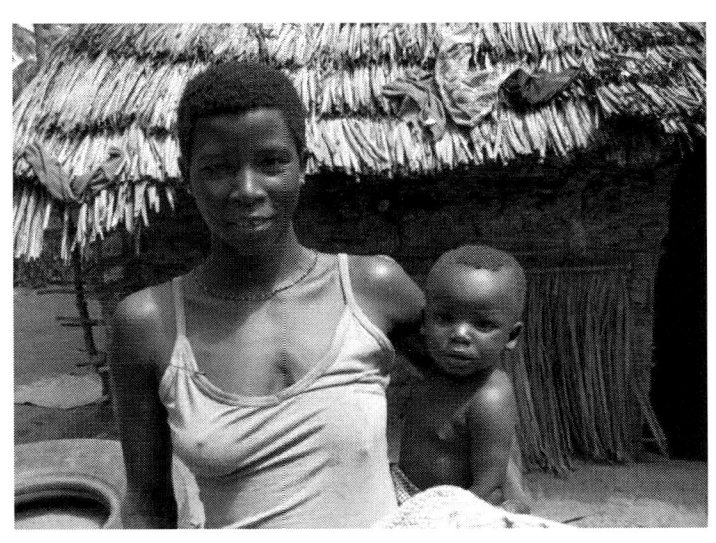

As you can see from the background, this Kenyan woman's living conditions are quite different from those of your clients

Whatever your clients' situation, it is likely to be quite radically better than that experienced by women elsewhere

Bill Bryson, an American travel writer, reported on the conditions that many women experience in his book *African Diary* (Doubleday 2002), which was commissioned by the charity CARE International. Here's an extract:

> To step into Kibera is to be lost at once in a random, seemingly endless warren of rank, narrow passageways wandering between rows of frail, dirt-floored hovels made of tin and mud and twigs and holes. Each shanty, on average, is ten feet by ten and home to five or six people. Down the centre of each lane runs a shallow trench filled with a trickle of water and things you don't want to see or step in. There are no services in Kibera—no running water, no rubbish collection, virtually no electricity, not a single flush toilet. In one section of Kibera called Laini Saba until recently there were just ten pit latrines for 40,000 people. Especially at night when it is unsafe to venture out, many residents rely on what are known as 'flying toilets', which is to say they go into a plastic bag, then open their door and throw it as far as possible.
>
> In the rainy season, the whole becomes a liquid ooze. In the dry season it has the charm and healthfulness of a rubbish tip. In all seasons it smells of rot. It's a little like wandering through a privy. Whatever is the most awful place you have ever experienced, Kibera is worse.
>
> Kibera is only one of about a hundred slums in Nairobi, and it is by no means the worst. Altogether more than half of Nairobi's three million people are packed into these immensely squalid zones, which together occupy only about 1.5 per cent of the city's land. In wonder I asked David Sanderson what made Kibera superior. [David is CARE International's regional manager for southern and western Africa.] "There are a lot of factories around here," he said, "so there's work, though nearly all of it is casual. If you're lucky you might make a few dollars a day, enough to buy a little food and a jerry can of water and to put something aside for your rent."

There are simple reasons for the 500,000 unnecessary deaths in developing countries

Kibera is by no means the worst slum

"How much is rent?"

"Oh, not much. Ten or twelve dollars a month. But the average annual income in Kenya is $280, so $120 or $140 in rent every year is a big slice of your income. And nearly everything else is expensive here, too, even water. The average person in a slum like Kibera pays five times what people in the developed world pay for the same volume of water piped to their homes."

"That's amazing," I said.

He nodded. "Every time you flush a toilet you use more water than the average person in the developing world has for all purposes in a day—cooking, cleaning drinking, everything. It's very tough. For a lot of people Kibera is essentially a life sentence. Unless you are exceptionally lucky with employment, it's very, very difficult to get ahead."

Every day around the world 180,000 people fetch up in or are born into cities like Nairobi, mostly into slums like Kibera. Ninety per cent of the world's population growth in the twenty-first century will be in cities.

Bill Bryson

Is it surprising, given this environment, that the developing world has such poor birth statistics? Incidentally, if you would like to support the work going on to improve living conditions for people in places like this, go to www.careinternational.org.uk

---

There are also other reasons for the 500,000 maternal deaths in developing countries—the figure reported by the UN Department of Public Information in 2005:

EARLY MARRIAGE

In certain regions of the world, especially sub-Saharan Africa and the Middle East, adolescent marriages are very common. This is a particular problem because with insufficiently grown bodies, girls aged 15-20 who get pregnant are twice as likely to die in childbirth as those in their twenties. Girls under the age of 15 (who are also married off in many countries) are five times as likely to die in childbirth. Young girls who survive pregnancy and childbirth often suffer another problem because of their size—they are often left with a fistula. (As you must know, this is a rupture in the birth canal which occurs during prolonged, obstructed labour, which leaves the girl incontinent and ostracised from her community. Although 9 out of 10 fistulas can be successfully repaired surgically, this rarely occurs simply because of a lack of funds and trained surgeons. (The UNFPA-led Campaign to End Fistula is working in 40 countries to rectify this situation.)

DISASTERS, SHORTAGES, POLITICAL UPHEAVAL & WAR

Maternity services may be dramatically affected by natural disasters, accidents, terrorism, shortages, politics and war.

A shortage of skilled midwives dramatically affects outcomes in many countries

PREVENTABLE MEDICAL CAUSES

According to UNICEF, the UN Population Fund (UNFPA) and WHO, more than 80% of maternal deaths take place as a result of medical problems which could be solved through additional funding. These preventable causes include haemorrhage, sepsis, unsafe abortion, obstructed labour and hypertensive disease in pregnancy. Haemorrhage alone, which may well often be caused as a result of ritual disturbance occurring before the third stage of labour, accounts for 21% of the 500,000 deaths occurring each year. Although this and other problems can be treated in the UK—e.g. by the use of oxytocics, blood transfusions and other skilled midwifery or obstetric care—they are rarely treated in poorly resourced places, simply because of a lack of skilled personnel (especially midwives), a lack of roads, clinics, blood banks, to mention only a few reasons.

LACK OF EXPERTISE

Without skilled professionals teaching family planning, attending births and acting when problems occur during labour, any problems which do arise quickly result in deaths.

Requests for home birth

Even if you agree that our circumstances in Britain are much better than those in other parts of the world, you may still not be very happy about the idea of supporting a woman who comes to you asking to have a home birth. What kind of risks are we dealing with here?!

Actually, nowadays, homes are usually such sanitary places and hospitals are harbouring so many infections that the idea of giving birth at home is not a romantic one. If you feel disinclined to believe this, consider that in 2003 the *Reader's Digest* reported that an estimated 100,000 people were picking up an infection in hospital (in Britain) each year. In the same article they stated that hospital-acquired infections killed more than 5,000 patients and that they contributed to the deaths of some 15,000 more. Has the situation changed so dramatically since then? Is it realistically possible for hospitals to become places which are 'cleaner' than houses, given that their main purpose is to serve people who are sick? Even in maternity wards, bugs can collect on catheters, intravenous lines, computers, watches, curtains and male doctors' ties—not to mention hands which are not washed thoroughly.

Carol Walton is one midwife who can still recall the circumstances she sometimes encountered after cycling to a home to attend a woman in labour in the 1960s. In one home she recalls that the kitchen was full of unwashed dishes and clothes. On another visit she found a child in the gutter, eating out of the dustbin. She recalls how one toilet served three flats—and of course only a few decades ago many families in Britain still had outdoor lavatories.

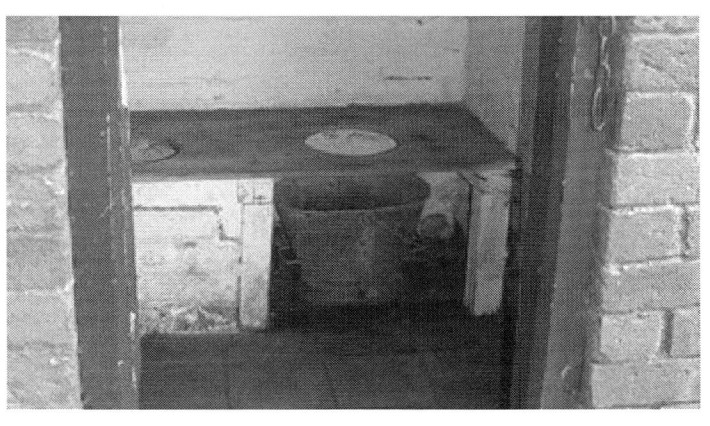

Even recently, home birth would have been a very different prospect for most people. This photo is a simple reminder of how far we've come in the last century in the United Kingdom. [Photo courtesy of the Beamish Living Museum in Co Durham, UK]

A visit to one of Britain's 'living museums' serves as a good reminder of how much things have changed over the last century. At the Beamish Living Museum in Co Durham, it's possible to stroll around houses which are as they would have been in 1913. Not only are surfaces all difficult to clean and cleaning products simpler, fabrics were more challenging to launder, rooms couldn't be heated as quickly or easily, and water had to be pumped. Drugs, expertise and technology were also not readily available and of course, most of what was used at that time hadn't been subjected to randomised controlled trials. All in all, women giving birth at home in the early 1900s—just a hundred years ago—were in a completely different situation to women giving birth in the first decade or two of the 21st century. Modern women not only have better homes, they also have quick access to phones, roads are better, more vehicles are available (and they're more reliable), medical facilities are more developed and numerous drugs and technologies can be used to treat a range of conditions quickly and efficiently.

Thinking back to Africa and the poorer countries of Asia (to consider only two parts of the developing world), given the open drains, the poor sanitation, the slums, the water shortages and the inadequate health facilities, which are usually inaccessible to many women in any case, we need to realise we're in a very different situation in the developed world. Our homes and infrastructure are entirely different.

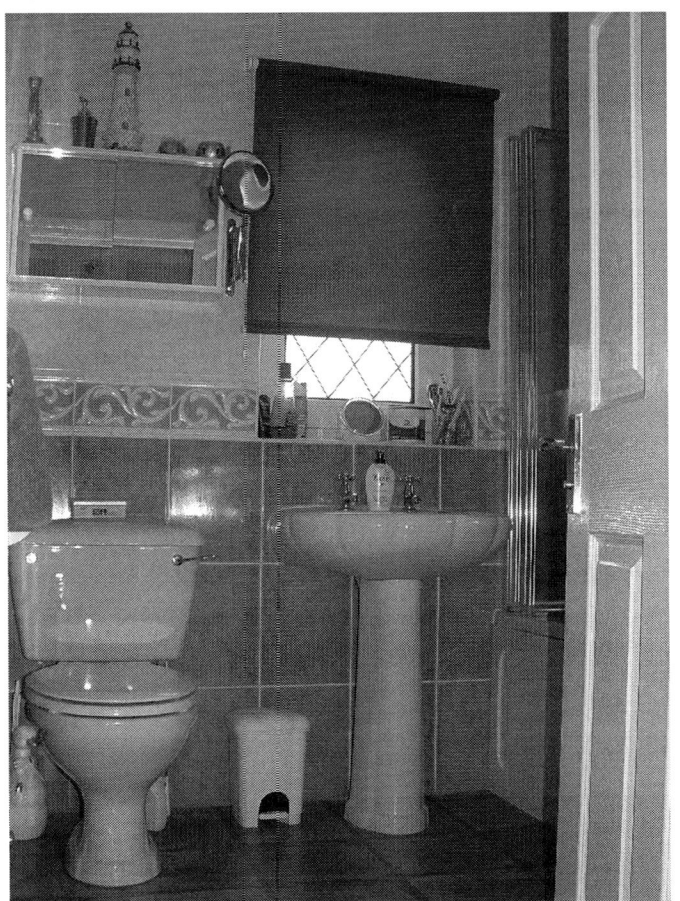

Modern homes are usually clean and comfortable, with good amenities. If they're within easy reach of emergency facilities, they can be the ideal place to give birth.

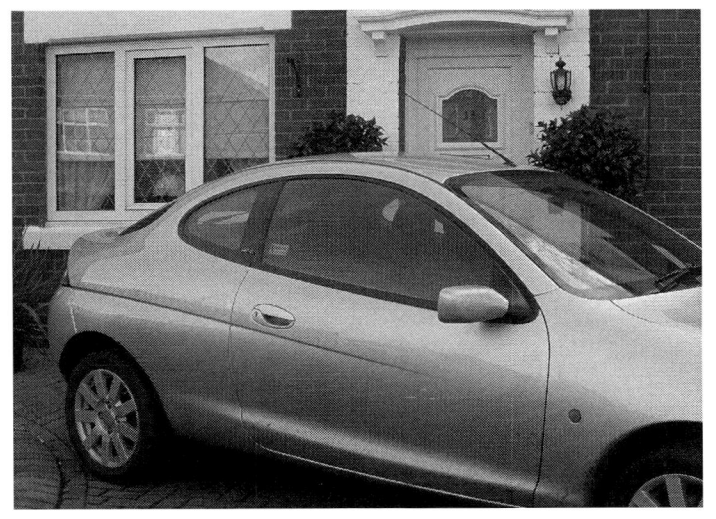

Nowadays, even when things go wrong, most women have easy access to health care and they are able to get there in plenty of time, provided they have skilled midwives who can assess risk

The risks of risk assessment

From the very first appointment onwards, you may well feel negative about a woman's chances of having a physiological birth because of risks you perceive. Like many women nowadays, your new client may be over 35 (i.e. 'elderly'), or she may come to you with a tale of woe about her first experience of birth. Instead of thinking how her previous birth might have been *disturbed* by her previous care providers (perhaps even at the woman's own request), you might immediately assume that this woman is incapable of having a physiological birth, unencumbered by drugs and interventions.

Actually, I think optimal birth is possible in many more situations than many people expect. It is actually a *safer* option than a birth which involves the use of drugs for induction, augmentation or pain relief, or which includes interventions which are initially not primarily carried out for safety reasons. In Michel Odent's opinion, the same principles apply to low and high risk labouring women: the amount of disturbance a woman experiences and the extent to which she feels safe are most important. In other words, leaving the labouring woman undisturbed might be more important than close monitoring because it will give the woman and her unborn baby the best possible conditions for successfully orchestrating the cocktail of hormones necessary for a safe birth.

In any case, it's very unfortunate when a woman is labelled 'high risk' early on in her pregnancy... From that moment onwards she will inevitably worry about the birth, which will change her entire experience of pregnancy. Instead of being a time of joy, discovery and expectation, it becomes a time of dread, anxiety and tension. Since psychological reactions so often have a physical impact (taking into account the close link between emotions and hormonal production), this is a real tragedy... especially if the pregnant woman was wrongly labelled 'high risk' in the first place!

Perhaps many midwives have very low expectations of women's safety prospects because they are accustomed to scenarios which involve the use of drugs (usually for pain relief or induction/augmentation). Many have not attended births of 'high risk' women who choose to avoid drugs and interventions, if at all possible. As many professionals have found, if the physiological processes are not just left undisturbed, but are *facilitated* (with the midwife creating an atmosphere around the labouring woman of confidence, security and privacy) beautiful outcomes are usually the result.

In *BIRTH: Countdown to Optimal* (the companion book to this one, for pregnant women), I include many birth stories about women who would normally be labelled 'high risk', who went on to have extremely successful—and joyful—physiological births. These births were truly optimal because as well as being safe, they were beautiful.

- **Elderly primagravidas** Of course, at 38 I was an elderly primagravida in Sri Lanka. Michel Odent's former partner was not only an elderly primagravida, she also had MS. Nevertheless, she had a very straightforward birth after a three-hour labour. Pascal, the 'baby' is now studying for his PhD, following in his father's footsteps! Rachel Urbach (who we met in Birthframe 5) also had an entirely undisturbed physiological birth (with an NHS midwife in attendance) at the age of 38. (Other women, of course, who were multiparas—myself among them—gave birth entirely successfully too, physiologically.)
- **Previous births that went wrong** Maria Shanahan (who we read about in Birthframe 4) is just one of many women mentioned who had a straightforward physiological birth for a second baby after a bad first experience. Pauline Farrance (Birthframe 23) is another. The key to these women's success—in Michel Odent's opinion—was the complete privacy and lack of disturbance they experienced while they were in labour the second time round. The hormones needed to give birth safely were produced very smoothly because the labouring women really did enter that strange state of mind we've already described.
- **Twins** There are many accounts of twin births which were entirely physiological. The midwife Debbie Brindley (who we met in Birthframe 11) collaborated with her colleagues to ensure that her hospital birth would be as undisturbed as possible. While her consultant and the paediatric consultant waited in the corridor, she had a very private birth in a warm, dark hospital room, next to the pool room. Olga Mellor, a Russian woman—(see p117)—unexpectedly gave birth to twins at home, having chosen a homebirth in order to avoid pressure from care providers in a hospital. Another Russian woman, Tanya Kudrayshova, discovered she was expecting twins after an ultrasound scan. She also chose to have a homebirth because she wanted her babies' first moments after the birth to be 'good and happy'. Another woman, a 40-year-old British primagravida, who was told she was expecting twins, went to a lot of trouble to find midwives and consultants who would support her in an entirely physiological birth at her local hospital (Birthframe 10). Another British woman, Kathryn Clarke, also chose a hospital-based birth for her twins, even after she was told that Twin 2 was breech. Helen Arundell, gave birth vaginally to her twins when they were 10 days overdue. Another woman, who went to a lot of trouble to prepare herself psychologically (through rebirthing), had her twins naturally after a 15-hour labour. (When she wrote her account the twins were 4 years old and she was still breastfeeding them!)
- **Triplets** I managed to find two women who'd had physiological triplet births. Mave Denyer, a third-time mother, gave birth to her triplets in hospital in 1961. Janet Hanton had her triplets in a London hospital in 1999.
- **Breech position** Elise Hansen had a natural breech birth in France in 1977 (mainly because it hadn't occurred to her to have a caesarean). Liz Woolley had a VBAC breech birth in hospital in 2001. Laura Shanley—whose account I include so as to promote discussion!—had an unassisted *footling* breech birth at home in the USA. Esther Culpin, a midwife, chose to have her fourth baby (who she knew was breech) at home, with Michel Odent in attendance.

Do you not think these cases might be replicated many times if more 'high risk' women were 'allowed' to give birth physiologically? With the infrastructure we have in Britain (roads, phones, facilities), as well as our expertise and resources, we can achieve much better birthing outcomes, respecting the possibilities of the undisturbed physiological processes, while being ready to intervene if absolutely necessary. In other words, if we and our pregnant charges choose to do so, we can have the best of both worlds.

Testing protocols

You are probably required to offer your clients many tests. In some cases, either you or the hospital will even assume that a woman is going to have certain tests, without even consulting her on her wishes or preferences. In other cases, you may well put pressure on pregnant women in your charge because you may personally feel that specific tests dramatically reduce risks for women. While this may well be the case, and while hospitals may be behaving extremely efficiently in assuming that all women will want tests, I would like to ask you here to reconsider these protocols...

REASSURANCE VS. WORRY

While some tests may reassure clients—because a negative test result is always pleasant to receive—the wait and/or a positive test result may have an altogether different effect. Of course, this is the reason that chorionic villus sampling is sometimes offered in preference to amniocentesis (since it can be offered earlier and the wait is shorter)... But is the test reliable enough in terms of identifying problems or predicting outcomes and might the worry caused by the prospect of side effects (e.g. the risk of miscarriage) outweigh the advantage of the reassurance the test seeks to give? Michel Odent has written about what he calls the 'nocebo effect', which is where procedures carried out by caregivers cause fear and worry in clients. Should pregnancy be a period of testing, waiting, worrying and relief (or discussion), or should we consider the advantages of a more hands-off approach instead? Even if tests continue to be used, how is it possible to safeguard the joy, anticipation and sense of discovery a pregnancy should ideally involve? What is your role as a midwife? To what extent should you be a 'checker' and to what extent should you be a person who inspires and educates? How could you give women more choice in terms of the midwifery style they experience?

THE INVASIVENESS OF TESTS

There are usually clear-cut views amongst medical professionals as to whether a test is 'invasive' or not. It seems to me, though, that the boundaries are blurred. Why should we call a test (such as an ultrasound scan) non-invasive when we cannot be sure of its effects? In fact, we can guess that a scan definitely has an effect on the growing fetus (so is actually invasive in a sense) because many research studies have detected changes which appear to have resulted from the repeated use of scans. And what about the psychological impact of each individual test? Somehow this should also be the focus of research.

THE OUTCOME OF A 'POSITIVE' RESULT

In a case where the result of a test is positive it is obviously only useful if it influences treatment. If a woman has decided in advance that she wouldn't have an abortion *anyway* why offer her tests which check for Down's syndrome, etc.? Do you spend enough time discussing *outcomes* of test results with women before they agree to have the test in the first place?

If a dating scan is carried out to confirm the EDD, what use is this if the woman feels strongly about the idea of induction in any case?

Here's an extract from one of Michel's articles:

In many countries about ten antenatal visits is routine. Each visit offers an opportunity for a battery of tests. These traditional patterns of medical care are based on the belief that more antenatal visits mean better outcomes. They are not based on scientific data.

Studies made in the UK failed to find any association between late enrolment in antenatal care (after 28 weeks' gestation) and either adverse maternal or neonatal outcomes or between the number of visits and the onset of eclampsia. This casts doubts on the efficacy of such protocols.

I asked Michel for more specific comments...

What advice would you give someone who's just discovered she's pregnant?

I rarely give advice. It's not in my nature to give advice. Hmmm. I suppose I'd say, if you know that you are pregnant and if you know when you have conceived your baby and you think that everything's OK, doctors can probably do nothing for you. Women need to realise that the role of medicine in pregnancy is very limited. Really, if a woman feels she's in good shape, the only thing doctors can do is to detect a gross abnormality and offer an abortion. That's all. And even then, there are false positives. What's important is for a pregnant woman to be happy, to eat well, to adapt her lifestyle to her pregnancy, to do whatever she likes to do. If a woman has a passion for her job, perhaps it's better for her to go on working... I think that's what we have to explain to women. They have to realise that doctors have very limited power.

A comment from a mother of three born 1967-72, and grandmother of seven, born between 1984 and 2006):

> It seems there's a lot more worry involved in being pregnant for women nowadays. Pregnancy was an awful lot simpler in our day without all the antenatal testing. There was a lot less worry. Since there weren't any tests, we just had to trust that everything would be fine. You can always find people who will tell you horror stories about what can go wrong, but you just have to block them out and believe that the best will happen. Most of the time, it does.

A comment from another contributor, who was an elderly primagravida:

> I was 36 and didn't want a lot of medical intervention so I didn't go to the doctor until at least 14 weeks were up, just in case the fetus dropped out beforehand. I used to be a nurse and had delivered babies in developing countries, and knew that the medical system in the UK is not very good at reducing stress in the mother. In fact I knew that lots of trips to the hospital, clinics or even antenatal yoga classes would make me more anxious. Pregnant women are forever being told what to do and not do, loads of prohibitions on what we must eat, drink, smoke, work at, etc and treated as if we are to blame for everything that might go wrong. I figured that if it was so hard to have a healthy baby there wouldn't be an over-population problem in the world, although most first-time mothers are a lot younger than I was.

Monitoring procedures

Monitoring is another aspect of antenatal care which needs to be thought about because it can lead to additional tests, interventions and radically different birthing experiences. The way in which it's conducted can also dramatically affect any individual woman's 'emotional landscape', which in turn may have an impact on hormonal processes—because, as we've seen, these are intrinsically interlinked. (As we've already noted, it's no coincidence that we produce adrenaline when we're afraid and oxytocin when we're having a meal with a friend or partner.)

It's even useful to consider the *definition* of 'monitoring'. Personally, I prefer a broad definition: it can be anything from a few questions and palpation to the use of ultrasound. Obviously, the idea is to track both maternal and fetal progress and intervene with additional checks when any concerns arise, all so as to ensure positive outcomes.

Let's consider some typical forms of antenatal monitoring so as to gain a greater understanding of them:

- **Blood pressure and urine check** While the aim is to check and record the woman's blood pressure and urine, does anything else happen at the same time? Since women are told by their midwives that these checks are carried out so as to check for symptoms of pre-eclampsia and the life-threatening condition eclampsia, which very occasionally follows it, many (if not all) women are likely to travel a psychological journey. I well remember my feeling of anxiety each and every time these checks were performed on me when I was pregnant and the sense of relief I experienced when I heard I'd again 'passed' the tests. The importance of distracting and reassuring women while carrying out these tests is clear. And if ever you discover a high blood pressure reading late on in a woman's pregnancy, it's worth remembering that this alone needn't necessarily constitute a problem. In fact, research shows that a woman's blood pressure is *supposed* to rise later on in pregnancy (back up to normal levels)—and that the rise is associated with good outcomes! Also, while remembering that few medical treatments are available to effectively reduce a woman's blood pressure, simply advising a woman to lie on her left side might help to reduce any pathological rise.
- **Palpation** While the objective is to establish fetal size, positioning and the amount of amniotic fluid, again there can be a psychological effect on the woman. If an unusual position is discovered, although there is value in informing the woman, it's obviously also important to give her information about the likelihood that the fetal position may well change later on in her pregnancy. Also, as we noted in an earlier chapter, it's also helpful to give her advice on how she might be able to influence the position of her baby, through the day-to-day positions she adopts (see pp 12 and 16). While measuring the 'bump' manually (with a tape measure), it's also important to remember that bumps also grow outwards at the sides, as well as at the front! If ever you suspect the fetus may be SGA, consider whether or not it's really constructive offering ultrasound in a case where the woman has refused scans before, or when she is unlikely to accept an induction.
- **Auscultation** It's worth remembering that a) many women might prefer to have this carried out without the help of ultrasound (using a Pinard) and b) it can be done with the woman sitting up, rather than lying on her back.

I decided to ask Michel Odent about auscultation...

Michel, why is auscultation a routine part of antenatal care? Obviously, it's to listen to the fetal heartbeat... but why? A dead fetus would be detected, but the woman would have found out a few days later anyway, since presumably she would go into labour if that were the case. Since auscultation is carried out only once a month/once a fortnight/once a week (depending on the stage of pregnancy), the chances of catching a fetus while in distress, but early enough to carry out an emergency caesarean, seems remote. So what's really the reason that auscultation is carried out? I can understand it better in labour—but even then, a minimum of disturbance to the labouring woman seems ideal—hence your preference for the Sonicaid, of course, which allows more discrete auscultation.

Sylvie, you are right. Prenatal auscultation is not a very useful ritual and cannot change outcomes. Here is a list of studies regarding electronic fetal monitoring. References 2, 6, 8 are about non stress test, which simply means prenatal auscultation. None of these studies could detect an effect on the birth statistics. Reference 13 is about admission cardiotocography (a 20-minute trace when the woman in labour enters the maternity unit). Once more, no detectable effect on statistics.

- Brown VA, et al. The value of antenatal cardiotocography in the management of high-risk pregnancy : a randomised controlled trial. Brit J Obstet Gynaecol 1982; 89: 716-22.
- Flynn AM, et al. A randomized controlled trial of non-stress antepartum cardiotocography. Brit J Obstet Gynaecol 1982 ; 89 : 427-33.
- Haverkamp AD, et al. A controlled trial of the differential effects of intrapartum monitoring. Am J Obstet Gynecol 1976; 126: 470-76.
- Haverkamp AD, et al. The evaluation of continuous fetal heart rate monitoring in high risk pregnancy. Am J Obstet Gynecol 1976; 125: 310-20.
- Kelso IM, et al. An assessment of continuous fetal heart rate monitoring in labor. Am J Obstet Gynecol 1978; 131: 526-32.
- Kidd LC, et al. Non-stress antenatal cardiotocography – a prospective randomized clinical trial. Brit J Obstet Gynaecol 1985; 92: 1156-59.
- Leveno KJ, et al. A prospective comparison of selective and universal electronic fetal monitoring in 34,995 pregnancies. New Engl J Med 1986; 315: 615-19.
- Lumley JC, Wood C, et al. A randomized trial of weekly cardiotocography in high-risk obstetric patients. Brit J Obstet Gynaecol 1983; 90: 1018-26.
- McDonald D, Chalmers I, et al. The Dublin randomised controlled trial of intrapartum fetal heart rate monitoring. Am J Obstet Gynecol 1985; 152: 524-39.
- Prentice A, Lind T. Fetal heart rate monitoring during labor – too frequent intervention, too little benefit. Lancet 1987; 2: 1375-77.
- Sky K, et al. Effects of electronic fetal heart rate monitoring, as compared with periodic auscultation, on the neurological development of premature infants. New Engl J Med 1990 (March 1): 588-93.
- Wood C. A controlled trial of fetal heart rate monitoring in low-risk obstetric population. Am J Obstet Gynecol 1981 ; 141 : 527-34.
- Impey L, Reynolds M, et al. Admission cardiotocography : a randomized controlled trial. Lancet 2003; 361: 465-70.

So should the use of ultrasound be abandoned in all cases? To what extent should you listen to women's concerns about side effects? How much information do you have yourself?

Ultrasound

Scans have quickly come to be seen as a non-invasive, routine form of monitoring even though many research studies have detected changes in outcomes when ultrasound is used. (For example, one study noted an increased incidence of left-handedness, which has been associated with behavioural disorders.) Although none of the changes seem to be specifically pathological, surely the fact that different outcomes have been detected in some studies should make us hesitate to use this technology unless it is really likely to change treatment offered and accepted? Shouldn't our memory of other recent mistakes— e.g. X-raying—give us reason to be more hesitant to use artificial technologies when they aren't strictly necessary? And shouldn't we note that studies focusing on how ultrasound has improved outcomes have so far drawn a blank? Here's an extract from an article by Michel Odent:

> Routine ultrasound scanning in pregnancy has become the symbol of modern antenatal care. It is also its most expensive component. A series of studies compared the effects on birth outcomes of routine ultrasound screening versus the selective use of scans. One of these randomised trials, published in the *New England Journal of Medicine*, involved 15,151 pregnant women. The last sentence of the article is unequivocal: "Whatever the explanation proposed for its lack of effect, the findings of this study clearly indicate that ultrasound screening does not improve perinatal outcome in current US practice".
>
> Around the same time, an article in the *British Medical Journal* assembled data from four other comparable randomised trials. The authors concluded: "Routine ultrasound scanning does not improve the outcome of pregnancy in terms of an increased number of live births or of reduced perinatal morbidity. Routine ultrasound scanning may be effective and useful as a screening for malformation. Its use for this purpose, however, should be made explicit and take into account the risk of false positive diagnosis in addition to ethical issues".
>
> It is possible that in the future a new generation of studies will cast doubts on the absolute safety of repeated exposure to ultrasound during fetal life. One of the effects of this might be to reduce dramatically the number of scans, particularly in the vulnerable phase of early pregnancy.
>
> Even in a high risk population of pregnant women, ultrasound scans are not as useful as is commonly believed. Evidence from randomised controlled trials suggests that sonographic identification of fetal growth retardation does not improve outcome despite increased medical surveillance. In diabetic pregnancies it has been demonstrated that ultrasound measurements are not more accurate than clinical examination to identify high birthweight babies.

An anonymous comment, gleaned from the Internet:

> I am appalled at the practice of renting hand Dopplers out to expectant mothers, some of whom are listening to their babies several times a day. Talk about exposure! Also, if a woman isn't really trained at using one correctly, I would assume that every time she can't find the heartbeat it causes undue distress.

Here's another comment from a woman who contact me:

> I have a currently pregnant friend who has had Weeks 8-20 of her pregnancy completely ruined by a false positive ultrasound which gave her all sorts of alarming 'news', none of which has now been found to be true.

WHAT IS ULTRASOUND AND WHY IS IT USED?

An imaging technique dating back to the Second World War, ultrasound involves the use of ultra-high frequency sound waves travelling at 10-20 million cycles per second. (Note that this is dramatically faster than audible sound, which only travels at 10-20 *thousand* cycles per second.) Initially developed to detect enemy submarines and later used in the steel industry, ultrasound soon became the focus of research conducted by a Glaswegian surgeon. In July 1955 this surgeon—Ian Donald—tried using it on abdominal tumours which he'd removed from his patients. Realising that different tissues gave different patterns of 'echo', he soon realised that it represented a new way of looking into the world of the growing fetus. The new technology quickly spread into clinical obstetrics and commercial machines were already available in 1963. By the late 1970s scans had become a fairly routine part of obstetric care.

When a sonographer carries out a scan the hand-held transducer emits ultra-high frequency soundwaves. The echo caused when the waves hit shapes inside the woman cause an image to build up, since hard surfaces (such as bone) cause a stronger echo than that produced by soft tissues. An ultrasound machine uses pulses of ultrasound lasting a mere fraction of a second each and uses the gaps to interpret the echo that is produced. Other devices, such as fetal monitors, Sonicaids and vaginal scanners use continuous waves, which mean the woman has longer exposure to the ultrasound.

Of course, you must be aware of the various uses for ultrasound in antenatal clinics nowadays. It seems, though, that ultrasound is only really useful for confirming whether or not a woman is expecting more than one baby, for determining whether or not a baby is breech, very close to 40 weeks, and for checking for placenta praevia. (Of course, you can identify breech and multiple pregnancies through palpation too.) As you probably know, in 19 out of 20 cases placenta praevia diagnosed by scan is actually *misdiagnosed* because it's checked for too early: the placenta will effectively move up later in the pregnancy and will not cause problems at the birth. In any case, a study conducted in 1990 concluded that detection of placenta praevia by scanning is not safer than detection in labour. Finally, using scans to check fetal growth also seems unnecessary: research shows that dating by ultrasound may be inaccurate, especially for scans later in pregnancy. As an article in the *British Medical Journal* pointed out (summarising research), the best way of checking fetal growth is still palpation.

Scanning for abnormalities, although widespread, also seems to be unreliable. Apparently, only between 17% and 85% of the 1 in 50 babies that have major abnormalities at birth are identified in advance. A recent study from Brisbane showed that ultrasound at a major women's hospital missed around 40% of abnormalities, and major causes of intellectual disability such as cerebral palsy and Down's syndrome are unlikely to be picked up on a routine scan, as are heart and kidney abnormalities. Of course, ultrasound scans, like other kinds of testing, also produce false positives. A UK survey showed that, for 1 in 200 babies aborted for major abnormalities, the diagnosis on post-mortem was less severe than predicted by ultrasound and the termination was probably unjustified.

In this survey, 2.4% of the babies diagnosed with major malformations, but not aborted, had conditions that were significantly over or under-diagnosed. There are also many cases of error with more minor abnormalities, which can cause anxiety and repeated scans, and there are some conditions which have been seen to spontaneously resolve.

As well as false positives, there are also uncertain cases where the ultrasound findings cannot be easily interpreted and the outcome for the baby is not known. In one study involving women at high risk, almost 10% of scans gave uncertain results. This can create immense anxiety for the woman and her family, and the worry may not be allayed by the birth of a normal baby. In the same study, mothers with 'questionable' diagnoses still had this anxiety three months after the birth of their baby.

In 1975 a study of scanning unborn babies using Doppler ultrasound was published in the *British Medical Journal*. The researchers didn't tell the mothers whether the scan machine was switched on, but when it was the fetuses were found to move about much more. In the UK in 1993, the Association for Improvement in Midwifery Services' journal, the *AIMS Quarterly*, published a selection of comments from mothers about their babies' responses to being scanned. They included:

> The baby was moving around so much the technician could not take any measurements...

> It had both hands up to its ears, fist fashion.

> The gynaecologist got very frustrated because he could not get a clear picture because she (the baby) would not sit still. At first she would move to a totally different part of my womb, then when she was bigger, turn around and around.

> [The baby] was extremely active when we wanted a picture of her. Then she put her head as low as possible in my pelvis where the ultrasound seemed to have difficulty getting a clear picture.

And what of the known effects of ultrasound? I learnt from Sarah Buckley, a GP from Australia who has researched this area, that ultrasound waves are known to affect tissues in two main ways. Firstly, the sonar beam causes heating of the highlighted area by about 1 degree Celsius. (Apparently, this is presumed to be non-significant, based on whole-body heating in pregnancy, which seems to be safe up to 2.5 degrees Celsius above normal.) Secondly, ultrasound apparently causes 'cavitation'. This is where the small pockets of gas (which exist within mammalian tissue) vibrate and then collapse. In this situation, according to the American Institute of Ultrasound Medicine Bioeffects Report (1988) "temperatures of many thousands of degrees Celsius in the gas create a wide range of chemical products, some of which are potentially toxic. These violent processes may be produced by micro-second pulses of the kind which are used in medical diagnosis..." The significance of cavitation effects in human tissue is unknown.

Several studies give cause for concern

A number of studies have indeed suggested cause for concern. Studies not involving humans have shown that cell abnormalities persist for several generations, that the myelin that covers nerves is damaged and that rates of cell division are reduced, while 'aptosis' (programmed cell death of the small intestine) happened twice as often.

Studies on humans exposed to ultrasound have shown various possible adverse effects

Studies on humans exposed to ultrasound have shown that possible adverse effects include premature ovulation, preterm labour or miscarriage, low birth weight, poorer condition at birth, perinatal death, dyslexia, delayed speech development and less right-handedness. (Non right-handedness is, in other circumstances, seen as a marker of damage to the developing brain.) One Australian study showed that babies exposed to five or more Doppler ultrasounds were 30% more likely to develop intrauterine growth retardation—a condition that ultrasound is often used to detect.

For Sarah Buckley, ultrasound represents yet another way in which the deep internal knowledge that a mother has of her body and her baby is made secondary to technological information that comes from an 'expert' using a machine. She says this is how the 'cult of the expert' is imprinted from the earliest weeks of life. She feels that by treating the baby as a separate being, ultrasound artificially splits mother from baby well before this is a physiological or psychic reality.

For these reasons, Sarah urges all pregnant women to think deeply before they choose to have a routine ultrasound. It is not compulsory, even though scans are often pre-booked for women in the UK on the assumption that all pregnant women will want them. Sarah says the risks, benefits and implications of scanning need to be considered for each mother and baby, according to their specific situation. She encourages pregnant women to seek out experienced and highly-skilled operators and suggests they request that the scan be performed as quickly as possible. If an abnormality is found, she advises pregnant women to ask for counselling and a second opinion as soon as is practical, remembering that it's her baby, her body and her choice at stake.

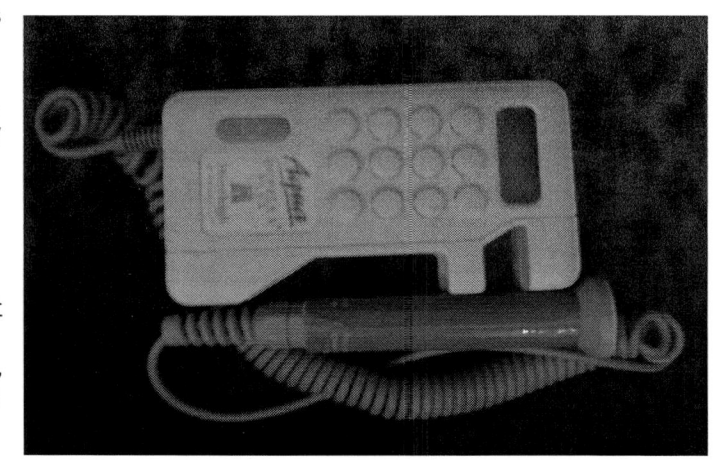

How often do you use a Sonicaid (or Doptone, Doppler, carotid Doppler, Dopplex)... To what extent do you explain and discuss its technology with your clients? And how often do you consider the possible implications of regularly using ultrasound on fetuses?

Antenatal checks

There are two other commonly performed tests which seem to cause a great many pregnant women a great deal of worry! Treatment for a positive result seems to be fairly standard, but it is actually quite controversial...

- **Anaemia check** As you know, it's a routine part of antenatal care to check the amount of red blood cells pigment (the haemoglobin concentration). This is because there is a widespread belief that this test can effectively detect anaemia and iron deficiency. In fact, it cannot diagnose iron deficiency because the blood volume of pregnant women is *supposed* to increase dramatically. The haemoglobin concentration indicates primarily the degree of blood dilution, which is an effect of placental activity. In fact, a large British study, involving 153,602 pregnancies, found that the highest average birth weight was achieved in the group of women who had a haemoglobin concentration between 8.5 and 9.5. These are the women who would normally be called 'anaemic'! Michel Odent says that although health professionals tell women they are at risk of anaemia unless their haemoglobin concentration is above 10.5, when the haemoglobin concentration *fails* to fall below 10.5 research shows there is an increased risk of low birth weight, preterm birth and pre-eclampsia! He says it is a regrettable consequence of routine evaluation of haemoglobin concentration that women are told they are anaemic—when they aren't—and are given iron supplements. There is a tendency both to overlook the side effects of iron (constipation, diarrhoea, heartburn, etc) and also to forget that iron inhibits the absorption of such an important growth factor as zinc. Research has shown that iron supplementation can also exacerbate lipid peroxidation (a process which leads to the development of free radicals, which is obviously bad news) and it can even increase the risk of pre-eclampsia!

- **Gestational diabetes check** Another test which many practices give routinely is for so-called gestational diabetes. Michel Odent says this diagnosis is useless because it merely leads to simple recommendations that should be given to all pregnant women, i.e. they are told to avoid sugar (including soft drinks, etc.), to choose complex carbohydrates (brown pasta, bread, rice, etc) and to make sure they get enough physical exercise. A huge Canadian study demonstrated that the only effect of routine glucose tolerance screening was to inform 2.7% of pregnant women that they have gestational diabetes; the diagnosis did not change birth outcomes. This issue should be of particular concern when we consider how anxious women become when they are identified with some kind of 'illness' during their pregnancies. Although common sense suggests it must be more difficult to give birth to larger babies (which may result from women who fail the glucose tolerance test) there are plenty of accounts which suggest that size is not the issue since all babies heads tend to have a diameter of no more than 10cm. Even if the risk of shoulder dystocia really is higher, would it not be better to take another approach, which does not involve unhelpfully labelling women? Is it not time that more nutritional studies were conducted to determine how nutrition during pregnancy might affect a growing fetus? Should we perhaps even evaluate the Russian practice of fasting one day a week and eating plenty of fruit and veg other days?!

This all leads us to a very important question: what can a health professional do in order to influence outcomes? Over to Michel again...

Since prematurity is a major preoccupation, let's focus on what medical care can offer in order to reduce the incidence of preterm births. Recently, considerable research has focused on how useful antibiotics might be to prevent this. A large multi-centre randomised controlled trial involving 6,295 women did not support the use of antibiotics. Another study concluded that the treatment of vaginal infection in early pregnancy does not decrease the incidence of preterm delivery. Cerclage of the cervix, although widely used to reduce the risk of premature birth, has now also been called into question: research into this technique is inconsistent but has shown that the risk of postpartum fever is doubled as a result. Medical interventions also do not reduce the risk of having a small-for-dates baby. Finally, even bedrest restrictions have been shown to be useless and even harmful.

From the point of view of the expectant mother, the primary question should be: "What can the doctor do for me and my baby, since I already know I am pregnant and I can feel the baby growing?" The doctor should answer with humility: "Not a lot, apart from detecting a gross abnormality and offering an abortion."

We should not conclude that there is no need at all for medical visits in pregnancy: we cannot make a comprehensive list of all the reasons why women might need the advice or the help of a qualified health professional before giving birth. It is the word 'routine' that should be discarded. It is easy to explain why current habits are a waste of time and money; it is also easy to explain why they are potentially dangerous. It is dangerous to misinterpret the results of a routine test and to tell a healthy pregnant woman that she is anaemic and that she needs iron supplements. It is dangerous to present an isolated increased blood pressure measurement as bad news. It is dangerous to tell a pregnant woman that she has 'gestational diabetes'. In general, it is the very style of medicalised antenatal care, constantly focusing on potential problems, which causes problems by making pregnant women worry.

The fall of routine medicalised antenatal care should take place alongside a rediscovery of the basic needs of pregnant women. I well remember the atmosphere of happiness that accumulated at singing evenings in the maternity unit at the Pithiviers hospital, in France. These singing sessions probably had a more positive effect on the development of babies in the womb than a series of ultrasound scans. Pregnant women need to socialise and share their experiences. It is easy to create occasions for this: swimming, yoga, antenatal exercise sessions... Let us dream of the potential of specialised restaurants for parents-to-be!

Psychological preparation for birth

Perhaps it's easy to underestimate the importance of your role in terms of preparing women for birth. In the case of high risk births, preparation could help many women avoid anxiety and confusion, which might have an impact on the decisions they make and postnatal bonding, not to mention the hormones they produce! As we've already mentioned, great sensitivity is required particularly since your priority should always be to avoid inculcating feelings of fear or panic in your clients, since these emotions are likely to have an effect on their pregnancies. (Here, as elsewhere, the link between emotions and hormones must not be forgotten.)

It's vital to help pregnant women prepare

Birthframe 23

When women don't think ahead the outcome is often far from ideal, as the next account shows. Sometimes, tragically, life gives us no second chances.

No family history on either side of multiples... I suppose history has to start somewhere. I continued to work full-time in a leisure centre on my feet all day. Felt well throughout. A little breathless on dog walks up hills. Sickness always at tea time. I didn't feel I got very big but people tell me otherwise. I would have to roll off the settee, though!

Hospital appointments—scans took longer to ensure they didn't do the same one twice! I never bothered to learn any doctors' names as I did not see the same person twice. My named obstetrician was on 'long-term sick', I later discovered. Three heart monitors across my bump was always long-winded. One doctor said it was a waste of time because of interference between them... It didn't stop them doing it.

The local midwife eventually made contact. We had been overlooked. She talked about antenatal classes. I was aware the kids would probably come at around 33-36 weeks. But there seemed no sense of urgency from anyone. I never heard from or saw the midwife again. So a rapport was never made with any professional. We seemed to be continually 'overlooked' or forgotten about.

At 28 weeks (only 10 weeks after finding out I was expecting triplets) I went into premature labour and had an emergency c-section.

I had another week at work before maternity leave started. I had been at work all day. Came home in the evening and couldn't get comfortable. At 10pm I noticed a pink tinge going to the loo and had 'period pains'. Called the hospital for advice and they said, "Come in." The journey was very uncomfortable. John wanted to drive quickly but every bump in the road jarred. Arrived 11.30pm-ish. Heart monitors x3 and internal examination. "You are 4cm dilated. Do you know what an epidural is?" I was then shaved. Very uncomfortable. It all happened very quickly with no suggestion of trying to stop labour. I was wheeled into the operating room with John. At 1.49am, 1.50am and 1.51am Friday Triplet 1, 2 and 3 were taken out of me. As far as I'm concerned, I didn't give birth. We were not shown the babies. Not even a quick lift up over the screen to see. Not a "One boy, OK." Nothing. Didn't hear them cry. John saw them four or five hours later. My first look was Polaroid photos in my ward room. Taken down to Intensive Care to see them later Friday afternoon, about 12 hours after having them. They were pointed out to me. It felt like: "That one, that one and that one are yours." 2lb 3oz, 2lb 5oz, 3lb 1oz birth weight. All wires, netting around the heads, feed tubes down the noses. They could have pointed to any incubator in the room and said it was mine. I felt nothing. Which one do you look at first? What are you supposed to do? What are you expected to do? That was the start of three months' hospital care.

I was given a breast pump. Express, bottle, label, fridge. This continued in the hospital and with a double electric pump on loan at home as well. I came home Monday—two nights after having them. The nurses care for them 24 hours a day. In an attempt to involve you, they hold back. How am I supposed to know what they want or need when walking in for only a few hours? An idea of timing for you: April, wedding—May, pregnant—July, found out triplets—October 15, had kids—October 22, moved house—January, kids come home.

Bill developed hydrocephalis. We were told he was going to have another lumbar puncture—we didn't know he had had the first one! He needed a series of six. This was to reduce pressure and stop the head diameter increasing. If it didn't work a shunt would be required. He was OK. Nine months later we were told he had cerebral palsy.

As they improved and gained weight, and were able to breathe without help, they were moved from Intensive Care to High Care, then Special Care. We were going through the motions of caring for these kids—learning how to do everything. Still no feeling of bonding or attachment.

The day before bringing them home John and I spent the first night alone—in charge—in control—responsible for our children. Hard work, no sleep, but satisfying. Our departure from the hospital involved being let out one door and being asked to bring the cots back. Not escorted or helped to the door. Three car seats. One three-door car. John in the back, jammed between two babies. Me driving with another alongside. No looking back. (I wouldn't go back 'to visit' if you paid me.) Life can start now. Note: Need another car before our backs give out. ▶

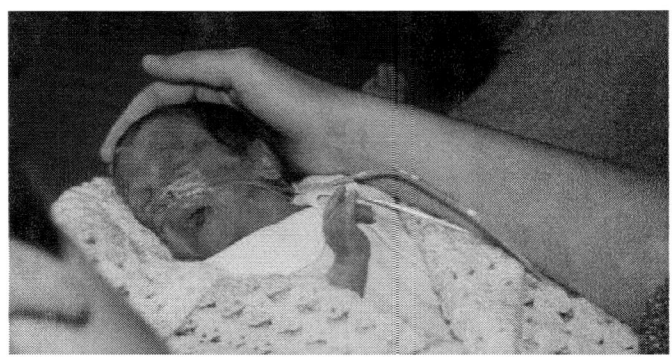

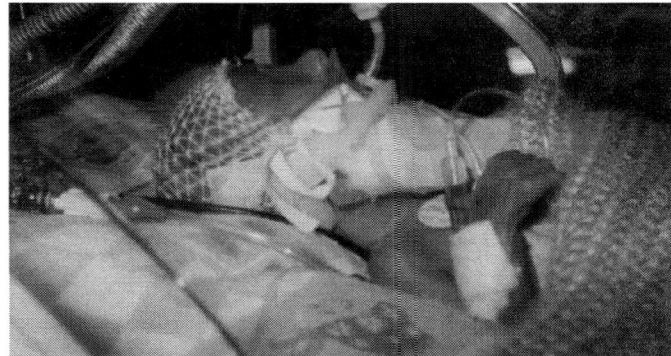

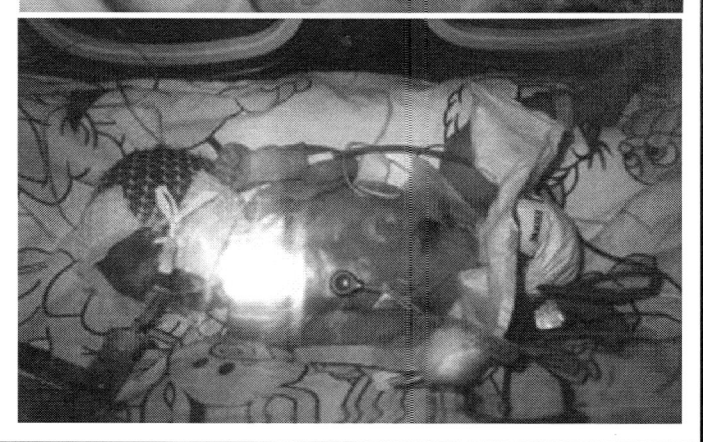

Right: *Shortly after the birth*

◀ We put a big whiteboard on the wall in our lounge. This kept track of who had been fed and changed and when. No sleep, not eating proper meals, needing help but not wanting it all resulted in postnatal depression. I asked for help from our health visitor three or four months after the kids came home. I was given antidepressants. For a couple of days I felt dizzy but began to feel more 'myself'. I took one course or packet, but didn't go back for more. I didn't like needing help. I should have kept with them—they really did make a big difference.

Three and a half years on. We still go through the motions of caring for our children. We have a bigger family than we wanted. We have never had a rush of love for them. We still look longingly at parents with singletons, seeing all the things we couldn't, can't and will never be able to do. I feel the whole premature birth and experience described has played a huge part in this lack of emotion.

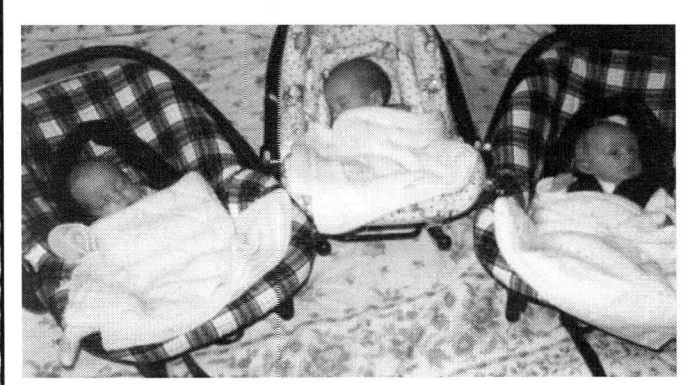

3½ years on we still go through the motions of caring for our children

Things I wish other women pregnant with triplets could do:
- Go and see a Special Care Baby Unit now—just in case. Ask about 'kangaroo care'. It was never mentioned and now I think that skin-to-skin contact with each child may have helped 'connect us' a little. [See Birthframe 50.]
- Rest and read as much as possible now. Pregnancy, birth and ideas for later. You won't get time when they arrive.
- Arrange help, especially regular week in, week out (same time, same day). It's a lifeline. Knowing when someone is going to walk in is great.
- Go outside with them. Being stopped and asked questions is much better than being stuck indoors.
- Try and make time to have a bath or shower!
- Do something for yourself.

Come to terms with the fact you will never be able to sit and chat with other parents in the same way as parents of singletons. You

We've never had a rush of love

Left: *Going home*
Below: *Seth, Alan and Bill, aged 3—names have been changed*

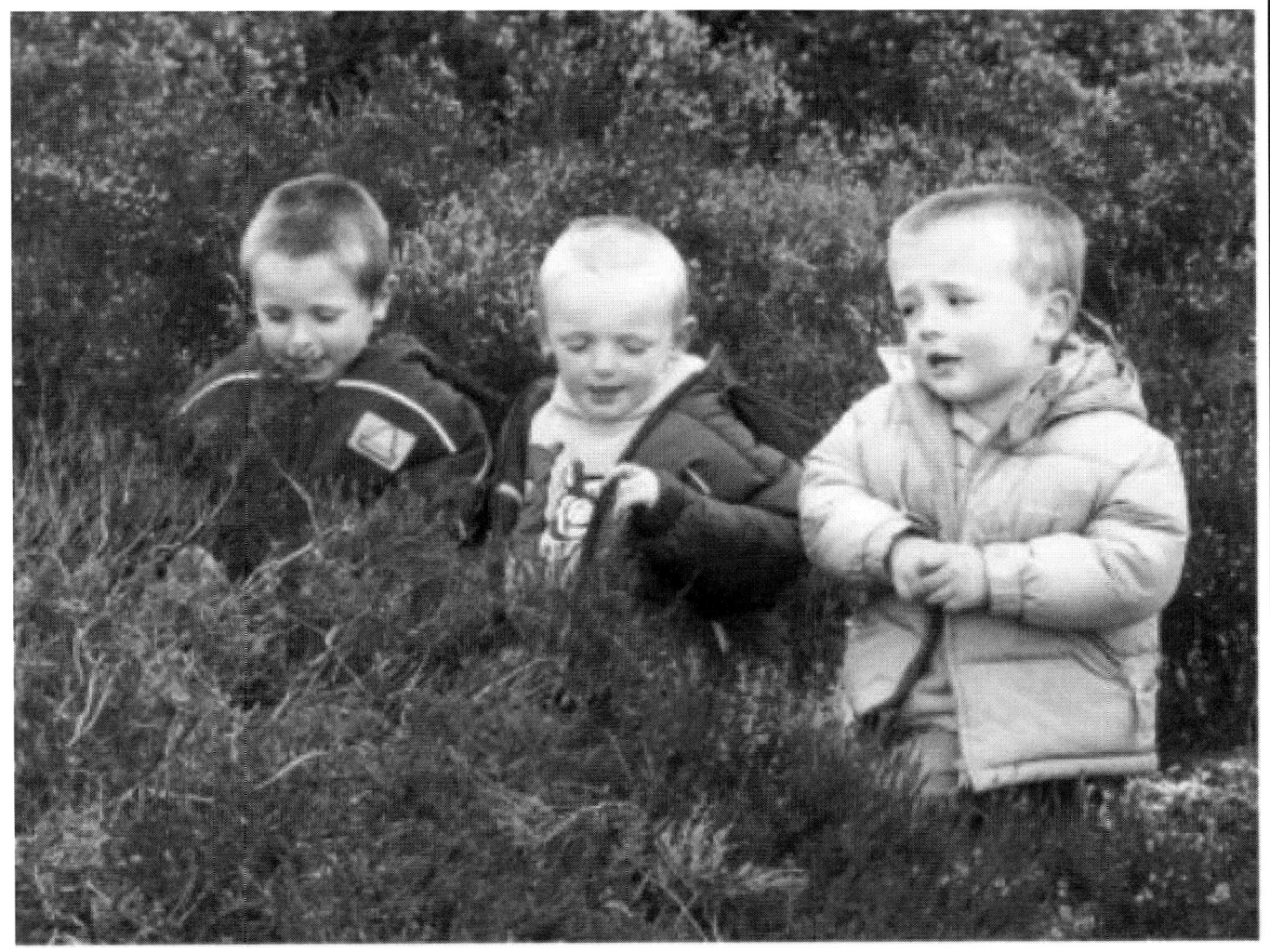

The importance and role of birth plans

REACHING AGREEMENT

Anybody who's ever had a boyfriend or been married will understand the importance of communication. In cases where it's easy to assume understanding, sadly we find it's often not there at all. Rapport is all very well, but sometimes we find we also need words.

Communication, discussion and agreement is particularly important when it comes to preparing for birth because preferences can vary so widely. In this book I'm assuming you're supporting women who are choosing to give birth physiologically, but how does each individual woman understand that? How do you? There is, of course, wide scope for variation, so details need to be discussed.

In cases where there is any disagreement, some kind of compromise needs to be reached. If this is impossible, it will of course be necessary for your client to find another midwife. However, just as *she* has the right to choose her caregiver, so you also have the right to limit what you do... or extend it beyond what some women would want! For this reason, there's no reason to be upset when a compromise cannot be reached. In any case, most of the time it should be possible to reach agreement.

Doing this preparatory planning will, of course, help your client to feel secure when she goes into labour. She will know that her midwife is fully behind her wishes, ready to support her or help her if there is any kind of problem. She will also know—if she has opted for a physiological labour and birth—that her midwife will do everything possible to facilitate her birth so as to optimise outcomes in all respects.

WRITING THINGS DOWN

Writing things down is useful so as to clarify issues and also so as to create a document which can be referred to by other people, if necessary. Another midwife (or consultant) might need to look through a woman's birth plan, as well as her husband or a doula. Of course, having something written down means that the woman's preferences can be conveyed with a minimum of fuss or explanation and there is no danger of any key details being forgotten.

When your client does this, I would encourage you to advise her to call the document not a *birth plan* but a 'care guide'. I've coined the term care guide because the words 'birth plan' often seem to trigger negativity in care providers and the words perhaps unhelpfully give women the idea that birth really can be *planned,* right down to the last detail. (Later on I discuss how we should all be positive about unexpected eventualities and not consider everything a disaster if it has not gone to plan...)

To summarise, a care guide should do the following:
- It should facilitate constructive discussion as to care during labour and birth
- It will remind you of any one client's precise wishes when she goes into labour
- It will communicate your client's wishes to your colleagues, if you can't attend any particular woman while she's in labour and giving birth
- It will confirm agreements reached about the kind of care you will provide during the woman's labour and birth

TIPS FOR SUCCESS

Like any other document, a care guide can be useful or a waste of paper, depending on how it's prepared and used. Here are a few ideas for optimising the effectiveness of any one care guide:

1. Make sure it's typed so it can be easily and quickly read.
2. Encourage your client to consider how to express her preferences most effectively. (Various approaches are exemplified in the companion volume to this book for pregnant women *BIRTH: Countdown to Optimal.*)
3. If you find anything vague or confusing, help your client rewrite it so it doesn't cause anybody else confusion.
4. If you disagree with any points in the care guide, be very honest with yourself about the reasons for your disagreement. Discussing feelings and problems openly is likely to result in much stronger agreements and better relationships.
5. Express any concerns about risk cautiously, remembering the very real (and immediate!) risk of inculcating fear and worry which wasn't there before, and which wouldn't be helpful.
6. Sign the care guide when it's confirmed so as to indicate clearly to your client that you agree with it and accept it.
7. Ask your client to make several copies of her care guide.
8. Encourage your client to give a copy of the care guide to anyone who might be present at the birth, e.g. her mother, her partner, a doula, a friend, or her consultant.
9. Encourage your client to keep a copy of the care guide on her person at all times (e.g. in her handbag) in case she suddenly goes into labour.
10. If your client is having a home birth, suggest she stick a copy of her care guide on a door near the front door of her house so that it will immediately be seen by any midwives arriving to attend her in labour.

A few comments from mothers:

> It wasn't really the risk of haemorrhaging, he finally admitted, that was preventing him from agreeing to a completely physiological third stage... He simply didn't want to have to hang around waiting for the placenta for what could be a very long time. Enormously respectful of his honesty, I then tentatively suggested we limit the time to two hours, which he agreed to.

> Twice I prepared birth plans, and twice my births proceeded as I wished. There were small differences, small unexpected eventualities, but nothing proceeded against my wishes and after each birth I felt strong and satisfied. My midwives were very happy too, although somewhat astonished!

> Stating in my birth plan that I wanted no pain relief meant that none was offered to me while I was clearly in pain. This was important because I would have been more likely to have 'given in' if I had been offered things.

Finally, remember that in helping your client to prepare a care guide, you're collaborating for success. Both you and your client will be hoping for positive outcomes and this is one way of facilitating them.

INTRAPARTUM CARE

Of course, your own institution will have its own protocols and guidelines, probably including a decision tree for watchful waiting, and these should all be informed by NICE guidelines. However, since there is enormous scope for variation it's important to consider what's important and also what's *possible,* so as to optimise in-labour care.

The importance of non-disturbance

I get the impression many people think that nothing much constitutes a disturbance when it comes to birth. All kinds of people are invited along to watch a labour and birth, cameras and even camcorders are used, and medical personnel pop in and out, frequently with no respect for the woman's privacy. People freely talk to the labouring woman, unaware that this might have a profoundly negative effect. Midwives and consultants interrupt the labouring woman whenever they perform vaginal examinations or listen to the fetal heartbeat and they sometimes suggest hooking her up to an electronic fetal monitor, which usually limits her movements. Many midwives issue commands or make suggestions, they offer drugs and other options for pain relief and if they actually administer any they completely change the woman's internal chemistry. They touch the woman and usually catch the baby, they offer comments and information without being asked (e.g. on the baby's gender) and they often interrupt early mother-baby interactions. All these things are done without any real concern that disturbance is a possibility. Insensitivity on top of—or instead of—all this disturbance can also result in poorer outcomes, as we saw in Birthframe 23, because mother's negative reactions can severely affect bonding.

Although at times there are excellent safety reasons for stepping in, sometimes carers, relatives or friends disturb things out of impatience. Sometimes their speech or actions are prompted by worry or fear; sometimes carers are not really following protocols at all, but doing things out of habit. At times it may even be a desire to control a seemingly wild experience which prompts someone to cause a disturbance. And, of course, very often the processes of labour and birth are disturbed by attempts to alleviate pain. The idea that a woman is entirely capable of giving birth without anyone else's help is shocking to many people... and the idea that it's possible to help prompts many people to action.

However, as I've stressed before, I really do believe that the processes of birth are so delicate that many things can disturb a labouring woman and consequently make her labour slower and more dangerous. Just as one small jolt changes the pattern in a kaleidoscope or one mistake at work might have enormous repercussions, affecting numerous people, even one inappropriate action, comment, intervention or therapy can have a dramatic effect.

If you personally question this, please remember the link between emotions and hormonal production... It may cause a dramatic chain of negative developments. The link between speech and the 'wrong'—non-instinctual—state of mind explains why even simple one-word interventions can be very disruptive. Furthermore, disturbance is particularly likely because of the sexual nature of birth. As you may know, even a mistimed comment or wrong movement during a sexual experience can take a person 'out' of the mood. If a person outside the experience should also come along... well that might *really* change outcomes.

States of mind are very important and things seem to proceed most smoothly if the labouring woman is allowed to drift off into a different, totally absorbed state of mind. To do this, a feeling of privacy and security is necessary... It's worth noting that first of all, as a midwife, *you* are the person who can create both a sense of privacy and security for the labouring woman. You have enormous power in this respect, even if it may seem rather Zen-like! (It's not exactly inaction but *considered* action or refraining from action from a standpoint of wisdom.) It's also worth noting that in not disturbing the labouring woman you're not handing over all control to her. As one experienced antenatal teacher (with first-hand experience of physiological birth) pointed out to me, it's not a question of handing control to the labouring woman, it's a question of *not controlling her.* As you know, while she's in labour and giving birth physiologically, she's going to seem well and truly out of control—totally wild!—so the issue of control seems a pretty irrelevant one really.

Here, in an adapted extract from *Birth and Breastfeeding* (Clairview Books 2007), Michel explains why our minds need to remain undisturbed and how it is that our bodies tap into their instinctual knowledge about giving birth:

The activity of the primitive brain prevails during the process of birth. We share this primitive or archaic brain with all the mammals. It is old also in the sense that it reaches maturity very early on in our lives, at the age when we are still dependent on our mothers. It cannot be dissociated from the hormonal system and the immune system, with which it forms a complex network. This network itself represents the adaptive systems involved in what we commonly call 'health'. The archaic brain, which governs the emotions and instincts, can also be looked on as a gland releasing the hormones necessary for the process of birth, inducing efficient uterine contractions, and protecting against pain as well.

The archaic brain, which governs emotions, releases hormones too

The process of birth is all the easier when the other brain, the new brain, takes a backseat. This new brain—the neocortex, whose huge development is the main feature of human beings—does not reach maturity before adulthood. Its activity during the process of birth only hinders the activity of the old brain. All inhibitions come from the neocortex during a delivery (and in any other event of the sexual life, as well). That is why, in a very spontaneous birth according to the method of the mammals, there is a stage when the woman seems to be cut off from our world, as if on her way to another planet. This changing level of consciousness is obviously related to a lesser degree of control by the new brain. Then the mother-to-be is freed from any sort of inhibition. She dares to scream out; to open her sphincters; to forget about what she has learned, what is cultural, even what is decent. That is why the best way to make a birth longer, more difficult, more painful (and more dangerous) is to stimulate the neocortex where all the inhibitions originate. The labouring woman needs to be protected from any sort of neocortical stimulation.

The neocortex can be stimulated by light, or by having to listen to people talking logically and rationally, or by being surrounded by people who behave like observers. A feeling of privacy, on the other hand, accompanies a reduction in neocortical control. The need for privacy, along with the need to feel secure, is a basic mammalian need in the period surrounding birth.

Birthframe 24

To illustrate how this non-disturbance might work in practice, here is an account by a first-time mother from London, Jenny Sanderson. Her account provides some clues as to how the physiological processes can be facilitated effectively. As you will see, Jenny started out planning a hospital birth and she only started considering a home birth when she learnt about typical hospital procedures. Labouring undisturbed with Michel in attendance, Jenny experienced typical optimal births.

When I was pregnant with my first child, and in a state of almost total ignorance about childbirth, my husband Tim and I attended Active Birth antenatal classes. I retained very little of the information we were given but will never forget the assertiveness role-play we did. It seemed that a hospital birth would involve countless interventions that had to be resisted—and I knew that I would not be able to resist them.

Then a friend told me about a lecture by Michel Odent that she had attended and suggested I phone him; he lived in London, and delivered babies at home. So as not to disappoint her, rather than anything else, I called and made an appointment. My appointment took place at his home, during early pregnancy. Over about one-and-a-half to two hours we discussed my work, education, childhood, Tim's work, where we lived, hobbies, etc. He asked if I knew anything about my own birth—I didn't—and was interested to know about my mother's experience of stillbirth; he felt it would not be a good idea for her to be present for my labour. We went over my pregnancy to date and he listened to the baby's heartbeat and felt its position.

It was all very straightforward—my pregnancy was normal, he was available around the time I was due and, almost before I realised it, we had arranged for him to deliver me at home.

My Active Birth teacher, surprisingly, was concerned. How would I cope just with my husband, Tim, as a labour companion? Did I know that Michel would pretty well leave us to it? This didn't seem like a problem to me compared with the treatment I seemed certain to get and the battles we'd have to fight in hospital.

My Active Birth teacher, surprisingly, was concerned about my plans...

About a month before the EDD Michel visited Tim and me at home, mainly to meet Tim, see the house and our heating arrangements and where the bedrooms and bathroom were. He again listened to the baby's heartbeat and felt its position.

A week before the EDD, Michel sent a letter to me, with a copy to my GP and the hospital. It confirmed his intention to attend me at home during labour.

Here's her account of the birth itself:

On the morning of my EDD I didn't feel too good, not very well, a bit tummyish—but not bad enough to cancel friends who were coming to lunch—an arrangement deliberately made for this date, on the assumption that the first baby would be 'late'. I ate a normal breakfast.

Our friends arrived about 11.00am. Soon after, I began to feel that I didn't want to sit still and went round the garden and up and down the house. We rang Michel; I spoke to him but he wasn't anxious, especially when he heard about the breakfast. By lunchtime, I didn't want to be sociable or to eat anything and went upstairs. Tim phoned Michel again and everyone had lunch, leaving by early afternoon just as Michel arrived. He saw that I was not in 'hard labour', felt the baby's heartbeat and pronounced everything to be normal.

During the afternoon and early evening I spent some of my time walking round the bedroom but mostly in the bath or on the loo. Later on I found leaning against the towel rail useful but I didn't want to use Tim for support and the one time I tried lying down on some cushions felt stranded and found the contractions harder to manage. I spent a good deal of time on the loo, though I'm sure my bowels were long since empty.

During this time Michel listened to the baby's heartbeat several times with his Doppler machine and confirmed that the mucous plug had been ejected into the bath. He spent most of the time upstairs in the spare room with a book and occasionally talking to Tim.

Shortly after 8pm Michel could hear that my breathing had turned to grunting and suggested that I move out of the bath into the bedroom. Tim supported me for two or three contractions before Rebecca was born at 8.25, by candlelight.

Michel laid her on a towel and used his mucus extractor. [This was simply the funnel of a hand-held stethoscope. The procedure is explained in detail on p107 of *Birth Reborn* (Souvenir Press 1984).] Then Rebecca and I lay down on some cushions. She didn't want to suck but didn't cry much either. Michel lay on our bed for half an hour or so; Tim made tea. At about 9pm I delivered the placenta into a hastily found casserole dish; we did not eat it! Michel weighed Rebecca (8lb) and did the necessary paperwork before leaving us to a leisurely meal.

The following morning he returned and we phoned the hospital, my GP and the community midwives. Both Michel and the midwife visited for most of the following ten days.

Here's Jenny's account of her second labour:

About three days after my second baby was due I went out to tea with Rebecca (my first daughter), experiencing occasional indigestion-like twinges. By the time Tim came home I thought I was probably in labour but didn't mention it until about 6.30 or 7.00pm. We put Bec to bed and I phoned Michel at around 8.30pm; this time he said he'd come straight away. Tim and I then had supper, though I ate only moderately. After Michel arrived we had a cup of tea. Tim and I went for a short walk and when I returned I went at once to the bath, where I stayed for most of the rest of the labour.

From about 10.15pm contractions were getting very strong. At approx. 10.40pm I thought I needed to go to the loo, but after straining for a bit, I reached down and felt the head.

Rosamund was born all in one go with the next contraction, at 10.45pm; Michel caught her as she came and laid her on a towel.

I lay in the bathroom with the baby for half an hour or so and then squatted to deliver the placenta with no assistance. Michel checked me, weighed Ros (7½lb) and did his paperwork before leaving us together.

This labour was certainly the shortest; I was out visiting friends at about 5pm when I felt the first early contractions and Ros was born just over five hours later. There obviously was a second stage but it was very short and I didn't need to do any strenuous pushing as I did for the other three. But it was quite a shock for the baby to be born so quickly.

Jenny Sanderson

By 1995 Jenny had had not just two, but four entirely physiological births. (In her own words: "No continuous monitoring, no vaginal examinations, no episiotomies, no tears, no syntometrine, no hospital food...")

Here are some photos of her family.

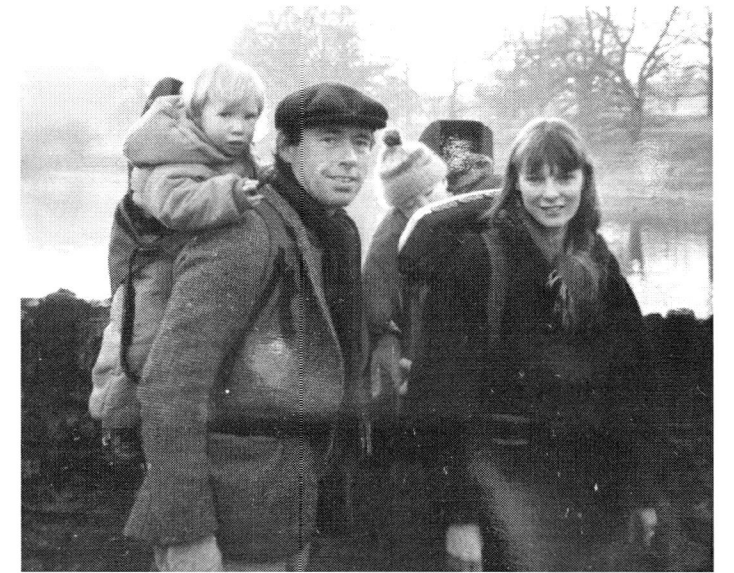

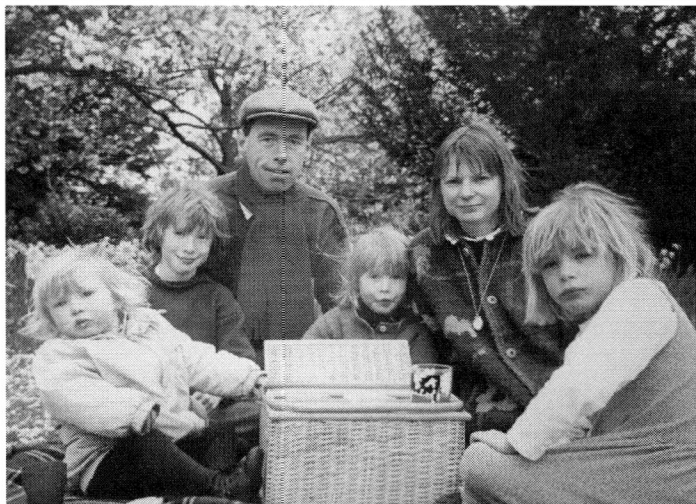

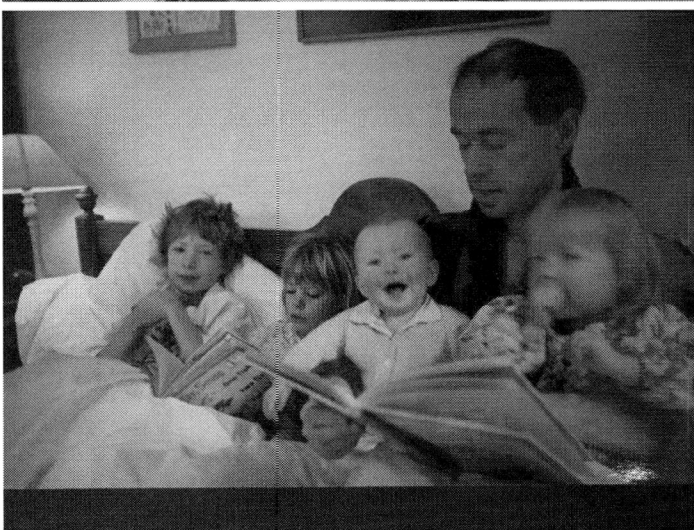

I can't remember where I read it—and this could be an extremely unscientific titbit!—but I'm sure I read somewhere that women who give birth naturally tend to have more children. Food for thought...

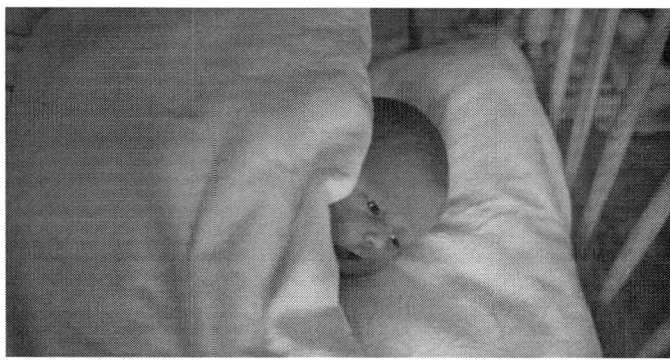

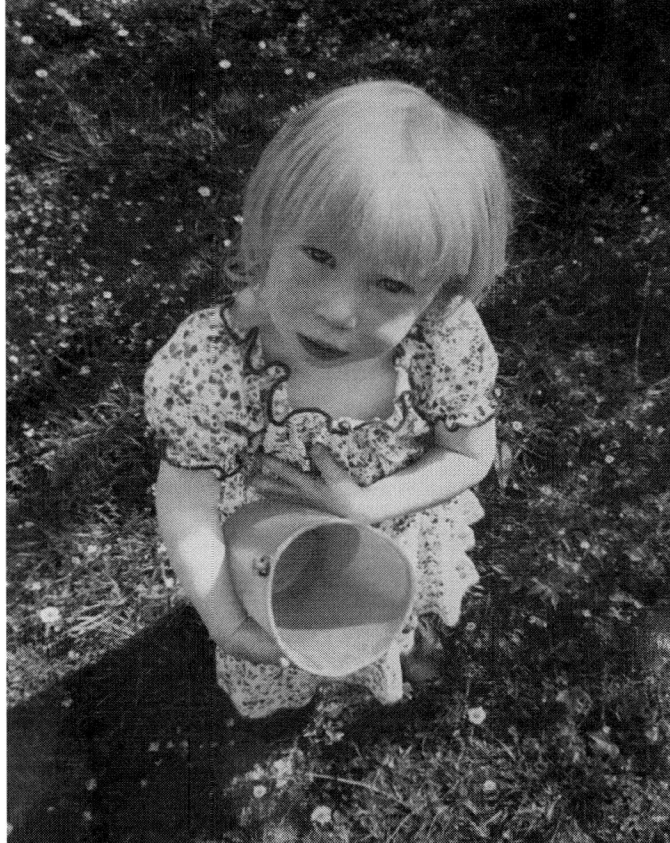

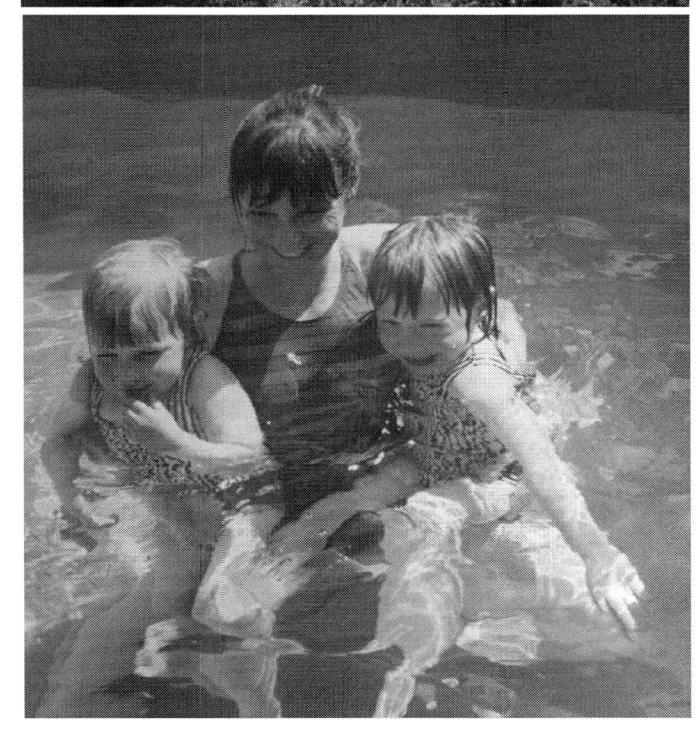

Disturbance vs. negligence

It's important to note that I'm not advocating a completely laissez-faire attitude. As we know, things *do* sometimes go wrong during labour and birth and things can be done to prevent maternal or fetal mortality or morbidity. That's where the decision tree comes in... along with your years of experience, which will help you interpret it, and your sensitivity, which will help you relate to the labouring woman entirely silently and without disturbance.

In the text on the previous page Michel Odent is talking about a complete lack of disturbance, not a situation in which there is a lack of care or inappropriate care—where a woman's labour is disrupted, neglected or mismanaged.

I remember once speaking to a very bitter German woman who'd given birth in Japan. Not speaking any Japanese, she'd nevertheless communicated her wish to have a natural labour. After three days in labour, she gave birth to a brain-damaged baby. I listened carefully to what she said and it was only after much reflection that I realised that there were various things that were odd about her account. Certain comments she'd made indicated clearly that her birth had not been at all 'natural'. For example, she'd mentioned in passing that she'd had to drag her drip, on its stand, to the pay phone, and had said what a nuisance this had been. This must have meant either that she was being denied all food and drink and had therefore been put on a glucose drip, or—a more likely scenario—that she was being administered pitocin in order to accelerate or induce her labour. It's very sad that she insisted on continuing in this situation for a full three days, before finally giving birth. She'd clearly had interventions, so the natural processes had been disturbed. Her labour was then neglected at her own insistence.

Perhaps this is not such an uncommon scenario, not because of the communication difficulties which were obviously a factor in this birth story, but because lack of understanding on the part of women or care givers as to what really constitutes disturbance. Very often, midwives will talk about or suggest procedures which disturb the labouring woman, without realising that they are doing anything disruptive. The labouring woman will then insist on continuing in a disturbed situation because of a misguided view about natural birth. This is sad because really we have a choice between leaving nature alone completely, or disturbing it and having a very 'managed' labour. Unless we are extremely lucky, there is usually no middle road.

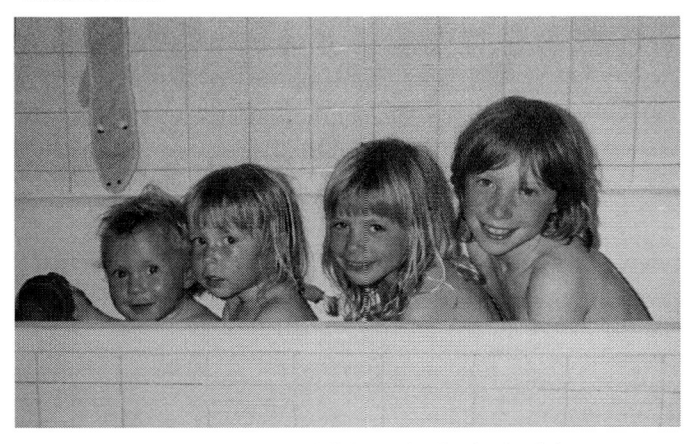

Anyone who's ever let children play in the bath knows the difference between disturbance and negligence...

The prevalence of accidental disturbance

I've often come across cases where women have told me they wanted a natural birth, but it didn't work out. After listening to them I usually found it easy to pinpoint the disturbance which occurred in their labour and in almost all the cases I've come across it was a disturbance which wasn't at all necessary from a safety point of view. I have been amazed by the predictability of this element in 'failed' natural births.

What has saddened me is people's apparent unawareness of disturbance. Again and again, the assumption that nothing can possibly 'disturb' birthing processes emerges. In one article I read in a popular women's magazine, a woman expressed disappointment and sadness at not having the natural birth she'd wished for *after being induced*. What did she expect? Induction is an enormous intervention! In the same way, I've been repeatedly amazed that women who've had epidurals have then expected the natural processes to proceed smoothly. After any major intervention, such as induction or the use of pain relief, medical management is essential for the sake of safety. In his book *Birth Reborn* (Souvenir Press 1994) Michel Odent commented that the more medicine gets involved with childbirth, the more complex and difficult everything becomes.

It's no wonder that the phenomenon of the 'cascade of interventions' has become so well-known. Very often what started out seeming 'helpful' ends up being a trigger for another problem and another intervention. By definition, disturbing things means changing them in some way, and this is particularly the case with birth.

Does this all surprise you? It's true that sometimes things do proceed towards a happy conclusion despite any number of disturbances... but usually they don't. We can only be sure women will produce all the right hormones at the right moment if we leave the processes of pregnancy, labour and birth undisturbed.

On this topic, an email exchange I had with Michel Odent is very relevant...

I attach a twin birth story which is full of interventions, along with detailed questions about each intervention. Was all this intervention really necessary?

You cannot imagine the number of e-mails and phone calls I have about twins. Midwives practising home birth before 'the industrialisation of childbirth' were not scared by twin births. In general those who know about privacy as a basic need in labour are not scared by this sort of birth. It is the art of doing nothing. First you wait for the first baby. Then you wait for the second baby and finally you wait for the placenta. The point is to make sure that there is not too much excitation around after the birth of the first twin, so that the mother is not distracted and has nothing else to do than to look at her baby in a sacred atmosphere. The same after the birth of the second one, while waiting for the placenta. It is important to know that a twin delivery is often less violent, less intense and longer than a singleton delivery. Those who don't know about the importance of privacy are so scared about twin births that they create a cascade of interventions... if they have not chosen the easy way, that is to say a caesarean section. Today many practitioners are right to prefer a caesarean section. Giving birth without any privacy among scared people can be dangerous. This twin story you sent me is one among many others. You know my answers to all your questions.

Birthing without privacy can be dangerous

The reality of working within protocols

Modern antenatal clinics and hospitals don't usually provide an ideal environment for lack of disturbance. Many medical professionals intervene for the reasons suggested before and more... Perhaps they feel they need to 'manage' the process of pregnancy, labour and birth, perhaps they are afraid of the processes, perhaps they simply lack faith in them, or perhaps they feel they need to be seen to be 'doing something'. Maybe health care providers offer drugs or treatments because they mistakenly believe they will prevent, relieve or eradicate pain. Some even claim their main motivation in operating as they do is a fear of litigation: by tracking everything (irrespective of whether it causes disturbance) they at least have extensive records of the trouble they took, which they feel is helpful in a court case, even if the truth is that it made the birth less safe. And to make matters worse, relatives tend to come in with their camcorders...

> My first baby was a planned hospital birth. I expected to just turn up in labour, have the baby and come home. I did not really take on board the 'cascade of intervention' which can and does happen in hospitals to upset the natural balance of a labour that is going well.

> At some point in transition or second stage, the second midwife arrived—this is normal procedure, just in case both mother and baby need attention after the birth. Next, the contractions became more spaced out, and more painful.

> My husband took some video immediately after the birth. I stopped him filming the birth, even though we'd planned to, because it felt like an intrusion.

> I was put under a lot of pressure to deliver the placenta after Kiz's birth. They had their arbitrary time limit of an hour and were planning on pulling on the cord if I hadn't managed to push it out when I did. I'm sure the fact that they had me sitting on a bed pan on a chair (extremely uncomfortable) meant that it took longer than it would otherwise. I had to lean on my hands to keep all my weight off the bed pan, which meant I couldn't hold Kizzy to breastfeed her. She suckled for the first time—held in position by the midwife—just before I pushed the placenta out.

Maybe sometimes it's the women who should say 'No'...?

Birthframe 25

As we've already noted, women often fail to have the birth they want because they don't understand where things could go wrong... where the processes could be disturbed. The following birth story is an unhappy example of this.

'A woman's intuition' is something that's often mentioned, but usually dismissed. In this case, the woman in question had a strong feeling that her upcoming birth needed to be natural. Unfortunately, though, she did not realise that in order for this to be possible she would have to say 'No' at one or many points in her pregnancy and labour. Not refusing one seemingly small intervention—allowing her waters to be broken—led to a cascade of interventions because her babies clearly were not ready to be born. In a way this woman did have the 'natural' birth she wanted, but it was one which made a mockery of what nature really has to offer. The writer of this birth story has submitted it and approved it (including this blurb and my commentary on the next page) because she wants her story to help other women. Incidentally, when I spoke to her over the phone she said she was glad she avoided a caesarean, even though she did not have quite the vaginal birth she had hoped for. [Names have been changed here, but all other details are exactly as in the original account.]

I gave birth to twin boys, Jamie and Sean, on 24 April 1997.

Ever since I found out I was pregnant with them I always told my husband I was going to have them the most natural way possible, no matter what.

I went for an antenatal check-up at 38 weeks and they told me I was 4cm dilated. They told me I had probably been in labour for a week since my mum and sister took me on a ten-mile walk the weekend before, which gave me backache.

They decided to break my waters... I was not having any contractions

They sent me up to the labour ward to monitor the babies. Around 5pm, they decided to break my waters. I was adamant they were not going to intervene but for the babies' sake they had to. For some reason, I was not having any contractions. They found Jamie was the wrong way round, not breech but as the doctors put it 'face-to-pubis' and stuck! He was not budging. All I could think of was not having a section. Under no circumstances was anyone going to make me have these babies unnaturally, after all it may be the only chance I have in life.

I had an episiotomy, a spinal and forceps

I was given an episiotomy but still Jamie was not budging. A while later they took me to theatre. I told them I was not having a section so they decided to give me a spinal injection and as I was hooked up to a contraction monitor because I couldn't feel the contractions, I was told to push when I had them. Jamie came out with forceps at 4.39am and then Sean followed at 5.15am, after forceps and suction. I guess that was as natural as they could have made it for me.

I did not start to bond with them until they were about 12 months old. I had a difficult time after it all. The doctors told me it was probably because of the birth. Because of what my body went through, it just rejected the boys. I guess it makes sense really.

I did not start to bond with my babies until they were about 12 months old

Let's consider the interventions which occurred:
- There was no need for the vaginal examination at the 38-week check-up. These 'internals' have become common in some obstetric practices but they often create more problems then they solve. After all, what useful information do they really provide?
- There was no need to break this woman's waters. The waters help to cushion the presenting baby's head as it is pressed against the cervix and as soon as an amniotomy has been performed, since there is a risk of infection, the woman is under pressure to give birth.
- The electronic fetal monitoring, made necessary by the amniotomy, was unhelpful for two reasons. Firstly, the very fact of monitoring in this way must have created anxiety in the labouring woman, whose state of mind must be safeguarded at all times. It's hardly surprising her contractions stopped. Secondly, it would have compromised the babies' oxygen supply because women who are being monitored are almost always asked to remain immobile in a supine or leaning-back position. The fetal distress which the equipment is aiming to detect actually creates it! What's more, a supine or lying-back position would have done nothing to help the babies get in a good position for birth. Leaning forward positions and moving around would have been much more helpful from this point of view.

Was there really a need for intervention?

- The episiotomy clearly did nothing to help the birth of the first baby, so constituted another unnecessary intervention and would have caused the woman additional, unnecessary distress, not to mention pain or discomfort at best, for weeks or months after the birth.
- The spinal would no doubt have relieved the woman's pain but the anaesthesia would have made it difficult, if not impossible, for the woman to perceive what was happening within her as her babies descended the birth canal. Given that she was so keen to give birth naturally and spinals and epidurals, etc are well-known to increase the caesarean rate, precisely because of the lack of sensation that results, this woman might well have refused the spinal if she had not felt so disempowered during her labour and if she had realised the possible consequences.

So this woman's labour and postpartum experiences might have been very, very different if nature had been left to take its course. Left to her own devices, this woman probably would have gone into established labour spontaneously hours or even days after her 38-week antenatal appointment.

The reality of non-disturbance

Birthframe 26

In case you're blasé about the possibility of a labour being disturbed, let me remind you about two forms of disturbance which have become commonplace in our society: cameras and partners. We need to be very aware of the potential of these two very human kinds of disturbance and remember that we basically have the same needs as other mammals.

Here's an account from Michel...

A week ago on Sunday, I was at a conference in California. I was a keynote speaker. My topic was provocative. It was why and how we should dehumanise childbirth. There were two organisers, two midwives, Iona and Laura. Iona was pregnant and due quite soon—this month—and expecting her first baby. Laura, who herself had three children, was at the same time Iona's partner as a practising midwife, and also her midwife for this birth.

I gave a keynote speech about why and how we should 'dehumanise' childbirth

Iona introduced me on Saturday at about 11.30am and while I was speaking some people noticed that she was often touching her back. Then at about 3pm she had a rupture of membranes at the conference. So she went back home, which was about 20 minutes from there, with Laura. Luckily there was a third midwife involved in the organisation of the conference.

In the end, real labour started in the middle of the night and Iona gave birth on Sunday morning exactly a week ago. And I just heard before leaving (because I left on Sunday afternoon) that she had had a baby boy. But I called her yesterday to find out more. She told me an interesting story.

The two main conference organisers disappeared... one of them was in labour! Luckily, a third midwife was also involved

She told me there was a time when many women—when the baby was not far away—used to say, "Do something! I can't do it. I can't do it!" But Laura told her, "You can do it. You're a mammal!" [Hearty laughter.] Because of my lecture they had changed their approach. Originally, she had planned to give birth in front of some BBC television cameras but then she heard me talking about privacy and cameras. I'd also said that it was important to be careful about the presence of the baby's father. So in the end she had much more privacy than she'd expected to have. It was her first baby and it was wonderful. And Laura had said twice, "You can do it! You're a mammal!"

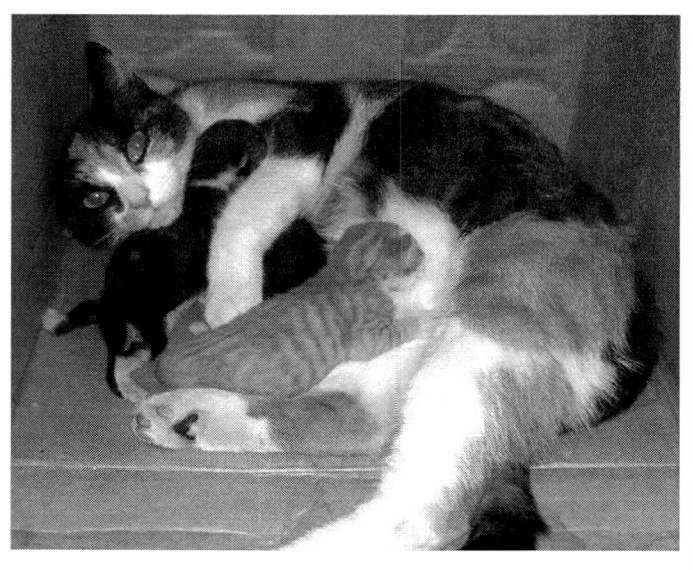

An example of a mammal... cats know how to give birth!

Despite our discussion of principles on p82, I can imagine you're thinking, 'Hang on a minute! Surely this doesn't apply to women who are categorised high risk?!' I asked Michel about this to check:

I have read that you have said the higher risk the woman the more important it is that she remains undisturbed during labour. The conventional approach seems to be the opposite—i.e. women who are high risk are told they will be monitored very closely. Do you think it is important that all women are left to labour undisturbed, or would you make exceptions in certain cases? If so, in which cases would you make an exception?

This is the basis of the art of midwifery: to know what is happening without disturbing. I wrote chapters about that, particularly in my book *Birth and Breastfeeding* (Clairview Books 2007).

So I assume you're saying that this can be achieved if (1) the midwife observes without giving the labouring woman the feeling of being observed, if (2) he or she uses a Sonicaid to monitor the fetal heartbeat—or nothing if conditions seem to be good, if (3) the midwife makes sure there is no disturbance from anyone else between first and second stage and then again between second and third stage... and if (4) the midwife stays out of the way at these times too, i.e. throughout the length of the natural process—for example, by remaining in an adjoining room while the mother-to-be labours and gives birth alone. Have I forgotten anything?

Do you think it's always best if the mother-to-be gives birth alone, without the help or support of a midwife or other attendant?

The key word is privacy. It does not mean loneliness. Privacy is compatible with the presence of somebody who does not behave like an observer or a guide.

Note, by the way, that I mention the use of the Sonicaid here. The reason is actually quite simply, if a little surprising. In the last section I was discussing the use of ultrasound in non-essential cases. I chose to ask my own midwives to use Pinard throughout all of my pregnancies precisely so as to avoid ultrasound and because the Pinard represented an equally effective means of checking the fetal heartbeat.

During labour the situation changes, of course, because the priority is to disturb the pregnant woman as little as possible. Instead of auscultating while chatting, it's helpful if you can either use watchful waiting (e.g. listening to the sounds the labouring woman makes and observing her movements), or aim to auscultate extremely discretely, without your client even noticing. Of course, since most midwives find it hard to auscultate with a Pinard in any position apart from lying down, they will almost inevitably cause a disturbance if they use the Pinard during a woman's labour. This is where the Sonicaid comes into its own because it can not only be used discretely, it can even be used silently (with earphones, with the speaker switched off)—and some models will even operate underwater.

When I first started discussing this and other issues with Michel Odent, this was one of the two issues we disagreed on. (The other was optimal fetal positioning, which he refuses to accept simply because there's no research evidence to prove it yet.) After hearing him explain the advantages, though, and after considering that the baby's exposure to ultrasound would be minimal and at a time when he or she is fully developed, I relented! So if I were to have another baby, I'd probably ask you to use a Sonicaid.

To be very specific, this means:
- Don't talk to a woman while she's in labour, while she's giving birth or before the placenta has been born. If your client addresses you make your responses absolutely minimal or even ignore her comments, only responding nonverbally, aiming to be reassuring. If you need to talk to your colleagues, move well out of earshot so the labouring, birthing or postpartum woman can't hear what you're saying.
- Stop anyone else from talking to the woman too.
- Leave the woman (and baby) alone, without making her feel abandoned. (Quietly make your presence felt, while not intruding.) Of course, if your client specifically requests something (e.g. candlelight, a bowl, a hot bath, or some specific music) silently meet her request. Ignore any request which you know to be unhelpful (e.g. administering an enema, performing 'yet another' internal or breaking her waters), remembering that some requests will be made out of a lack of confidence. Your role is to reassure the woman and give her a quiet feeling of protection and confidence. Words are not necessary to achieve this, of course—silence and a reassuring smile are more effective than words. Remember she will find her way if allowed to 'go to another planet'. Her courage is likely to return after a few moments.
- Create a feeling of privacy and ensure there are no cameras or camcorders around until well after the birth. Nonverbally shoo people out of the woman's way!
- For safety reasons, don't approach the woman just as she's given birth (unless you've caught the baby). Leave her completely undisturbed (still no talking!) until after the placenta's been born. Don't let anyone enter the room at this point either, because that would also be a disturbance. Don't ask any questions or make any comments and *definitely* don't look yourself to find out the baby's gender. Let the woman do that herself in her own time. Only step in to help you if you observe that either the woman or the baby is experiencing difficulty. The initial Apgar scoring can easily be calculated by distant observation. (Of course, as at other times, this non-disturbance at this stage relates to safety because disturbance would dramatically increase the risk of postpartum haemorrhage, which used to be a major cause of maternal death.)

I've heard Michel Odent talking about a midwife needing to behave like a cat: it knows what's going on but it's discrete!

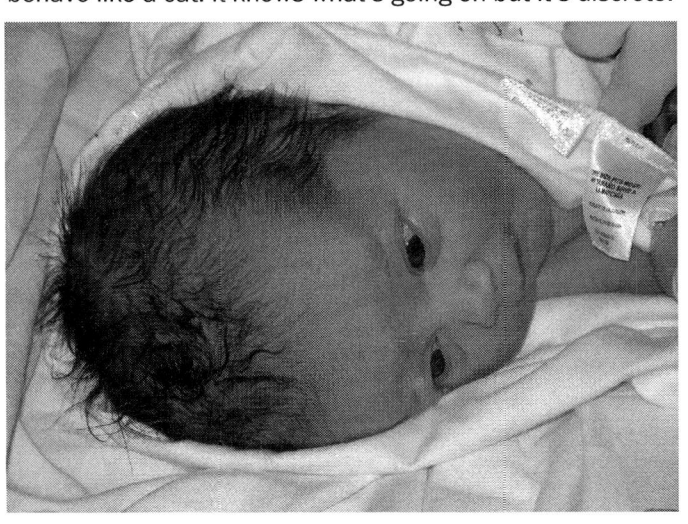

A physiologically-birthed baby, two hours after her birth

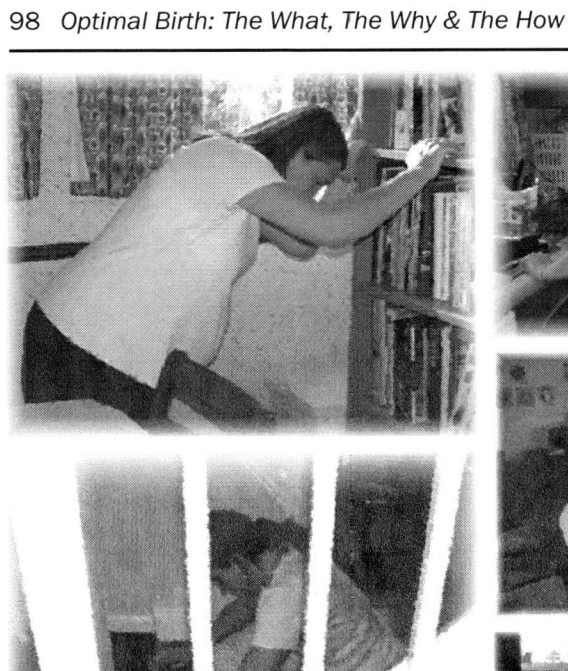

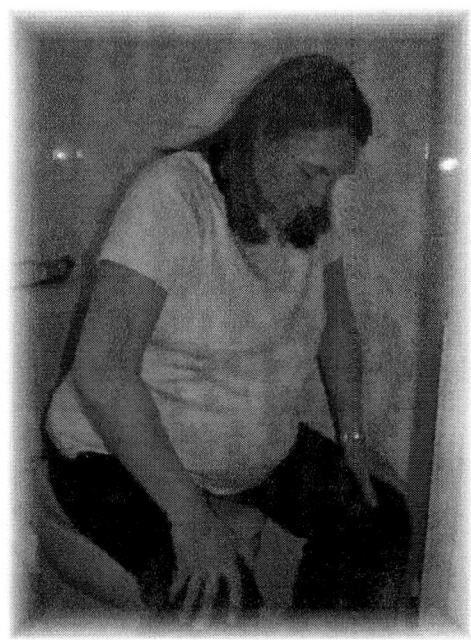

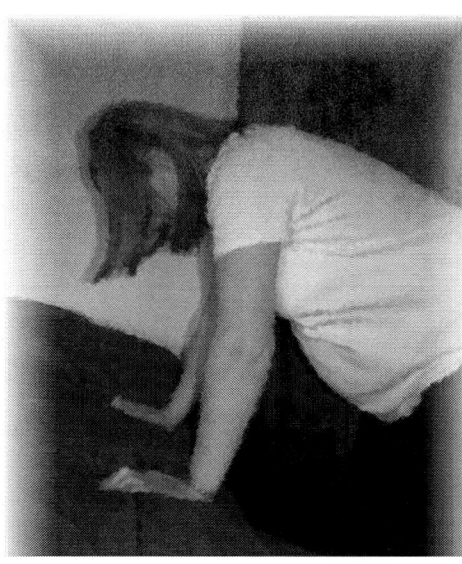

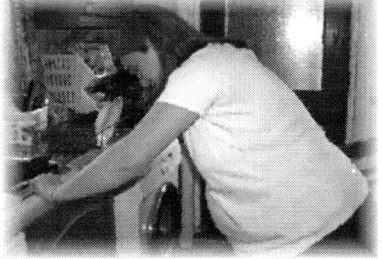

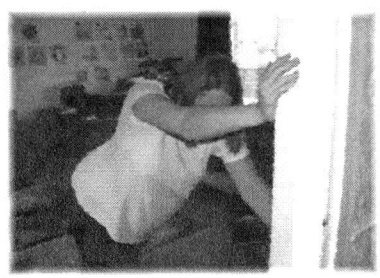

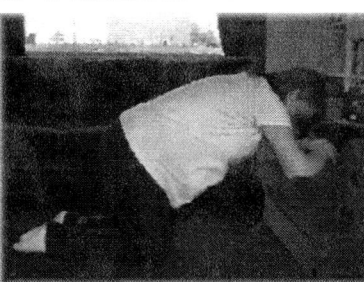

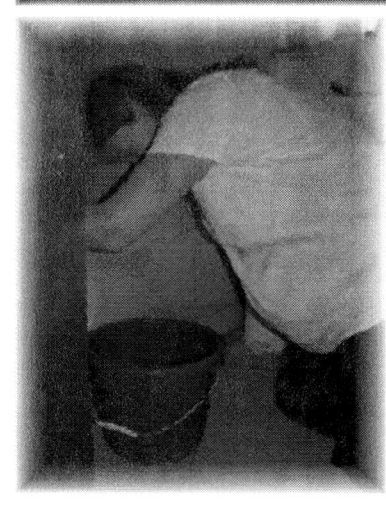

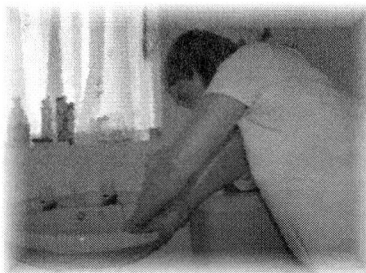

Special thanks to Linda who modeled this fake labor when she was 36 weeks' pregnant!

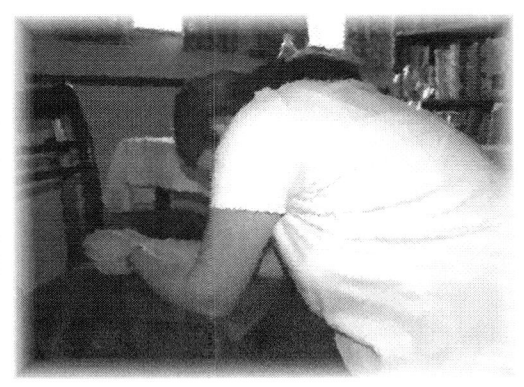

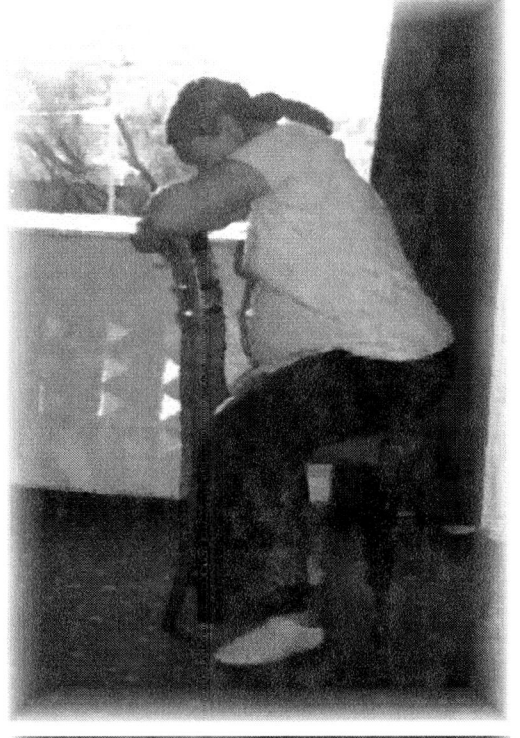

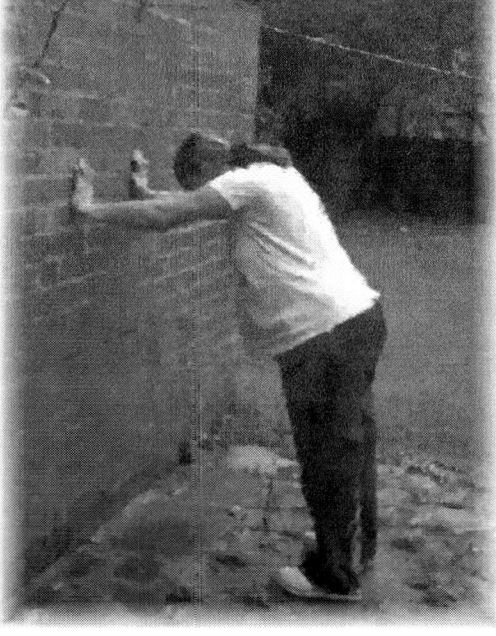

During watchful waiting when active labour is progressing well you will probably observe your client adopting a range of leaning forwards positions, as depicted here. Of course, these positions are ideal for the baby because they ensure there is no pressure on the vena cava, so fetal distress is much less likely. Moving around also helps the baby to get into a good position for the birth.

Using water

What if your client asks for a water birth or at the very least to use the birthing pool? Here are some comments from women on their experience of using water in labour:

> I tried the bath but found it too limiting in terms of movement.

> I found the bath perfectly adequate. I leant forward during contractions then slumped down for a dreamy, sleepy rest between each one. After an hour or so like that, I suddenly wanted to get out and a few minutes later, I gave birth.

> I got into the water and instantly the pain halved. It was beautiful. Mum stroked my head, and Dave my back. The lights were low, the music was on, the water was a giant woman-god warmly holding me together.

> Get a birth pool if you can. They're wonderful.

> I was a little scared that I would have no official pain relief once in the pool. But I didn't need it—the water was amazing. I could just move around and get into really good positions whenever I had a contraction.

> My partner started to fill the pool, as I'd chosen a water birth. It was so hard for me to get downstairs at this point to the pool in our living room. I just didn't want to move, but with my partner's encouragement I did, and felt so much better for being in water. It just felt the most natural place for me to be.

> Water is fantastic pain relief. Stepping into the birth pool felt like a miracle. Instantly the pain disappeared. No, it was still there, but suddenly it was manageable. I could have stayed in the pool all day.

> Personally I found no need for any analgesic intervention as when I entered the water the pain I was feeling was substantially reduced. I wanted to labour, and possibly give birth, in a birthing pool because I was worried about suffering perineal trauma and, although there is conflicting evidence on the subject, I felt sure that the water would work as an aid in softening my perineum, thereby reducing tearing.

> Before the second stage started there was a complete lull in the contractions. The lull felt like about 20-30 minutes and in this time I just dozed in the pool. When the contractions started up again I wanted to push and my second daughter was born within minutes under the water.

> Baby was born in the water, and I gently brought her to the surface with the midwife's help. She was soft and velvety, purple, wonderful-smelling and crying. I sat there holding and feeling and looking for ages, and then was moved to check she was a girl after all, only to find she had a willie! "It's a boy," I was the one to announce.

In case you're new to birthing pools and reluctant to use them, here's a summary of information I've found which is geared towards increasing the optimality of outcomes. I'm including this here only because many midwives seem wary of using birthing pools, perhaps because they have had bad experiences for all the wrong reasons. *Not* allowing women to use water seems a shame because it is one form of natural pain relief which seems very helpful, provided a few guidelines are followed...

- Since women tend to need water suddenly, it's worth setting up a birthing pool in early labour, so that nobody's panicking at the last minute.
- Of course, extra hot water needs to be available in order to keep the water in the pool at an even, safe temperature.
- Putting folded towels on the floor of the pool is helpful because it gives labouring women a greater sense of security.
- Stop a woman from entering a birthing pool (or even a bath) before she is 5cm dilated. If she enters the water early, the hot water is likely to *delay* her labour, not help it progress, which is obviously not at all helpful. Of course, this may well be the reason some midwives have a poor view of birthing pools. Many midwives advise women to have a bath when they phone in to announce they're in labour, but this is not helpful, since the chances are the woman will be far less than 5cm dilated. As you probably know, if you're not checking dilation with internals when the woman is having contractions thick and fast (perhaps one minute apart), it's likely she'll be sufficiently dilated.
- If you see labouring women leaning back, gently encourage them to lean forward. One way of doing this is to silently take both her hands and pull her towards you, so that she ends up leaning against the side of the pool, rather than propped up against it. Of course, the idea is to avoid compression of the vena cava and subsequent fetal distress.
- Silently monitor the water temperature because excessive heat can be dangerous for an unborn baby. (Of course, your unit will have guidelines on this.)
- If a birthing pool is not available, consider preparing a bath for your client, because this could be equally beneficial. Even if she only gets in for a few moments, the hot water could have the same effect of hot compresses on her perineum and might decrease the risk of tearing.

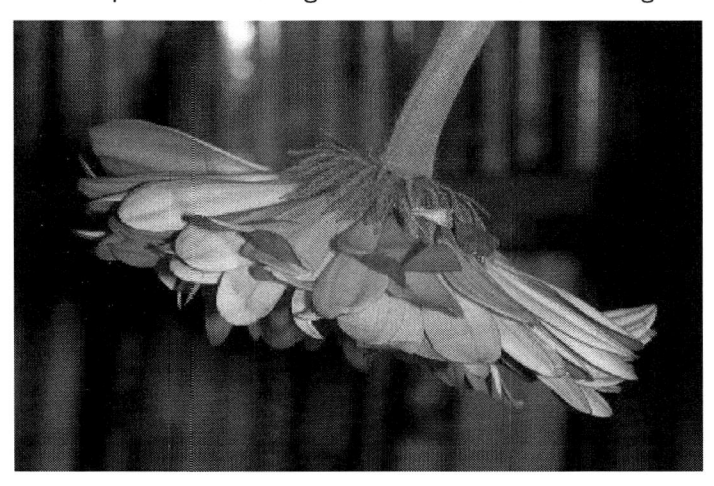

Warm water really can help your client open up like a flower so as to release her baby. The water can be extremely relaxing for a woman in labour.

What if labour goes on and on and on?

Michel Odent recommends using water to actually *test* whether labour is really obstructed or not. He calls this 'the birthing pool test'.

When a woman appears to be having difficulties, a birthing pool can actually be used to check whether or not a caesarean is necessary. It is particularly useful because a decision can be reached before fetal distress has occurred. I call this the 'birthing pool test'.

Carrying out this test is very simple: when the woman is in hard labour, she is immersed in water at body temperature for approximately 90 minutes. Usually, within this time period, something spectacular happens. (The period of time is approximate, of course.) By spectacular I mean, for example, if she enters the bath at 5cm she reaches full dilation, or if she enters at 3cm she reaches 7cm. If after an hour and a half in water nothing like that happens, if you can see no difference in dilation, it means something is wrong, that there is some kind of obstacle. So the best course of action is to do a caesarean section—waiting is not at all helpful in this case.

Birthframe 27

Michel told me two interesting stories to illustrate the 'birthing pool test'.

A woman was on a boat and I was with Liliana, the doula. It was obviously a big baby and we first went there early in the morning.

Around 2 or 3 o'clock in the afternoon she was in hard labour but just stayed at 4cm dilation. I suggested she get in the birthing pool. (Amazingly enough, they had rented a birthing pool for the boat!) She then spent two hours in the pool but after these two hours she was still only 4cm dilated. I said, "You know, you need to go to the hospital," because I was convinced she should have a caesarean section. I told Liliana to go with her because I could no longer be responsible for the birth.

After two hours she was only 4cm

At the hospital, the consultant put the woman on an oxytocin drip and ruptured her membranes. However, in the end she had a caesarean.

Knowing what I knew about her labour I would have done a caesarean immediately, when she arrived at the hospital at around 7pm. What happened was that they tried everything and finally she had a caesarean section the day after, in the morning. The baby was OK but it might have been better for both the baby and the woman if the caesarean had been done earlier.

Liliana diagnosed it with the pool test!

In the second case I was not there myself—it was Liliana who told me the story. It was at a hospital in London. The woman arrived in hard labour, even though she was only a couple of centimetres dilated. Eventually, she got into the birthing pool and no more progress was made so Liliana told them, "I think she needs a caesarean section." She probably mentioned my name but they didn't believe her in any case. Then, a senior obstetrician came along and she said it was a brow presentation—which is completely incompatible with the vaginal route. So without having any other way of diagnosing a problem, apart from through 'the birthing pool test', Liliana said it should be caesarean section. The senior consultant gave a reason for the diagnosis... but the result was still a caesarean section.

Birthframe 28

At times, with or without the use of a birthing pool, it really does seem clear that labour is obstructed. Sometimes, as the following account suggests, there may well be psychological reasons for this. In these cases of course it's possible that talking to the woman in labour might actually be very helpful. (It's the exception to the rule, if you like.) Have you read the many accounts in the American midwife Ina May Gaskin's book *Spiritual Midwifery* (Book Publishing Company 2002—originally published in 1975) where talking to the pregnant woman or getting her to laugh was often the solution? In the following account, as in some of the births Ina May describes in her book, the solution would perhaps have been to get the woman talking to her partner... although in the following case it was probably far too late by the time she was actually in labour.

While I was researching this book I got chatting to an old friend, who said she thought natural birth was all very well as long as it didn't last for five days, as had happened in her case! Five nights actually.

Her story was initially strange and perplexing: when she was 36 weeks' pregnant, for five nights in a row, she experienced strong contractions but each morning, as the sun rose, her contractions came to a complete halt. Eventually, her labour was augmented and her baby pulled out with forceps.

Since I know this woman quite well, I asked her if she'd mind if I asked some questions. Very quickly, I ventured to suggest why she might have had this stop-start labour... My friend immediately agreed with my interpretation. First of all, it was an unplanned pregnancy in a very well-established relationship where it had been agreed there would be no children. Her partner had reacted badly to the news of the pregnancy and had made no secret of his reluctance to go ahead with it. Apparently, even while she was in labour, this woman's partner had complained about her having a baby! Secondly, this woman had conceived just three months after the death of her mother, who she had been very close to; throughout her labour she said she had longed to have her mother's support. With so much emotional baggage, it's hardly surprising this woman couldn't relax into labour. And given the father's strong negative feelings, it was as if she felt she needed to have the baby in secret, in the dead of night, as it were. But on some level of her mind, she was not even allowing herself to have this baby.

This story does have a happy ending. The child is now a healthy and happy 8-year-old. After being looked after by her mother for the first year, her father became her main carer because this is what worked out best financially—although her mother continued to breastfeed her until she was 3½ years old. Despite the enormous change this new baby made to her parent's lifestyle, she is now much loved by both parents and they all make a wonderful family.

[The mother did check, edit and approve this account.]

Birthframe 29

Here's an account from Nuala OSullivan, the woman whose beautiful birthing photos you saw on pp 2, 26 and 29, which exemplifies the delicate balance needed between non-disturbance and vigilance. Although this was a difficult posterior labour, Nuala moved through the difficult moments in her safe but undisturbed environment and even managed to continue through to a face-to-pubis birth. (I know from my own first birth experience, just how difficult that can be.) Most importantly, although Michel Odent had been supremely focused on not disturbing Nuala while she was labouring and giving birth, he was clearly very much there when she needed him—to get her apparently lifeless baby breathing...

His faith inspired confidence

I booked Michel Odent for my second daughter's birth, having complete confidence in him and his approach to birth. I had first met Michel when I was being a birthing partner for a friend and watched her beautiful daughter emerging like a lithe Excalibur from the depths of the birthing pool. Michel had then helped me to deliver Ciara, respecting my labouring foibles. He not only accepted that I would soak anyone who came near me but also reassured the local beat police that in fact a child was being born and no-one was being murdered despite the scary screams! His gentle consistency and faith in the labouring mother inspired confidence and allowed me to deliver as I had not believed I could.

Ciara had been 17 days late so when my due date of New Year's Eve came and went, and all the women in my yoga class delivered before me, I wasn't unusually perturbed. On Thursday, 14 January I made the journey to nursery with my toddler dancing forwards and back to keep pace with my slow gait. I was expecting that the 17 hours of Ciara's birth would be divided by three for this baby. Contractions were steady but only 10 minutes apart so I still felt safe and anyway knew people in the shops and houses all the way to nursery. Her key worker and other parents were all excited for me and still maintained their enthusiasm when a day later we had only progressed to 5 minutes apart as we made the journey even more slowly. On Friday afternoon we walked to Coram's Fields with the children and I sat on a see-saw with another parent to try to encourage contractions along. By the evening labour had become established.

I bathed Ciara walking around our tiny bathroom as she sang to me. Once she was asleep I called Michel, who came to see me, reminding me to ring at any time.

My dear friend, Fee, arrived and sat with me. With night and our relaxed energy there seemed to be a lull and, although they never stopped, the contractions didn't seem as powerful as they had been. All night we sat up awake but contractions weren't developing. We looked at the birthing space with the empty birthing pool dominating my bedroom. Located over a cement archway the bedroom was deemed the best room for taking the weight of a filled pool. I had scented oils, the same ones I'd used for Ciara and candles at the ready—remembering how light sensitive I'd been the last time and how I'd craved the cocoon of my room. The freezer had frozen lemon ice cubes for sipping later and there was plenty of cooled water in the fridge.

I was getting worried by the slow development of contractions but by 6am on Saturday contractions had re-established themselves more earnestly. Sally arrived early on Saturday followed by Danuta, my homeopath, and Jill Furmanovsky who had taken such precious pictures of Ciara's birth. Michel dropped in on his way for a swim, untroubled by what felt like established labour to me. I felt partially put out that my 'serious' labour didn't warrant any further attention and partially reassured that he was off for a swim, so delivery wasn't imminent.

In between contractions I dressed Ciara and she went off for the day with friends.

The day passed in a blur. I liked the sounds of the women around me as they talked, prepared meals and got on with other things somewhere on the periphery of my consciousness. I did not engage well with the group by this stage, didn't want people near me. All my social senses dulled, my need for attention became muted. Jill came and gave me a massage at the base of my spine as I had been rocking and could not get comfortable. It was welcome and comforting, and her gentle energy was calming. Mostly, I felt the need to be alone—to have them all somewhere near me, but as background rather than with me.

Michel seemed to materialise as stages progressed and then to fade into the background again. Fee came and sat quietly in the room, when she wasn't making tea for everyone. Sally cared for Ciara and timed contractions from the kitchen, attuned to my sounds. Danuta checked on me and monitored changes in mood and energy but only sporadically as Michel was keen for me to be left in peace. He instructed that no-one should make eye contact with me or disturb me unnecessarily. His protection of the birthing room was useful to me as I took myself out to deal with the contractions. I became acutely sensitive not only to light but even to whispering sounds from the other room.

Nothing was expected of anyone, so each found their own role.

I felt sick. The waves of nausea were welcome as they meant that my body was starting to work and would bring my baby to me. Contractions escalated and I was aware of how tired I had become after two sleepless nights so I began using self-hypnosis. As the contraction began I took myself out and when it released I came back in again. I begged to go into the pool and was heartened when I saw them filling it. It paced me through the next few contractions and gave me something new to focus on.

The light faded and Ciara arrived home. Sally bathed her and I kept going in and out to change her story tape over—I was driven by an odd duty to be there for Ciara, even whilst labouring.

Because of Ciara, I think, there was no screaming this time and the contractions waned when I shifted attention from them to her. Ciara's birth had been loudly vociferous. As a trained soprano I had released each contraction with treble notes, as round and powerful as the labour itself. My neighbours knew I was labouring and were unconcerned but a passing beat pair called in to ensure that no murderous assault was in progress. Michel had protected me from prying eyes and the presence of extraneous visitors. Although the police wanted to see me, to set their fears to rest, Michel reassured them that all was as it should be and that I was having a baby. They returned the next day to ascertain that a baby really had been born with the PC declaring that the sound had been 'bloodcurdling' and the WPC resolved never to have a baby after what she had heard! Yet Ciara's birth had been beautiful to me. ▶

To me, Ciara's birth had been beautiful

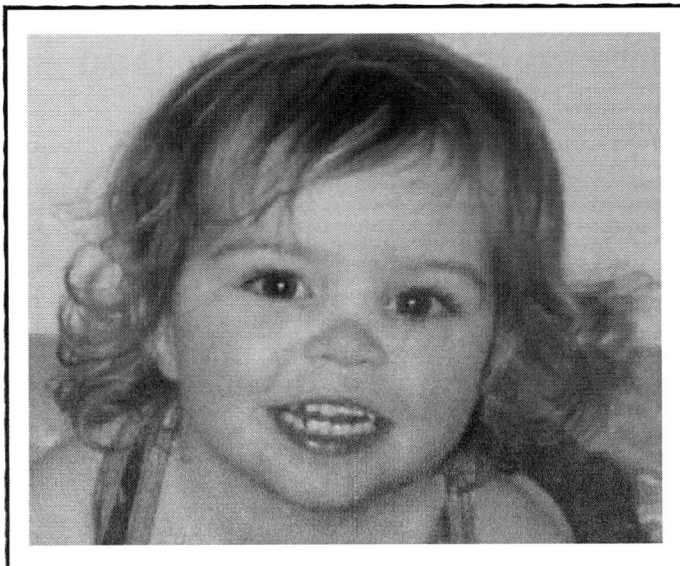

Isolda aged 14 months, enjoying a dip in the swimming pool

◀ Sally lay down with Ciara, and I could hear her telling Ciara about the night she was born and answering Ciara's questions until they both drifted off to sleep.

The landscape of pain established. If I had been told two hours or four hours more it would have helped me to put a shape and sense to it but there was no way of predicting. I was 5cm and in the pool. Contractions took me out and when they abated I floated. I kept telling myself I could do 'just that much' again. I drank and sipped ice cubes but couldn't communicate with anyone. I was glad they were there somewhere nearby, but not near me. I tried counting, moving, dancing, going in and out of the water until I was too tired to move from the warm waters.

Michel came and monitored me and told me the baby was fine and coping well. That was all I needed to hear. I could keep going if the baby was coping, so this time I stood still to allow monitoring and didn't drench anyone. I could feel my leg wriggling ready to move away. I found the enforced sedentary pose intrusive but I brought all my reasoning to bear on keeping still for long enough for him to take a good reading. Then he moved away again, quietly leaving me to my own space, the journey of my baby and me, unfettered.

Contractions kept challenging me. Just as I got used to one level a new one opened up, demanding my full concentration. Sounds became excruciatingly magnified as all my senses heightened. I shouted to them in the kitchen to be quiet even though my own sounds were louder and they had only been whispering. Still, all complied with the unreasonable request.

My waters exploded like a water bomb in the pool. Sudden, shocking. Danuta was topping up the pool and took the opportunity to ask me how I felt... I told her: "Everything irritates me". "Nox Vomica," she muttered, and went off to find a remedy. I heard the book pages flipping from the kitchen as she studied. It was all too noisy. The pages were like flapping sails to my ears.

Within an hour of taking the remedy I went from 5cm to 10cm dilation and delivered. The last hour I found exhausting. The baby was aligned along my spine and not my front as Ciara had been. The pool no longer comforted me and I wanted to get out. I felt hot, cold and unable to find the centre of the contraction anymore. My drive towards the birth and meeting my new baby wavered and I felt emotional and hesitant for the first time in over nine months. My 43-week pregnancy was drawing to a close. From nowhere I started to panic. I believed that I would not be able to bring my baby into the world. Then I felt the baby wasn't capable of going on this arduous journey.

Even as I crossed the bridge of transition I knew that if I could only get through it I would be able to deliver successfully.

Pushing started then and confidence returned. Here was a part I understood. I had a role and something to do with each contraction. I felt myself organising my body's responses and planning how I would greet the new contraction. I got out of the pool thinking that I needed to open my bowels and that once I had I could have my baby. Once in the bathroom I realised that the sensation was confused because my baby was on the base of my spine and was in fact crowning.

I called out to them: "She's crowning!" As I staggered back to the bedroom, I noted to myself that even I had started to adopt Ciara's 'little sister' notions. The different voices passing on what I'd said didn't irritate me this time

Michel materialised, allowing me to find my position and my own connection with the contraction. I leant my hands against the wall and pushed. A head emerged with the cord round its neck and an arm up beside it, making the top centile head even wider. Michel deftly slipped the cord over the head. Another contraction and the rest of the baby slithered out, caught by Michel as I collapsed in a heap.

Tired out but terrified.

Because there was no sound. No crying.

A little grey daughter with no muscle tone and no sound.

3.6kg, 59cm and inert.

Michel was cradling my baby and sucking out her nose and throat. I splashed water from the pool to baptise her, desperate to do something for her.

Then I heard the indignant sound of Isolda's own voice. Michel rewarded me by handing me my wailing daughter. Perfect.

Sally took her whilst the placenta was delivered. Despite having size 4 feet (related to the pelvis size?) and an 8lb (3.6kg) baby I didn't need any stitiches! Everyone came around me to admire and meet Isolda Lily, each loving face welcome to me now. I bathed with her and then Ciara woke to meet her 'little sister'.

Ciara is 17 and taking A levels now, hoping to study for a degree in Midwifery in September. Isolda is 14 and 5' 6", preparing for GCSEs and aiming to be either CEO of ICI or a catwalk model—whichever happens first! In the meantime, she is curiously delighted with how she has turned out... which is refreshing for a teenager.

Nuala OSullivan

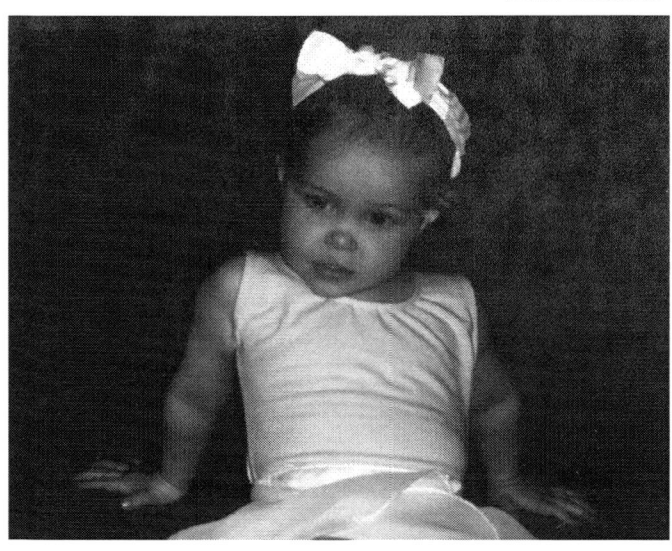

Taking a moment to reflect, aged 3, before a ballet class

What if your client has brought along a doula?

While some women—like Nuala OSullivan—may want a lot of people around them (even if they want them to stay out of the way!), other women may choose to have a qualified doula with them in labour. What is this likely to mean from your point of view? In case you haven't had much contact with doulas so far, here are two accounts which give some insight into how a doula might behave and the role she might adopt. Of course, in this case the doula in question is Liliana Lammers, who we met in Birthframes 9 and 20. (This account was originally published in *LLL GB News*.)

Right: *Liliana Lammers, the doula*

Birthframe 30

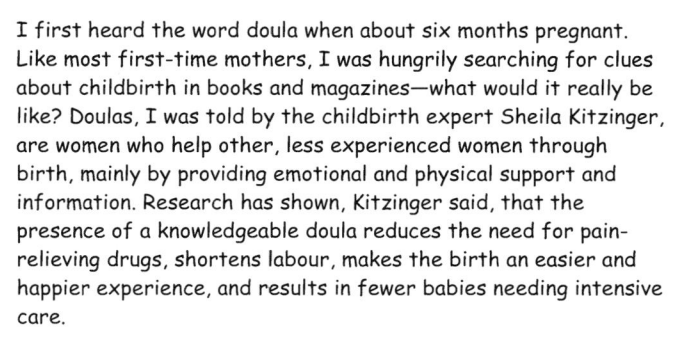

I first heard the word doula when about six months pregnant. Like most first-time mothers, I was hungrily searching for clues about childbirth in books and magazines—what would it really be like? Doulas, I was told by the childbirth expert Sheila Kitzinger, are women who help other, less experienced women through birth, mainly by providing emotional and physical support and information. Research has shown, Kitzinger said, that the presence of a knowledgeable doula reduces the need for pain-relieving drugs, shortens labour, makes the birth an easier and happier experience, and results in fewer babies needing intensive care.

Wanting as I did a drug-free, non-intervention birth, it all sounded good to me, but I thought no more of it until a couple of weeks before my baby was due. The baby's head had not yet engaged and this, I was led to believe by the London hospital where I was booked to give birth, might be problematical. A local acquaintance put me in touch with Liliana, a highly experienced doula who lived only five minutes away.

A few days later I was sitting in her kitchen eating homemade soup. At the time, I don't think either of us knew that she would actually be present at the birth but she gave me reassurance. Liliana told me about her own experience of giving birth to four children and, above all, advised me to have faith in my body; simply to let it do what it was programmed to do, leaving the intellect well out of it.

I had no real concept of the wisdom of these words until about a fortnight later when I went into labour. It was then that all the carefully laid plans for my partner Chris's involvement in the birth—offering lower-back massage, quiet encouragement and the sort of 'room service' you'd only ever expect in a five-star hotel—were summarily discarded. Once the contractions started forcefully to take over my body, I had no wish for communication with anyone; I wanted to focus unreservedly on the baby.

Liliana had said that she would come over once labour was established, that she'd be able to help us judge the 'right' time to go into the hospital—I wanted to leave it until the last possible moment. When she turned up, just before midnight, I was on my hands and knees in the candlelit sitting-room and contractions were coming quite strongly every three minutes. Liliana said hello and then almost immediately left the room. This was how she remained throughout the birth; a dreamlike comforting presence I was vaguely aware of from time to time, but there was never any direct contact or intrusion. About an hour after her arrival, Liliana warned Chris that, if the baby was to be born in the hospital as planned, we should leave at once. She then generously offered to accompany us.

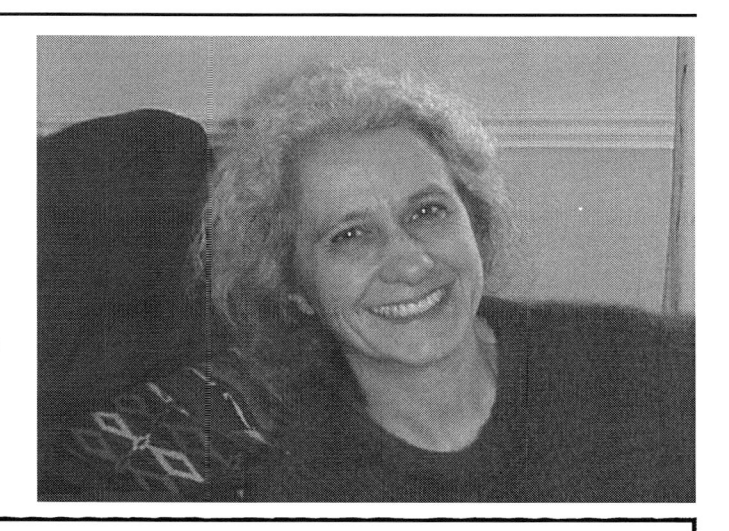

Above all, Liliana advised me to have faith in my body—simply to let it do what it was programmed to do

In many ways, Liliana's role—both at home and at the hospital—seemed to be that of a guard; discreetly, firmly she kept people (the midwife, Chris—the only others ever present in the room) away from me. She was sympathetic too to the feelings of Chris, who, far from participating in the birth of his child, as laid out in the birth plan, was snarled at every time he came near. Towards the end of the labour, by which time I had retreated to crouch in the total darkness of the lavatory, Liliana stood sentinel at the door, reassuring Chris that I was perfectly fine. I knew I was fine, she knew I was fine; for him it must have been perfect agony.

My daughter Bea was born in a birthing pool approximately seven hours after labour had started. She was still encased in the membrane or caul, so her appearance as she slithered out between my legs was awesome and ghostly. I held her and we looked at one another for a long moment, then she rooted immediately for the breast. While I delivered the afterbirth, squatting on a table in the delivery room, Liliana rocked and sang to Bea in the half-light, welcoming her to the world.

I couldn't have wished for a better birth for me and my daughter, except had I known then what I know now I probably would have opted for a home birth. I had wanted no interventions; I had none. I had wanted no drugs; I had none. I had wanted a gentle, natural birth for my child; and this I believe I achieved (though Bea is really the only person who can vouch for this). And all this in a typical hospital setting.

The only other thing I'd do differently now would be to make quite sure that, in the days and weeks after the birth, I had a doula at hand to mother me. A doula's role is often described as 'mothering the mother'. While I certainly didn't want mothering during the birth, I could have done with it after I took my baby home. A doula will come in to see a new mother for a couple of hours a day up to six weeks after the birth, offering support at a time when many women are at their most vulnerable. If I were ever Prime Minister for a day, I'd make this kind of essential care a provision of the state.

A doula 'mothers the mother'

Sarah-Jane Forder

Birthframe 31

This account gives even more information about how a doula can best support a woman in labour.

It was an eleventh-hour decision to have a doula at the birth of my second child. For eight months, my plan was to go to the Edgware Birth Centre, as I had for my first. And then as if by magic, a new trust arrived in me. One that told me I could manage at home. It really was a kind of magic. My head didn't convince me, or even my heart. Just as with my first pregnancy, an imaginary hand appeared—deep-down instinct I suppose—and I took hold of it.

As it turned out, that hand wasn't so imaginary. Two months before my due date, I attended a doula course with Liliana Lammers and Michel Odent. I found their ideas on birth exciting—at times breathtakingly so. I was especially fascinated by their belief in total privacy as being the key to a smooth birth and when Liliana helped me set up a home birth for myself, I knew she was the one I wanted by my side. As it turned out, she offered me more than that. This wonderfully calm and centred doula was more about and behind me, than beside me. Unseen, silent—but absolutely there.

I sometimes found Michel and Liliana's ideas on birth breathtakingly exciting

I was over two weeks late and pressure was mounting to get things going. Forget induction. Liliana had convinced me that even gentler nudges, like a sweep or reflexology were to miss the point. It must be the baby that gives the cue, she explained. "If the baby is ready, then the birth will go well." She urged me to feel for myself if everything was OK. Assured me that as the mother, I would know if something was wrong. I'd hang up the phone and feel a fresh energy. Something sure and strong and safe, guiding me. What Liliana was leading me to was my own instinct.

Liliana's ease was contagious

Finally, at 5am on a dark November morning, I felt the first twinge. By 9am, labour was really established and my husband Danny called Liliana. In true style, there was no urgency, no panic. She said she'd see to a couple of things, then cycle over mid-morning. Her ease was contagious. I did some cleaning, made some breakfast—calmly absorbing that most unabsorbable of notions. That at some point that day, I'd have my baby in my arms.

As soon as Liliana arrived, around midday, she made herself scarce—practising absolutely what she and Michel preached. I remember wanting to offer her tea, to make her comfortable, to talk—but she just shushed me and I closed my eyes. As I moved from room to room, from kneeling to standing and back again, I looked like someone alone. But Liliana was there all right. I could feel her unmistakable energy beaming through the walls. Could feel her listening—keeping an eye.

What I wasn't was being watched. I was totally private—and right inside myself as a result. Danny had made himself scarce, the house was silent, the room I'd somehow guided myself to, small and dark, and the world just fell away. I felt absolutely safe, wholly secure in my surroundings and with that in place, the chemicals just cued themselves up. I could almost feel the hormones firing, ratcheting up the pace—and my labour's progress.

A couple of times I asked Liliana a question: "The contractions pick up when I walk around, so should I keep walking?" She didn't reply. With a shrug, she simply handed the process back to me. Coaxed me back to myself.

After an hour, the pain accelerated and I needed a hand to hold. It was there. A silent squeeze. Liliana gave no encouragement, no commentary. Words would interrupt me, bring me back to thought when what I needed was this flow. My eyes were closed, but her support was surrounding. I could feel her focus on me—saw through half-shut eyes, that her own were shut too. It was as if she was moving through each contraction with me. So much birth assistance seems to tell the woman to turn away from her pain. But Liliana did the opposite. She helped me move to its centre.

It suddenly felt right to get into the pool. As with every stage, she got me to follow instinct—her trust in me made me trust myself, like a circuit. The pain peaked and I practically pulled Liliana in with me. Just then, the doorbell rang—the midwife had finally appeared. "Oh, I'm not trained for water births," she told Liliana. "Don't worry, it's happening anyway," Liliana replied.

It was almost a quarter to three and I'd begun to push. There was no cheering me on, no cautioning me to slow down and pant. "Your body knows how to get the baby out," I could remember Liliana saying on the doula course. And so it seemed. Two pushes, and she was there—my beautiful daughter, Pearl, had arrived.

Natalie Meddings

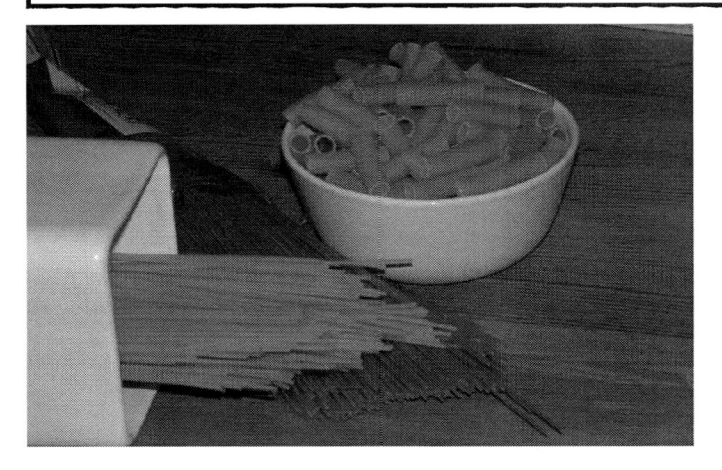

Left: *Some people say pasta's good to eat early on in labour*

On the subject of food, I was interested to come across some research which found that simple sugars can lower a person's pain threshold. (I'm afraid this was when I still had three under-5s, so I didn't note down the reference at the time. It will appear in a future edition.) If this research is valid, it certainly doesn't seem to be well-known because pregnant women are often encouraged (by family or friends) to 'keep up their energy' by having isotonic drinks (which contain high levels of glucose), chocolate or cake. If avoiding the use of analgesia and anaesthesia is your client's aim, it would surely be helpful to be able to advise her as to best foods? Clearly, that would be another valuable area for research.

The How 105

Typical birthing positions

As you probably know, these are some typical positions women spontaneously choose for giving birth, when they're not drugged or disturbed in any way.

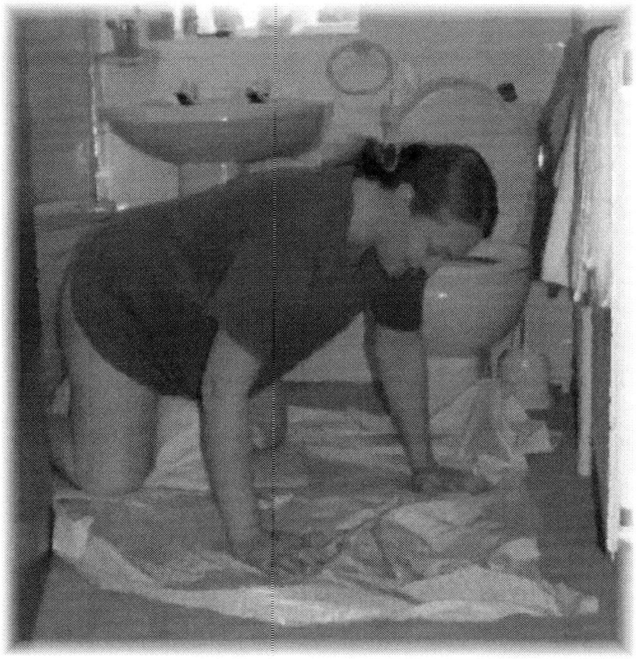

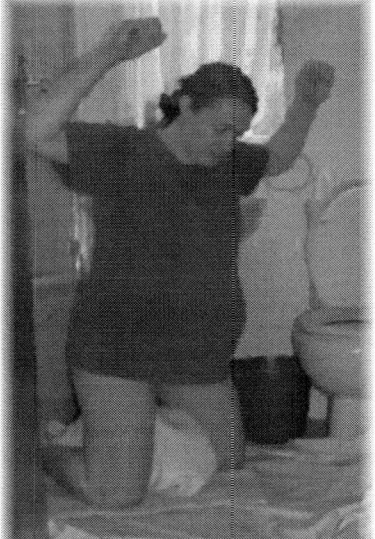

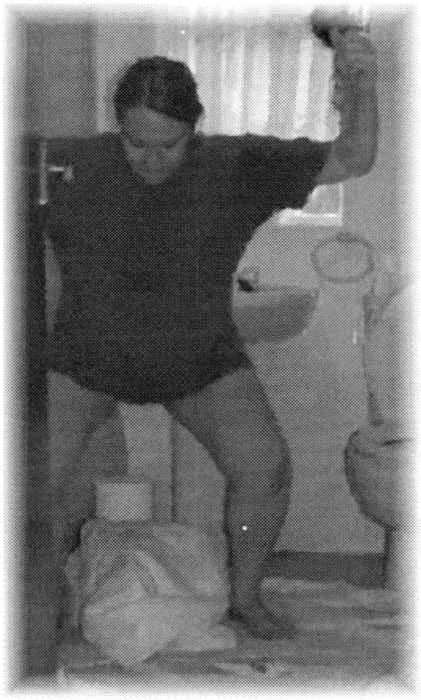

These are some typical positions for women who give birth fully conscious

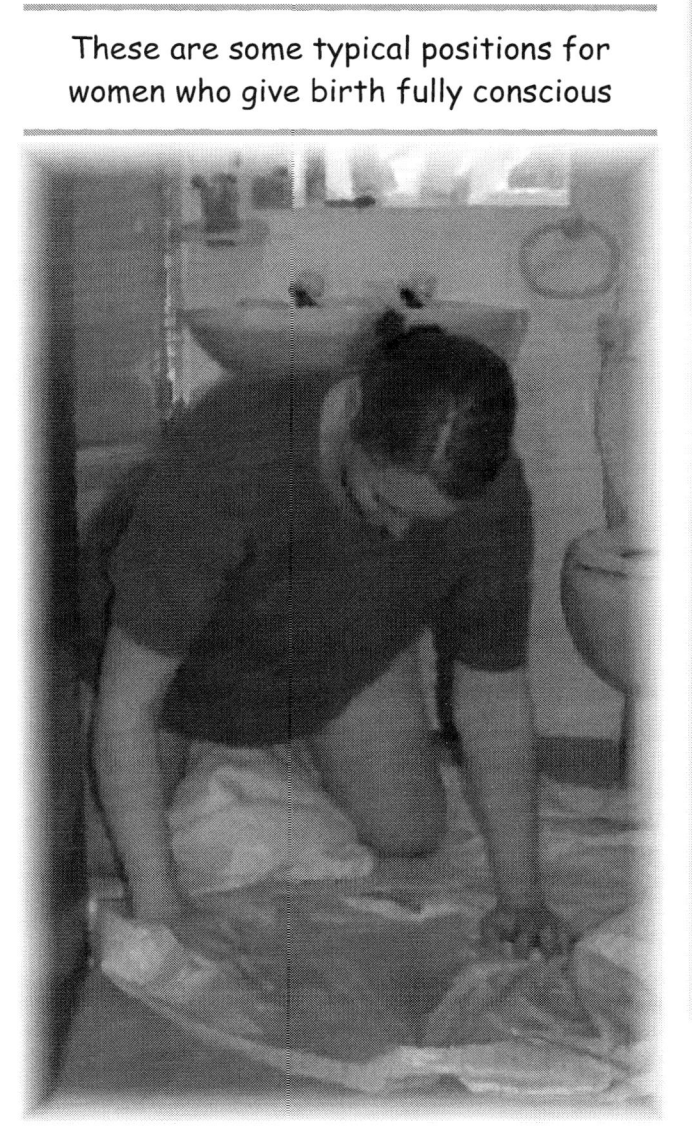

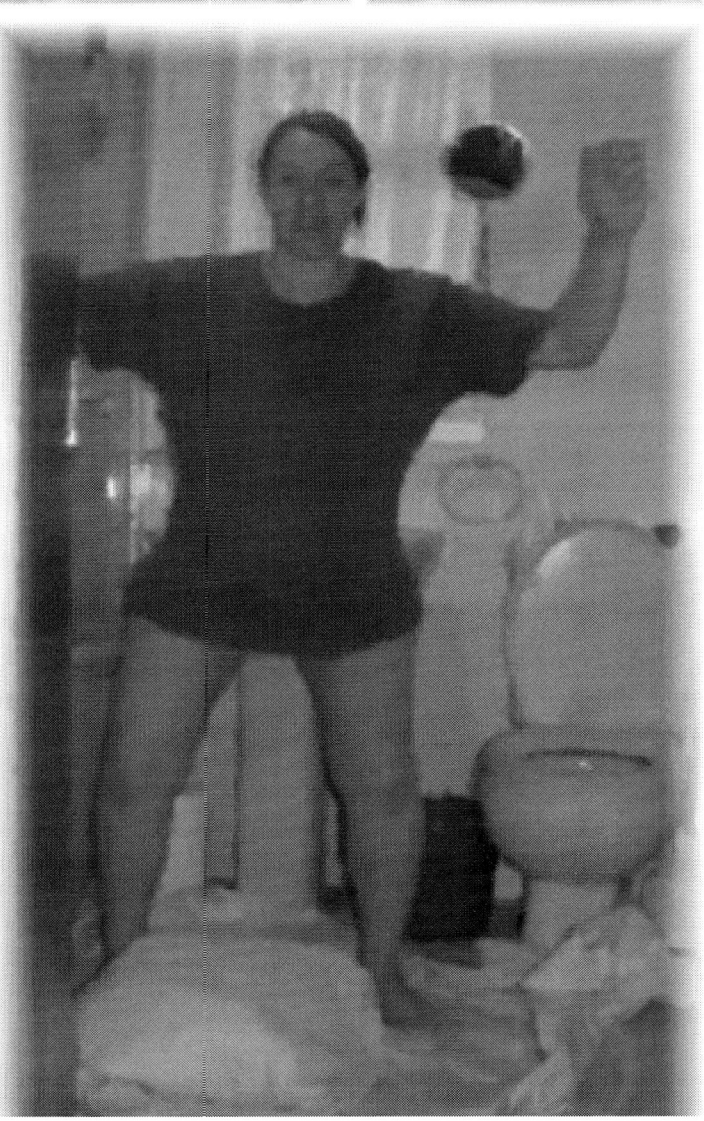

This is my favourite position! Standing like this, I gave birth to my second and third babies.

Unexpected events
Birthframe 32

Even when things go 'wrong' they don't necessarily need to go 'bad'... In my own pregnancies I became tired of meeting midwives who were full of doom and gloom. Please encourage your clients to embrace anything unexpected positively! I think both of the following accounts illustrate very well how *wrong* things can seem to go, while outcomes are still fine.

The first woman's labour took her by surprise. Although she briefly and reached for the TENS machine at one point, her labour was almost entirely natural. Even though it was not ideal that she should have so many interruptions between the birth of the baby and the birth of the placenta from a safety point of view, the third stage also went smoothly.

The players:
Me—Ruth
Adam—my husband
Ben—the star player
Eddy—our 2-year-old son
Sue—my midwife
Julie—my other midwife
Maggie—supporter for Ruth and Adam
Kerry—supporter for Eddy
Daniel—supporter for Eddy and also my brother

My first birth experience hadn't been as I had hoped. Due to a premature footling breech my plans for a home birth had been well and truly scuppered. So this time round I was twice as determined to have my baby at home. I was delighted when I discovered the baby was cephalic (a perfect LOA) and ecstatic once we got past that magical 37 weeks [after which point NHS midwives will cover a home birth]. In fact I was really excited about going into labour, no worries about anything... This was going to be good and everything that my last labour wasn't. My NHS midwives were supportive and we got on really well.

I was woken on 14 January at 5am by Eddy, who was crying. As I went in to see him I noticed a slight discomfort in my lower abdomen that was coming and going, I put this down to wind. After dealing with Eddy I went back to bed and listened to him singing and talking to himself until he went back to sleep at 6.15. All this time I was aware of the abdominal discomfort, only slight but enough to keep me awake (I am a light sleeper).

At 6.30 I decided that I needed to open my bowels. I thought I would feel better after this but I didn't, if anything I felt slightly worse. I wondered if, as this was six days before my due date, these were contractions and decided that if they were they must be Braxton Hicks.

At 7am I got up and fed the cats (all seven of them). The contractions were now coming about every 10 minutes and were getting stronger and longer but were easily bearable—I just breathed through them. I now also noticed a lower back pain but still did not think that I was in labour.

At 7.15am I needed the toilet again, this time it was much looser and I noticed a show. I wondered if this was the real thing as there were now four signs but I was not convinced.

At 7.30am I thought that maybe I should wake Adam. I told him I thought that I might be in labour; he said OK and did I need him, and then he went back to sleep. I decided I'd better phone the other people who were due to come over. Kerry had just got home from working a night shift and she had taken a sleeping tablet and was about to go to bed; she was not going to miss this for the world and set out to walk across town to our house. Daniel was on his way to work so I couldn't get hold of him. Maggie did not answer her phone (it was broken), so I rang her partner's mobile; he was half way across the country but managed to get a message to Maggie via relatives who live nearby. I got hold of Daniel at 7.55am, I told him there was no rush as he wanted to go elsewhere on the way.

By 8am Adam was getting out of bed. I saw him naked at the top of the stairs, and through bleary eyes he told me he needed to go to the toilet. I told him in no uncertain terms: "I need to go first." And once again I opened my bowels. My contractions were now very close together.

At 8.05am, still sitting on the toilet, I had the first really intense contraction. It was very different to the previous ones, which had all been really low down and opening-out type contractions. This one was from the top of my uterus, a really strong pushing contraction. My first thought was that this shouldn't be happening yet, I couldn't possibly be at this part of my labour as I hadn't had the painful bit yet. However my body was pushing and there was nothing I could do that was going to stop it.

I then decided that I needed to do my hair (which is down to my waist), so I unplaited it and asked Adam for my hairbrush. I also decided that I needed my TENS machine on; it was far too late for this but it seemed the right thing to do at the time.

After two or three more contractions I put my hand down between my legs and could feel something sticking out! I lifted myself off the toilet seat and asked Adam what it was... it was the amniotic membranes bulging out and was about the size of a grapefruit. At this point I decided that I needed a midwife rather urgently. She was the one person that I had omitted to phone when I made my calls earlier so she didn't even know I was in labour.

Adam went downstairs and called the labour hotline. He asked to speak to Sue. The person on the other end told him that she was a community midwife and he would have to call their office. He came back up to me moaning about this and how useless they were. "Did you tell them that I am in labour?"... "Oh... no". He went back downstairs and tried again.

At 8.25am Sue phoned back. She heard me shout out at the next contraction and suggested to Adam that he should be upstairs with me. I then shouted down that I could feel the baby's head. Sue said that she would phone back in two minutes once Adam had put the phone on the extension upstairs.

I instinctively kept my hand on the baby's head from when I first felt it. The next contraction came and the head moved out a bit and then back in again. Adam brought the phone upstairs and began to spread a groundsheet on the floor so that I could get off the toilet. As he finished doing this I had another contraction. With this one my waters broke, out came the baby's head followed by his body. As I delivered my baby I lifted myself off the toilet seat, brought him up between my legs and cradled our second son in my arms as I sat back down again. Adam looked round and folded the groundsheet back up again. Then the phone rang, it was Maggie. Adam asked her the time, so we now knew our new son had been born at 8.30am. ▶

My waters broke and out came the baby's head, followed by his body

◀ Almost immediately the phone rang again. It was Sue, expecting to talk Adam through the birth. He just said, "Listen!" She heard the cries and asked if we were OK. She also asked if we wanted to call an ambulance or just wait until she got there. As we were fine we said we would wait and she said that she would get there as soon as possible. I offered baby my breast but he nuzzled at my nipple for a bit and then went to sleep.

She'd got dressed in a hurry and was wearing pink socks with her uniform

At 8.35am Eddy appeared in the bathroom doorway, he looked at me sitting on the toilet and said, "Baby!" and then came to join us. Adam got a big towel to wrap around baby and me to keep us warm and then decided that he'd better get some clothes on before everyone arrived; he'd had no time to dress up to this point and I had been wearing his bathrobe. I then asked Adam to take some photos while the cord was still intact. Kerry arrived first and took some photos of all four of us, she then looked after Eddy.

At 9.00am Julie arrived. She had got dressed in the dark in a hurry and was wearing pink socks with her dark blue uniform and she had also been stopped by the police for speeding on her way to me. (They let her go as soon as she explained the situation.) As the cord had stopped pulsating, I was happy for her to clamp it and Adam cut it. Baby was then wrapped in another towel and Adam had his first cuddle while Julie helped me off the toilet and onto the floor. Adam then put baby on the floor so that I could lean against him while the placenta was born. While I was waiting for the placenta I noticed my window cleaner cleaning the bathroom window! At 9.10 I had a contraction and felt the placenta move down. Two minutes later I had another smaller one with which the placenta was born. Julie examined me and told me that I had sustained a small tear, which I decided not to have stitched. I stayed sitting on the floor while baby was checked and weighed. He was 7lb 12oz.

By this time Daniel, Maggie and Sue had arrived; Sue was later than she had hoped because she had skidded on ice and put her car into a ditch. At some point another midwife arrived but I have no idea who she was and she left once Sue got there. Maggie ran a bath for me and made drinks for everyone. Adam stood on our back doorstep to have a cigarette and shook a bit—poor chap still hadn't been to the toilet. I took baby into the bath with me where he had his first breast feed for about 20 minutes. Eddy kept coming up to check on us and look at his new brother.

I was then dispatched to my bed even though I felt full of energy and not the least bit tired. I wanted to tell the whole world what a wonderful experience I'd just had; it was a total contrast to Eddy's birth. I was far too energetic and high to sleep, so Adam brought me the phone so that I could call all our friends and family to tell them the news.

It really was the most wonderful and empowering experience of my whole life. I thoroughly enjoyed my labour and birth and I wasn't the least bit worried or frightened about birthing my baby without a midwife in attendance. It was so natural and instinctive. All we needed now was a name for our son. One helpful friend suggested Lou! And Eddy offered Mr McGregor (he's a big Peter Rabbit fan). Our baby was three days old when we decided to call him Ben.

Ruth Clark

Clearly, unassisted births happen occasionally for no good reason. In most cases, they proceed very smoothly because a fast and relatively easy birth is usually also safe. For this reason, when you arrive at someone's house, where the woman has given birth a little early, why not encourage her and be cheerful, while ensuring that all is safe, of course? I received one account for *BIRTH: Countdown to Optimal* which described how negatively midwives had reacted in this situation. They transformed what had been a very positive, uplifting experience into a negative one.

Of course, so as to avoid unassisted births from a safety point of view, it's a good idea if you encourage your clients to be well organised in terms of phone numbers, etc well before she goes into labour. I think it's interesting and surprising how otherwise well-organised women can fall apart at the prospect of collecting all the relevant information and making sure it's easily and quickly accessible, wherever she may be when she happens to go into labour. As well as sticking a card up on the wall (perhaps for her partner to see), she should carry one in her bag, so it's accessible at all times.

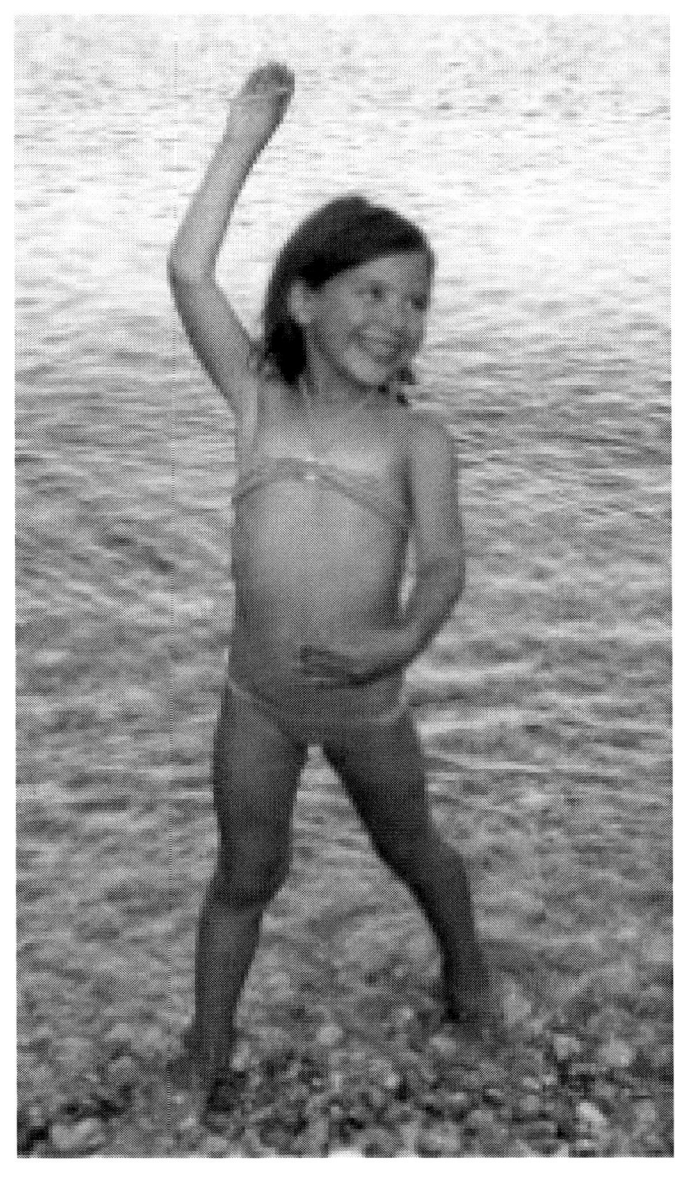

Sophia Zaphiriou-Zarifi at the age of 5—a 'fast baby' whose birth is described in BIRTH: Countdown to Optimal

Birthframe 33

My own third birth experience was not actually what I'd expected. All kinds of things 'went wrong'... but there was nothing that couldn't be dealt with.

First of all I went into labour at rather an inconvenient time. Not only was my husband about to go off to work (where he was rather busy), I was also supposed to be taking my other two children along to a morning playgroup. I went ahead as planned, stopping in the street on my way to and from the playgroup, as each new contraction made it impossible to walk for a few seconds.

All kinds of things 'went wrong' but it was all absolutely fine too

I hadn't felt comfortable with the idea of asking my new friends to help out with the children (since we'd only recently moved to the area). An hour or so after we got home, I eventually decided to phone my husband...

The next 'problem' was that it was broad daylight and we had no curtains in our bathroom. I'd had visions of a candlelit labour and birth because births always take place in the middle of the night, right? Oh well, I'd just have to carry on. Had to stay in the bathroom because I was merrily being sick, and somehow sitting on the loo seemed the most comfortable position a lot of the time!

As I turned on the water to have a shower and run myself a bath I discovered there was no hot water. Aaaargh! What could have gone wrong? A cold bath was hardly likely to have the same effect... I decided to ask my husband if he could prepare me a bath using the kitchen kettle. ("Hot, but not too hot!")

It was broad daylight and we had no curtains in the bathroom... so much for the idea of using candlelight

The next minor blip was the midwives. I'd called them as late as possible because I wanted to avoid all possible disturbance. When they turned up, not only did I not know them at all, I also found them rather overly 'brusque' and business-like. No problem—they'd just need to be locked out of the bathroom. Fortunately, Michel had suggested this idea to me as a possibility by email only that morning.

Perhaps *because* of all these hiccups, I was not as calm and composed as I had hoped. I was even wrestling with some unresolved psychological issues... It's all very well for pregnancy books and magazines to tell us we need to discuss everything with our partner, but what if he's busy or doesn't want to talk? Now hardly seemed the time. I just continued, moment by moment, moving through each contraction as best I could. Somehow the time would pass... I gently talked to my baby to coax her out.

Another thing at the back of my mind was my lack of clarity on what to do with the placenta. Was I going to be really natural and have a lotus birth? [See Birthframe 4.] This question was answered for me very efficiently...

The cord snapped as my new baby was born—she shot out with such enthusiasm. And no, I didn't manage to catch her. Landing on our thick-pile carpet covered by a plastic sheet seemed to do her no harm at all. (Giraffes apparently fall about eight feet when they're born!) The broken umbilical cord caused absolutely no problems—she breathed immediately and I myself lost only a small amount of blood. The placenta slipped out just then too.

She shot out so fast I didn't catch her!

Coming back to glitches in this labour and birth, the post-birth afterpains also took me a bit by surprise. My uterus seemed very intent on getting back to normal as quickly as humanly possible... Vomiting while breastfeeding was not exactly pleasant, but then again the aftermath did only last a few hours in total and I had long breaks between each bout of afterpains. At least the midwives who visited me postnatally were impressed with my retracted uterus, not to mention my intact perineum. (I'd only sustained a few scratches to my vagina this time—no doubt caused by long newborn fingernails!) Beyond the afterpains in the first few hours after the birth, as before I had no postnatal pain and I was full of energy.

All in all, it had gone well, but NOT as expected! Even after the birth there were blips... First, we couldn't agree on a name and the matter was complicated by my wonderful mother-in-law trying to insist on her 'suggestion'. (That ended up being the middle name!) Then—just two days after the birth—I caught a bug off a visitor's baby. As I was throwing up for the umpteenth time that night I did at least console myself with the thought that Jumeira would get my antibodies through my breastmilk. She was fine—and I was also back to normal a few hours later. After that I just had the usual problems of early motherhood—sleep deprivation, a messy house and a rather podgy body.

A few days after the birth, I realised my faith in the natural processes had been reaffirmed. Our bodies and our babies know what to do. We simply need to have the courage not to intervene or disturb the natural processes. We need to observe and move through the sensations as we experience them, even if we perceive these as painful. And we need to hold on to that faith in the natural processes. We can and we must work through these times for the sake of our babies, our children, and the society into which they are born. And we're helping ourselves in doing so because postpartum our lives are likely to be much, much easier than they might otherwise be, after an alternative 'managed' birth using so-called 'pain relief'.

18 months later: Since Jumeira's birth I've experienced no pain, no discomfort—just a little tiredness now and then because of broken nights. The intense but brief pain I experienced during my third labour and birth was just that... strong but short-lived. Jumeira's on my lap, contentedly breastfeeding as I type away at my computer. She's a lovely, lively, happy little girl.

THE PUERPERIUM

In order to ensure optimality, there are various issues to consider and reassess. First, the normal scenario...

Postnatal scenarios

As we've already noted, after most physiological births women typically start breastfeeding totally spontaneously. Your client may sit down wherever she is—on the toilet perhaps if she happens to be in her bathroom at home! By the way, notice the extension lead in the corner of the photo on the right. It's there in case an extra, portable heater needs to be brought in to warm up the baby... or the new mother, who may well be in shock and shivering.

After a while, if the placenta hasn't come out yet, the woman might transfer to a bucket (as in the photo below). Of course, she shouldn't sit in this position for too long as blood flow to the vaginal area may become restricted.

When the third stage is over, your client will probably want to rest with her baby in bed. It's still best for her to lie on her left side because her baby will be lying on his or her right side—which is apparently the best possible position from the point of view of optimising breathing and blood flow. Of course, the woman needs to keep her new baby's head off the pillow and just keep him or her warm with a baby blanket. Midwifery support at this time is essential because although all safety issues will have been dealt with, the new mum may well be feeling very insecure.

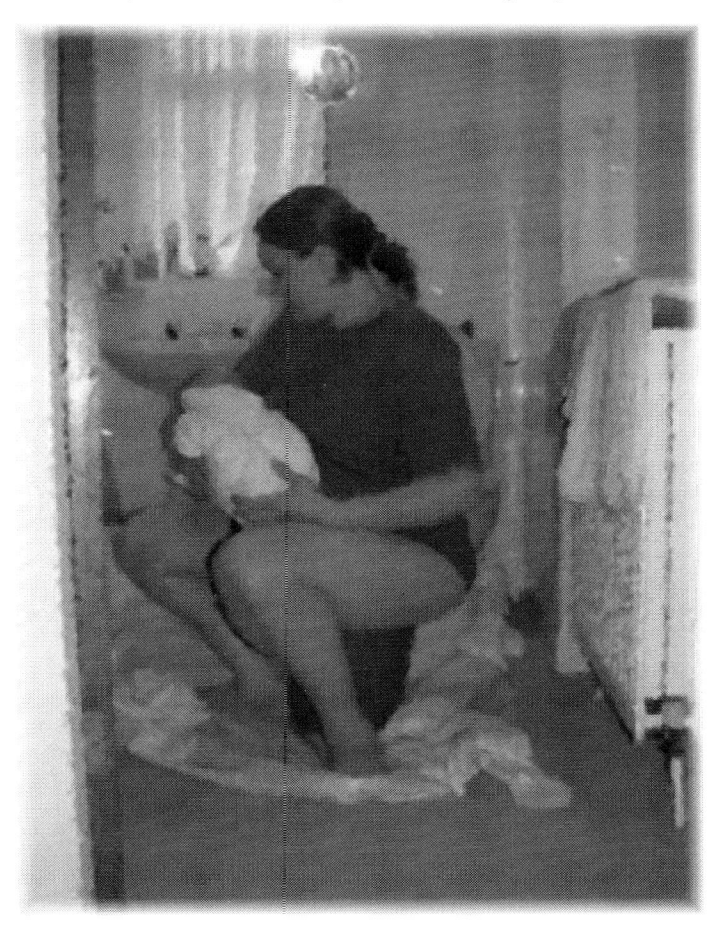

By the way, in case you're wondering... this is not Linda's real baby. It's a bald-headed doll borrowed from one of my children. And when she posed for these photos, Linda still had three or four more weeks to wait before her own big day.

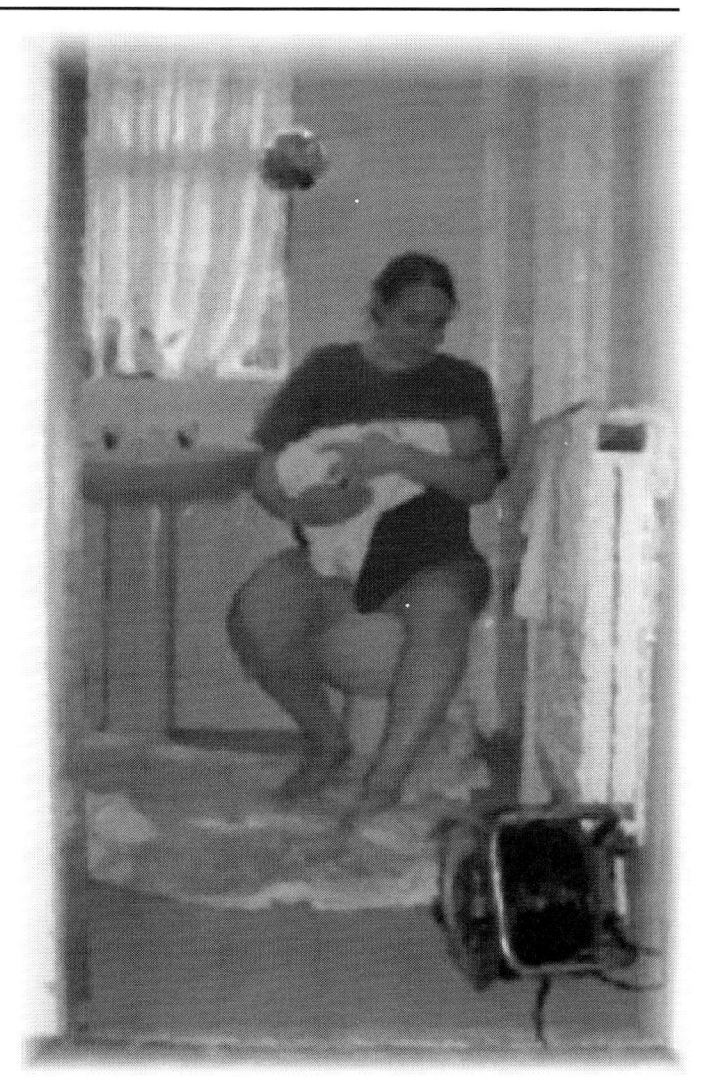

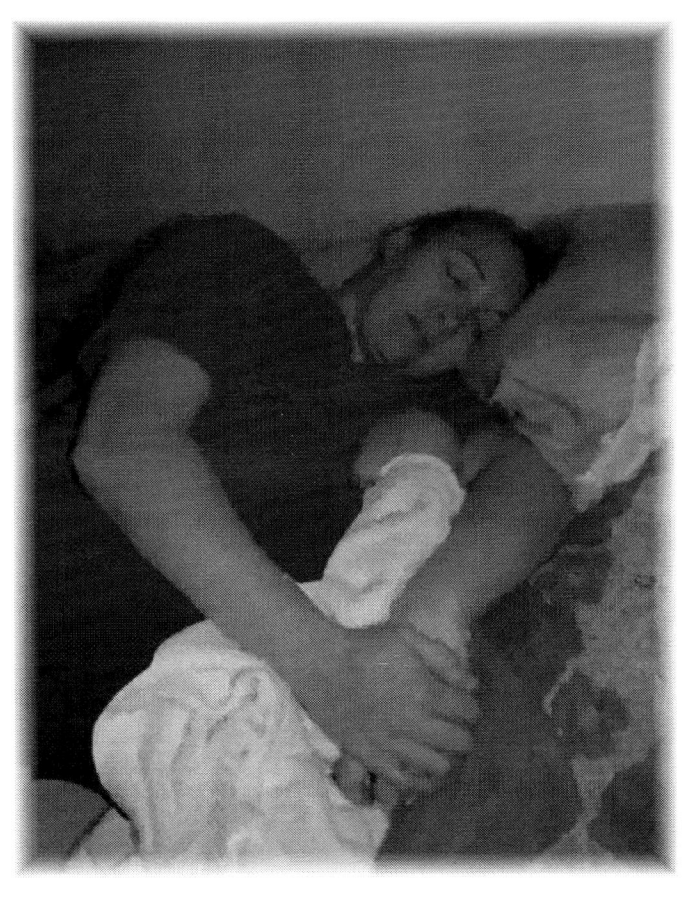

Cord-cutting

Of course, it is now widely accepted that delayed cord-cutting is advantageous because it ensures that the newborn gets its last 'dose' of oxygen from the mother's blood before needing to access it on its own, through breathing. Two research projects established this—one concluding that the baby receives some 43% of the blood left in maternal/placental circulation (Gunther M. The transfer of blood between the baby and the placenta in the minutes after birth. *Lancet* 1957;I:1277-1280; Wardrop CA, Holland BM. The roles and vital importance of placental blood to the newborn infant. *J Perinat Med* 1995;23(1-2):139-43.) Other studies (Kinmond S et al. Umbilical Cord Clamping and Preterm Infants: a randomized trial. *BMJ* 1993;306: 172-175; Piscane A. Neonatal prevention of iron deficiency. *BMJ* 1996; 312:136-7) questioned the assumption that it is either necessary or helpful to cut the cord at all as part of the third stage procedures.

In case you would like to follow up on this and support a woman who decides she does not want any cord-clamping how would you proceed? Some clues are given in the following account, in which a doula—Ashley Marshall, whose photo you've already seen on pp 22 and 24—had what is called a 'lotus birth'.

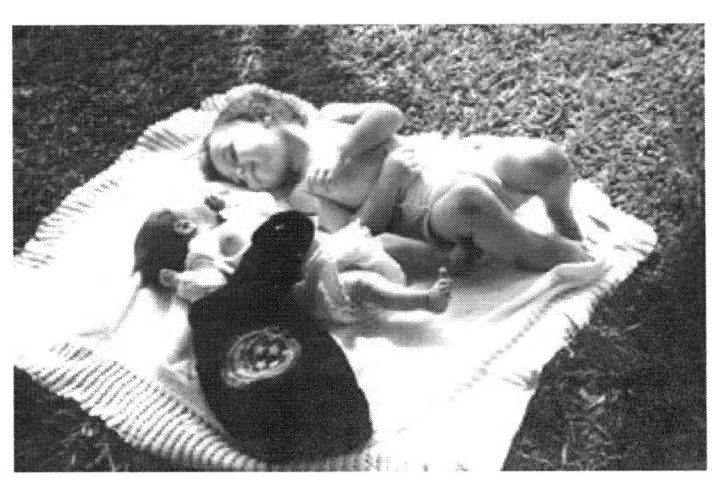

Big brother Caleb, baby brother Haper and Harper's placenta

We would never have another baby without having a lotus birth

Birthframe 34

Harper's birth at home was sweeter than I could have dreamt it. I laboured easily and powerfully with loving support from my husband, doula, and midwife. When Harper's bag of waters popped, birth energy rushed through me and soon his little head began to emerge. There was a slight case of dystocia and a tight umbilical cord but we were safe in the skilful hands of our midwife. Then, all of a sudden, there he was—pink, alert, and beautiful.

As I sat in awe of this perfect, wise being I rubbed the creamy coating of vernix into his delicate skin and knew we had made the right decision to give him a lotus birth. It was the most blissful beginning to follow the culmination of pregnancy and the sense of loss that often ensues.

Lotus birth is the process of leaving the baby's placenta attached via the umbilical cord until it falls off of its own accord. Its purpose is both physiological and spiritual. Physiologically, the baby receives 43% of the blood left in maternal/placental circulation.

Ever wonder why cord blood banking has become so popular? It is known that cord blood—or blood left in the cord and placenta that hasn't made its way to the baby—is useful in helping to fight childhood leukemia later in that child's life. Why not stop denying a baby this vital blood and allow it to pass to the baby after birth instead? Also, the placenta is the baby's life preserver before breathing is established. As long as the cord remains intact and while it still pulsates the baby is being oxygenated.

Long after the cord stops pulsating and the physical transference is complete, the spiritual transference has only begun. This quiet time is when the baby's aura, or spiritual presence, is being realised. The placenta originated from the same cells as the baby and because of this bond they are a genetic identical of one another. A lotus birth allows for a respectful goodbye to the baby's womb mate.

How does a parent care for an intact placenta? It was surprisingly easy. After Harper's birth my husband and midwife placed it in a colander and rinsed all of the blood clots out.

Then we rubbed it with sea salt and sprinkled it with lavender flowers.

Harper's placenta wore a cloth nappy just like he did and we changed it daily. We swaddled the 'placenta package' right along with him so we were free to pick him up, nurse and cuddle without the fear of tugging at his navel.

On the third day after his birth, Harper let go of his placenta. He was content and whole and ready to be free. We said goodbye to the organ that had nourished and protected our son for his first nine months but we will see it again when we plant it at Harper's first Blessing Way ceremony. In case you don't know, a Blessing Way ceremony is a Native American ritual used to mark significant life passages in one's life, frequently held to commemorate a birth, a marriage, a death or a woman's journey into motherhood. It is a more spiritual ceremony than the traditional American baby shower, where the focus is on showering the mother with gifts for the baby. A Blessing Way ceremony honours the mother and helps her draw upon her own inner resources that she will need to later give birth. My husband and I decided to offer our children a Blessing Way ceremony to celebrate their first year of life as well as my first year postpartum. We also planted their placentas at this time. (They were kept in the freezer up till then.)

On Day 3 Harper let go of his placenta

Harper is our second child to be born at home, but our first lotus birth. We now know that we would never have another baby without giving them a lotus birth. It was three very mindful days that enabled us to remain in that warped sense of time that follows birth. We were surrounded only by love and close family while Harper made his earthly transition. There was plenty of time for lively celebration later that week but I will always be grateful for those precious days when Harper was lotus-born.

Ashley Marshall

What if things go wrong or already have done?...

PPH

The World Health Organization estimates that every year a staggering 14 million women have a postpartum haemorrhage and that around half a million die as a result each year. It seems that the risk of PPH increases dramatically when women are disturbed between the second and third stages of labour. This is because their state of mind is irrevocably changed, which has dramatic physiological consequences. The following is an extract from one of Michel Odent's Primal Health newsletters.

Over the years I have come to the conclusion that postpartum haemorrhages are almost always related to inappropriate interference. Postpartum haemorrhage would be extremely rare if a few simple rules were understood and observed. I am so convinced of the importance of these simple rules that I have twice agreed to attend a home birth, even though in each case I knew the woman's previous birth was followed by a manual removal of the placenta and a blood transfusion. These rules result in an approach which is in stark contrast to 'expectant' or so-called 'physiological' management used in randomised studies.

First, it is important to create the conditions for the 'fetus ejection reflex', which is a short series of irresistible contractions which allow no room for voluntary movements. If this is done, the need for privacy and the need to feel secure are met. The fetus ejection reflex typically occurs when there is nobody around but an experienced, motherly, silent and low-profile midwife sitting in a corner and, for example, knitting. Knitting—or a similar repetitive task—helps the midwife to maintain her own level of adrenaline as low as possible.

When conditions are physiological, at the very moment of birth most women tend to be upright, probably because of a momentary peak of adrenaline. They may be on their knees, or standing up and leaning on something. After an unmedicated delivery, it only takes a few seconds to hear and to see that the baby is in good shape. Then, in most cases, my first preoccupation is to warm the room. In the French hospital where I used to work, we just had to pull a string to switch on heating lamps. In the case of a planned home birth, instead of a written list of what to prepare, I focus on the need for a transportable heater that can be plugged in anywhere and at any time (including practical details, such as the need for an extension cord). When the heater is on it is possible, within a few seconds, to warm up blankets or towels and, if necessary, to cover the mother's and the baby's bodies. During the hour following birth women rarely complain that it is too hot. If the mother is shivering, it is not psychological: it means that the place is not warm enough.

From that time my main concern is that the mother is not distracted at all and does not feel observed. I want to make sure that she feels free to hold her baby, to look into her or his eyes and to smell her or him. It is easier to avoid disturbances if the light is kept dimmed and the telephone unplugged. I often invite the baby's father (or any other person who might be around) into another room to explain that this first interaction between mother and baby will never happen again and should not be disturbed. Many men have a tendency to break the sacredness of the atmosphere that ideally follows an undisturbed birth.

During the first hour after the birth, I remain as silent as possible and keep a low profile. Either I sit down in a corner behind the mother and baby, or I disappear if there is an experienced doula present with personal experience of this situation. Minutes after giving birth many mothers are no longer comfortable in an upright position. This is most likely the time when their level of adrenaline is decreasing and when women feel the contractions associated with the separation of the placenta. The birth attendant may have to hold the baby for some seconds, in order for the mother to find a comfortable position, almost always lying down on one side. After that there is no excuse for interfering with the interaction between mother and baby.

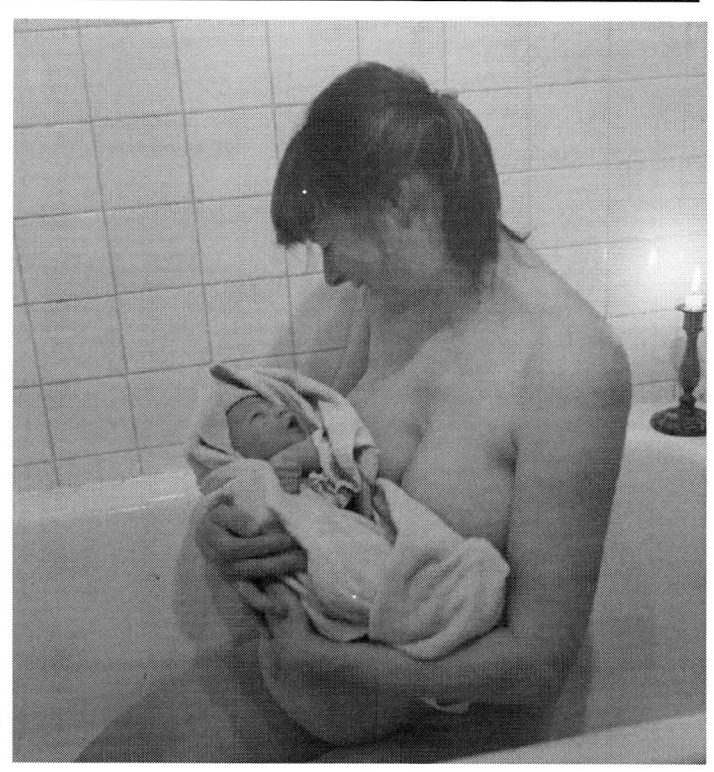

Immediately after the birth really is a magical time, which mustn't be disturbed—if only for safety reasons, quite apart from bonding

For an hour I don't go anywhere near either the cord or the placenta. Clamping and cutting the cord before the delivery of the placenta is a dangerous distraction. Suggesting a position to the mother is another unneeded distraction. Her position is the consequence of her level of adrenaline. When her level of adrenaline is low and she feels the need to lie down, it would be unkind and unphysiological to suggest an upright position.

It is only when an hour has passed after the birth—if the placenta has not yet emerged—that I dare to disturb the mother in order to check that the placenta is at least separated from the uterus. With the mother on her back I press the abdominal wall just above the pubic bone with my fingertips: if the cord does not move, it means that the placenta is separated. In practice, the placenta is always either delivered or separated an hour after the birth, and bleeding is minimal, provided the third stage has not been 'managed'. I have never had to inject a uterotonic drug to control bleeding.

Such an attitude, based first on clinical observation, is based on physiological considerations. An easy delivery of the placenta with moderate blood loss implies that, immediately after the birth of the baby, a surge of oxytocin has been released. It is well-known that oxytocin release is highly dependant on environmental factors. It can be inhibited by adrenaline. This is more than empirical knowledge. A team from Sapporo, Japan (Saito et al 1991) has studied the levels of adrenaline during the different phases of labour extensively by a non-invasive method (recording with a patch and analysing the skin microvibration pattern of the palmar side of the hand) and confirmed the findings of a previous study in which adrenaline levels were measured through indwelling catheters (Lederman et al 1978). The Japanese team clearly demonstrated that postpartum haemorrhages are associated with high levels of adrenaline. The release of oxytocin can also be inhibited by the activity of the neocortex. After a physiological birth, the mother is still in a special state of consciousness, as if 'on another planet'. Her neocortex is still more or less at rest so my advice is: "Don't wake the mother up!" Once again, I must emphasise the need for privacy and silence.

There's almost no blood loss with a fetus ejection reflex, which makes it very safe

Prematurity

How much do you know about kangaroo care? The following account will tell you more...

Birthframe 35

Here, an American woman Krisanne Collard explains how she came to use a very natural approach to supplement her new daughter's technological support system.

In July of 1994, my husband and I moved to the little town of Canon City, Colorado. We had no family in the area—in fact, we had no family within a day's drive. I found out I was pregnant within two weeks of the move. We were ecstatic! We had tried to get pregnant for three years and suffered a miscarriage eight months before. We were finally going to have the baby we had dreamed about for so long.

We were ecstatic I was pregnant! We'd been trying for three years— we were finally going to have a baby

I had my first antenatal appointment at the end of September when I was 11 weeks pregnant. The doctor asked me to provide a urine sample, confirmed I was pregnant and told me my due date would be March 4. He sent the rest of my sample off, so the lab could run all of the standard tests for new mums. He told me everything looked wonderful and I would be able to hear the heartbeat at my next appointment. I scheduled my next appointment for a month later, and my husband and I left the office overjoyed at the thought everything was fine. We went to Wal-Mart and looked at all of the pretty baby things, dreaming of what the nursery would look like.

The doctor called me three days after the appointment and asked to see me in his office later that day. He sat us both down and gave us the bad news. All of the standard tests he had run indicated that I no longer had a viable pregnancy. Our baby was probably no longer alive. He scheduled an ultrasound for Monday—just to be 'sure'. It was then Friday. All weekend we worried and panicked. By Monday afternoon, I had convinced myself that she was indeed dead—that we would have to try again. When I lay down on the table and told the technician why I was there, she had tears in her eyes as she prepared to take a look. For two agonising minutes, all was quiet. Then, she screamed, "Oh my God! Look! Your baby's moving!" Sure enough, there was my little fighter, mad at the world—wiggling and trying to get comfortable. Her heartbeat was strong. My doctor never had an explanation for the incorrect test results.

For the next two months, my pregnancy went by the book. I had some morning sickness and started to get the 'pooch' [a visible pregnancy tummy]. I felt her move for the first time on my birthday (November 14). We bought baby stuff and started to decorate the nursery. We were the happiest parents in the world!

But, on November 30, 24 weeks into my pregnancy, everything went black. I woke up with a dull ache in my lower back. I didn't think much of it till I started bleeding at about noon. I called my doctor and my husband, who rushed me to the local hospital. I was immediately hooked up to a fetal monitor and checked for dilation. I was already 5cm and her feet were in the birth canal. She was coming breech. Next thing I knew, I was being prepped for an immediate c-section. I was sobbing, screaming and confused. No one had time to talk to me—no one would let me know how the baby was doing. My husband and I were terrified!

At 24 weeks I started bleeding

When I woke up, I was in the recovery room. All I can remember was asking for a drink of water. I didn't ask about my baby because I thought she was dead. I just started crying— mourning her already. After about half an hour, another nurse came into the room. I asked her, "Was it a boy or a girl?" She smiled at me and said, "You have a beautiful little girl!" I was confused. She hadn't spoken in the past tense and she was happy. My daughter was still alive!

I was moved into my recovery room and my doctor came to talk to me. He told me that my daughter had been born weighing only 1lb, 12oz and only 13½ inches long. He said she came out kicking and screaming, angry at the world, but she was VERY sick. They were transporting her to a level three NICU (Neonatal Intensive Care Unit) at Memorial Hospital, an hour away, in Colorado Springs. He told me that there was only a 30% chance that she was going to make it through the night.

I didn't get to see her before they took her away. As I recovered from the c-section, I called the hospital she was in three times a day to check on her. She had been put on a special oscillating ventilator, I was told, and required maximum oxygen doses to keep her saturation up. They said she had gotten an infection from me and was very sick. I had a bladder infection I didn't know about (I have always been symptom-less), and she had come early because she was too sick to stay in my womb. They assured me over and over that she was a fighter and was going to be fine. They encouraged me to talk to her through the phone— but I felt silly because I hadn't even met her yet. Since we now felt she was going to make it, we decided on a name—Kaia Michele. A strong Norwegian name for a very brave little girl.

When I was released from my local hospital, four days after her birth, my husband and I immediately went to visit Kaia. When I walked into the NICU, nothing could have prepared me for what I saw. She was the size of two Barbie dolls stuck together. She had the blue bilirubin lights on her and tubes and wires everywhere. Her skin was translucent and her veins showed through her skin. I looked around, hoping to see 'my' baby in another bed. I looked back at Kaia. The nurse urged me closer and turned off the blue lights so I could take a closer look. I was terrified. The nurse urged me to touch her and talk to her—let her know I was there. I hesitated. She looked like she would break if I touched her. I started to talk to her, but it took 15 minutes to finally get up the nerve to touch her. When I did, her alarms went off. I jerked my hand back as the nurse came over. She had to rub her till her heart started again. I couldn't handle it—my baby had rejected me—I left the nursery in tears and went home.

The next night, as we were eating dinner, I burst into tears. My husband took my hand and led me to the couch. He put my shoes on and said, "Let's go—Mummy needs a baby fix." We drove the hour to Memorial Hospital. All the way there, I told my husband that THIS time I was going to be strong. I was going to count her toes and talk to her and let her know how loved she was. I was so excited!

▶

But, when I got to her side and touched her, her alarms sounded again. The nurse had to start her heart yet again. I just sat there for the next 30 minutes and looked at her, crying. Why didn't my baby love me? I wondered. A nurse specialist named Theresa Kledzik (nicknamed 'The Whisper Lady') came over to talk to me. She asked me if I had held my baby yet. I just laughed and said that Kaia couldn't tolerate me touching her—I would kill her if I tried to hold her. Theresa just smiled at me and asked me to follow her into the other room. She gave me a gown, told me to take off my bra and shirt and put the gown on with the opening in the front. I was in shock as I changed.

When I walked back into the nursery, there were three nurses getting Kaia ready to be transferred to my chest. It took about 15 minutes for them to get her ready and I got more and more nervous every second. I changed my mind about ten times, but the nurses didn't pay me any mind. I sat down in a strange-looking chair. (I learned later that it was specially designed to be used with babies on oscillating ventilators.) They laid Kaia on my chest, on her tummy, skin-to-skin with me. Her head was resting above my heart and her tiny feet were curled up in my hand. The tubes and wires were taped to my gown. I stared at the monitors as she wiggled into a comfortable position. I knew they were going to sound. I held my breath. She calmed down after about five minutes and stopped moving. I thought she was dead. I tried to make sense of the monitors. I called Theresa over and asked if I had killed her. She just laughed and said, "No, she's happy!" I looked down at Kaia and noticed the peaceful look on her face. I looked back up at Theresa and smiled. My daughter had just made me feel like a Mum for the very first time!

I was able to hold Kaia every day for two hours. I couldn't get to the hospital fast enough every day to share that special time with her. Within a few days, I was able to transfer her to my chest all by myself, even with the tubes and wires everywhere. I was always disappointed when our time together came to an end. She responded very well to it, and her oxygen requirements lowered during every session. She never had any episodes where she stopped breathing (apneas) or periods where her heart stopped (bradyas) while I held her. She would just go into a deep, healing sleep and actually tolerated my touch when she was on the warming table. The future was looking very promising for her.

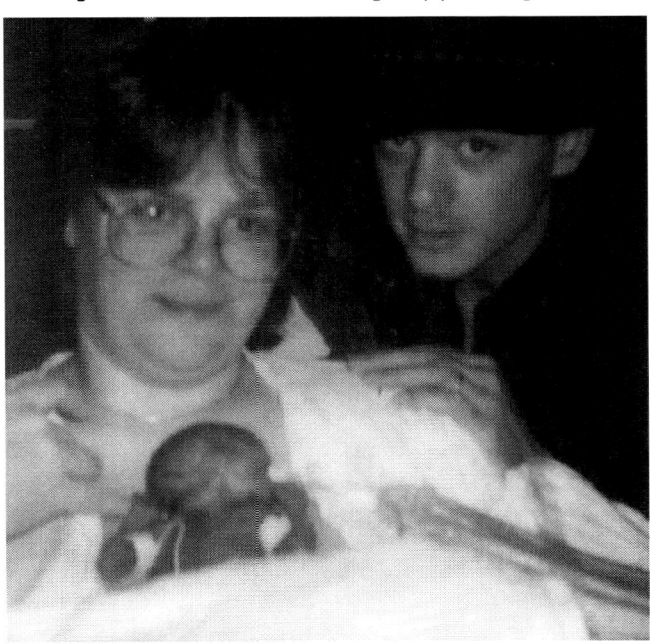

"No alarms. Yippee!" My first time kangarooing Kaia at 4 days old, with husband Gene.

When she was two weeks old, she had trouble getting comfortable on my chest. I wound up putting her back after only half an hour. I spent another hour with her, then headed home. When I got there, there was a message on my machine telling me to immediately return to the hospital. My husband and I rushed back just in time to say goodbye as they rushed her to the operating room. They had no idea what was wrong, and no idea how long we would have to wait. Four hours later, the Neonatal Surgeon came out and told us she was going to be fine. She had got a small perforation at the end of her large intestines and the surgeon had made a colostomy. We got to see her within an hour. She had a huge bandage on her tummy and they had given her paralysing drugs. She looked so little and sick. I cried as I held her hand for the next two hours. The nurses assured me I'd be able to hold her again in a few days. I missed her so much.

I visited her the next morning. She was very uncomfortable and was requiring maximum pain medication doses. She wiggled and cried (silently because of the ventilator tube in her mouth). Finally, after an hour of seeing her suffer, the nurse said, "Hold your baby, she needs you!" I leapt at the chance and got her out of bed myself—making sure not to put too much pressure on her tummy. The nurse came over a few minutes later to check on us. She smiled. Kaia was actually lying on her newly operated-on tummy, sleeping peacefully. I held her for the full two hours and she didn't even need her next dose of pain medicine! I was on top of the world. I had gotten to hold and comfort my child!

Kaia required another operation, at 3 weeks old, to modify her colostomy. She was moved to the Intermediate Nursery after two months, and came home on oxygen and a heart monitor a month later, on February 27, two weeks before her due date.

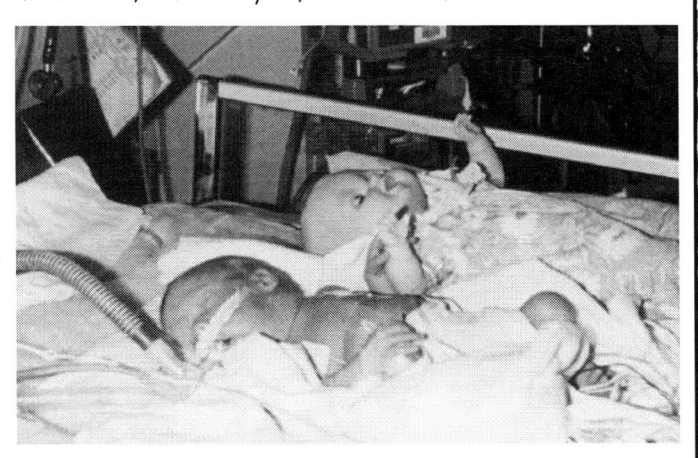

"Hold my hand. We'll do this together." Kaia, 8 weeks old, 2½lb.

She went back into the NICU two weeks later for eye surgery to correct ROP (retinopathy of prematurity), which is common in preemies who have been on oxygen for long periods of time.

A month after that—she was 4½ months old by this time—she had a **fundoplication** [an operation in which the top of the stomach is wrapped around the esophagus, creating a valve] to correct severe reflux. We had to feed her through a tube (called a G-tube) for the next four months.

When she was 8½ months old, she had her final surgery to reconnect her colostomy and take out the feeding tube. She remained on oxygen and a heart monitor, continuously till she was a year old. This meant lugging around a 15lb oxygen tank and a 10lb heart monitor everywhere. People were very curious. In the grocery and department stores, I was given strange looks or stopped and asked 100 questions before I could continue my shopping. We didn't get out much because it was such a hassle.

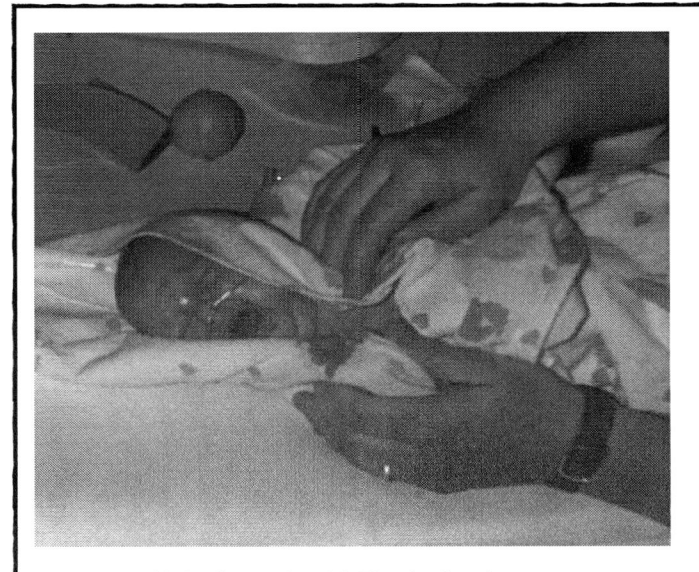

Kaia, 3 months old. First bath at home.

◀ That first year of Kaia's life was the most stressful year of my own life. There were so many things to do: doctor appointments, operations, therapy sessions, medications and colostomy bag changes. And so many milestones: first smiles, first words, first steps, first hugs! I was on a roller coaster that didn't seem to have an end in sight. I joined a local playgroup and an online preemie support group when Kaia was six months old. Both groups gave me so much love and support. They kept me from going insane. There are MANY premature baby support groups on the Internet and probably one in your own city or town. To find the one that's right for you, join several—don't limit yourself to just one. Every support group is different and unique. Your hospital will be able to tell you if there is a local support group in your area.

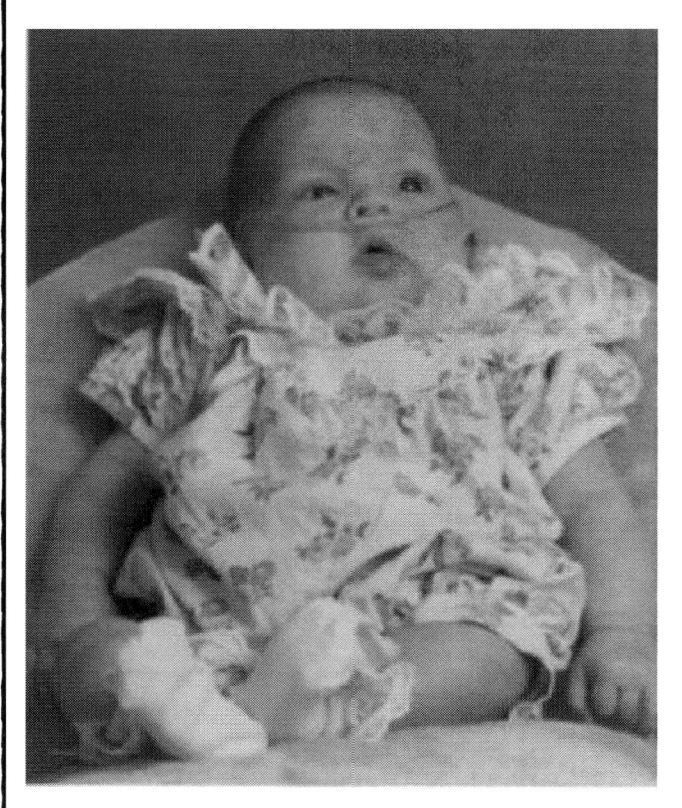

Kaia's first professional photo—4 months old

I was angry that more hospitals didn't embrace kangaroo care

At our NICU reunion party in August 1995 Kaia was 9 months old. I ran into the nurse specialist who had encouraged me to hold my daughter the first time, Theresa Kledzik. We talked for almost an hour about 'kangaroo care'. That's what she called the skin-to-skin contact I had with Kaia. I asked her if all babies were able to be kangarooed and she told me that I had been very lucky. Most parents in other hospitals weren't able to kangaroo their babies as soon as I was. Most parents had to wait till their babies were 'stable', off the ventilator or three pounds before they were allowed to hold them. I was shocked! Kaia would have been over two months old if I had had to wait. I couldn't imagine having to wait that long to feel like a Mum.

When I got home, I immediately told my online support group about what I had learned. Most wrote back asking what kangaroo care was and how they could do it. They had never heard of it before. I searched the Internet and found only one site that even mentioned kangaroo care. I was upset. How many other babies had to suffer without the loving touch of their parents? I emailed Theresa and she sent me all of the literature and research she had on the subject. ▶

How many other babies had to suffer?

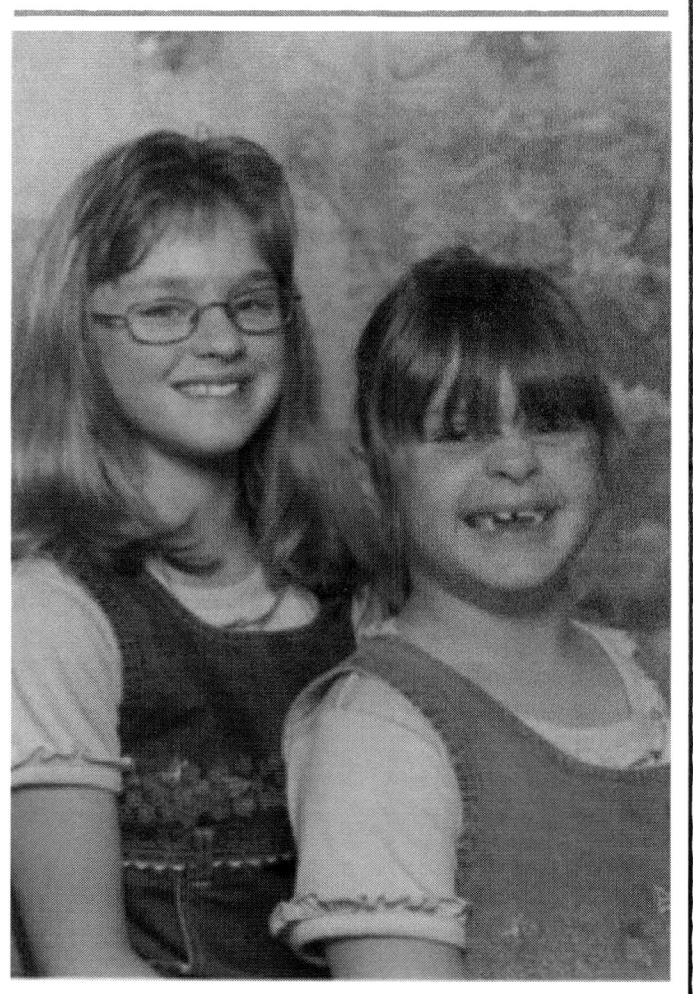

Kaia, aged 8, with her sister Katherine, aged 7

There was so much, it took days to go through it all. I was amazed at all I learned and angry that more hospitals didn't embrace kangaroo care. Here is just a glimpse of the amazing discoveries I made...

- Kangaroo care—originally called 'kangaroo mother care'—was developed in Bogotá, Colombia in July 1977 by neonatologists Edgar Rey and Hector Martinez. It received worldwide publicity in 1983 when the startling success of the approach became known. The mortality rate for premature babies in Bogotá had been 70% (39% in the US at that time) due to lack of power and reliable equipment (such as ventilators and incubators). After getting mums to carry their babies continuously in slings on their chests, the mortality rate decreased to 30%!
- Research has shown that mums and babies have a natural thermal synchrony. When Mum thinks her baby is getting too cool, her body heats up in response. When Mum thinks her baby is too hot, she cools down. Sorry, Dad, this only seems to happen with mums.
- The skin-to-skin contact helps in milk production and milk letdown. It is very important for mothers of premature babies to pump and store their milk for the time when the baby can start eating. The breastmilk of a mother who has given birth prematurely is tolerated by the baby's immature digestive system more easily than formula.
- Apnea (interruptions in normal breathing), bradycardia (severe heart rate decreases) and tachycardia (severe heart rate increases) decrease or disappear altogether because kangaroo care regulates breathing and stabilises heart rates. These episodes are VERY common in premature babies and can easily lead to death or lack of oxygen to the brain, which could cause brain damage.
- Kangaroo care stimulates the baby to gain weight more rapidly and be discharged up to 50% sooner because there are greater periods of deep sleep that enable the preemie's body to heal faster.
- Kangaroo care can also be done with full-term babies who have colic. Colic is believed by many to be a baby's inability to transition from one sleep-state to another. Kangaroo care allows babies to enter into the deepest sleep state with ease. Most preemies that are kangarooed never suffer with colic. Mine didn't.
- Preemies who are kangarooed during treatments (such as 'heel sticks' to check the amount of oxygen in the blood—an hourly requirement for preemies on a ventilator) experience far less discomfort and require no extra pain medication during these painful procedures. Kaia didn't even seem to notice the treatments if she was being kangarooed.

After telling my online support group about what I had learned, I was encouraged to set up a website to educate the world about the wonders of kangaroo care. One of my online friends helped me design the website www.geocities.com/roopage and several preemie mums wrote stories about their first kangaroo care experience. I received so many wonderful stories, I decided to compile them all into a tiny booklet that I could send to NICUs and parents across the world. *Kangarooing Our Little Miracles* lets parents, nurses and doctors share the emotional joy kangaroo care brings to babies and parents. Most parents shared with me that by writing down their emotions, it helped with their healing process. I gave away over 200 booklets within the first year and received at least 15 emails a month from parents, neonatologists and nurses who wanted to implement kangaroo care in their hospitals. It feels wonderful to be an instigator.

In October of 1996, I was asked to speak at the First International Congress of Kangaroo Care in Baltimore, MD. I was both flattered and nervous. I blew the minds of several nurses and neonatologists in the audience when I told them about my kangaroo care experience. They couldn't believe that I had been able to hold her on a ventilator (an oscillating one at that), or hold her when she was so unstable. They actually gasped when I told them about her reaction to being kangarooed after tummy surgery. They all cheered at the end of my speech when I told them that all babies deserve to feel their mother's and father's love and all parents deserve the opportunity to be parents, not visitors.

I blew the mind of several nurses and neonatologists when I told them about my kangaroo care experience

My 'preemie' is now 8 years old and going into 3rd grade. Where has the time gone? She is doing wonderfully in school and has no lasting effects of being born prematurely. She is sweet and kind and funny. She puts a smile on my face every day. The other day, when we were swimming at the local pool, another child asked her why her tummy was all messed up (she insisted on getting a bikini even though her massive scars showed). I held my breath, wondering if I should step in and help her explain. My eyes filled with tears as she said, proudly, "I was born the size of two Barbie dolls. I have these scars to show me how strong I had to be to live." I know that I helped give her that strength. I am so proud of her and thankful to Memorial Hospital of Colorado Springs for giving me the opportunity to be her mum!

We found out I was pregnant again in December of 1995. My pregnancy was uncomplicated. My doctor checked me every two weeks for bladder infections. (I was treated for two during my pregnancy.) My doctor informed me that the antenatal pills I took with Kaia might have played a role in her early birth because they contained a high content of iodine, which I am highly allergic to. He switched me to an antenatal vitamin that contained no iodine. With Kaia, whenever I had missed one pill, I spotted. After missing two, I had Kaia. I am still very allergic to iodine and have to watch which multivitamins I take and keep salt out of my diet as much as possible. Even though I showed no signs of premature labor (i.e. contractions or bleeding), my doctor put me on terbulatine (used to stop contractions) at 28 weeks to be sure I wouldn't go into premature labour. I strongly encourage women who have ANY problems with their pregnancy to talk to their consultant. Don't just let it go. Even a small problem could snowball and mean life or death for your baby.

My mum teased me as I went through the summer months uncomfortable and VERY pregnant. Every time I would complain about how miserable I was, she would laugh and say, "YOU are the one who wants to see what it's like to carry a baby to term. You are going the full 40, young lady!"

My doctor left for his first vacation ever on 1 August, a Friday, right after my 36-week appointment. He took me off the terbulatine and told me that I was NOT going to have her till he got back! I just laughed and told him that I wanted to have her that weekend. I did! I started having contractions within 24 hours of discontinuing the terbulatine and Katherine Elsie was born on August 4, Sunday, weighing a healthy 6lb, 15½oz by c-section. I was able to hold her within a couple of hours after she was born. I unwrapped her, counted her toes and fingers, and held her 'kangaroo care' style for hours as I slept.

◀ She has been perfectly healthy—I was able to actually enjoy her first year. However, Katherine is a real free spirit. The tantrums that child threw! WOW! Kaia tried to imitate her sister when she was about 3 years old. She lay down on the floor, spread her arms wide and said, "Mum, I'm angry!" I just smiled down at her and said, "You forgot to scream." She got up, dusted off her trousers and smiled at me. She never tried it again. I found out later that year that Kaia was short for Katherine in Norwegian. As they get older, I have noticed how ironic this is. They are as close as identical twins, but different as night and day. Just like their names!

The doctor who delivered Katherine suggested, after she was born, that I shouldn't have any more children. I was heartbroken AND relieved. My husband always wanted eight! He said that I hadn't healed well from my first c-section, and delivering Katherine had been very difficult with all of the scar tissue. It would be nearly impossible for him to deliver another baby safely. I was also told that I would never be able to deliver vaginally because I have a heart-shaped uterus (called a bicornuate uterus), which allows the baby only half the space to grow and no space in which to turn near the end of the pregnancy. (This had no affect on Kaia being born prematurely, incidentally.)

Today both of my children are healthy and happy—they are the lights of my life

---

Today, both of my children are healthy and happy. They are the lights of my life. I know I wouldn't be the person I am today without the experiences of having them and raising them. They have taught me so much and made me stronger. I am forever grateful. Thank you, baby girls! I love you!

Krisanne Collard

Note: There is some uncertainty as to when 'Kangaroo Mother Care' was first used. In some articles and websites it's given as being 1978. However, in the French translation of the first article by Edgar Rey, it is clearly given as July 1977.

I asked Michel about kangaroo care...
In what circumstances would you say it's appropriate to use so-called 'kangaroo care' with premature babies, instead of using conventional incubators?

In Bogotá they have used kangaroo care with babies below 1,000g. The baby just needs to be able to breathe unaided.

In Bogotá [Columbia, South America], they have used kangaroo care with babies below 1000g. The prerequisite is that the baby can breathe without any assistance. In Pithiviers [the maternity hospital for which Michel was responsible near Paris, France] we could not be as audacious as in Bogotá. We used this method for babies weighing more than 1700 or 1800 grams (and breathing easily). If a woman wants to use kangaroo care, it is better to start in the birthing room, without interrupting at all the skin-to-skin contact. It is difficult without the enthusiastic cooperation of the health professionals.

Breastfeeding

Of course, you don't need me to tell you that breastfeeding is the best approach to promote optimality postnatally, for both mother and baby.

In most cases, as I've already pointed out, women who've had completely physiological births breastfeed totally spontaneously. Often problems which have been predicted simply don't manifest because absolutely nothing has taken place during the birth to disturb the natural hormonal processes. Immediately after the birth both mother and newborn baby are primed to breastfeed.

Since many midwives may not have personal experience of breastfeeding successfully for long periods of time, here are a few guidelines so that you can offer new mothers the best possible support...

- Don't give the new mother any instructions at all in the first two hours postpartum. As we've detailed already, any kind of speech or communication can disturb the hormonal processes taking place at this time. This affects not only bonding, but also the safety of a physiological third stage.
- Remain behind the mother or away from her in a corner, making an effort not to intrude on her in any way. Also, make sure your phone is switched off and that you say nothing audible to other staff around you.
- After the third stage is completed and you're happy that the placenta is complete, do whatever you can to make the mother comfortable if she is showing signs of discomfort. (If she seems fine, just leave her to do whatever comes naturally. After my first birth I spontaneously started singing my new baby a very odd song when I started to breastfeed... Don't laugh!)
- After the first couple of hours are over, encourage the new mother to use a breastfeeding cushion (or pillow) to raise her baby to a comfortable feeding position. This will help her to get her baby well-positioned, which will prevent feeding problems and help her to avoid backache over the next few weeks and months.
- Encourage her to offer her baby a breast every time he or she murmurs or cries. (It's best she responds immediately if she wants to have an easy time!)
- Explain to her (if she doesn't already know) that she needs to offer both breasts every time her baby feeds, but that she needs to let the baby decide when to switch. The baby will show his or her readiness to switch over by unlatching from the first breast.
- Tell her that at each new feed she needs to put the baby to the breast the baby *last* fed from (because he or she probably didn't drain it completely).
- If she ever experiences any soreness or pain, tell her she needs to unlatch immediately and reposition her baby. To get the baby to latch on properly, tell her to touch the baby's bottom lip with one finger, then stroke one of the baby's cheeks to get him/her to turn his or her head. (At this point she zooms the baby in!)
- Explain to her that babies often want to suck a lot and that this is normal. Her body will adjust to her baby's needs and produce milk accordingly. (The baby's sucking stimulates milk production, so the baby should never be kept away from the breast if he or she wants to suck.) Also explain that as well as having huge needs for milk, babies take comfort in sucking while snuggled up to their new mums—and that's OK!

- Tell her there may be times when she feels she's breastfeeding round the clock, but that these times will usually be preparation for growth spurts or days when her baby isn't feeling 100%. She still needs to take her baby's lead.
- Tell her it won't be helpful for her baby to use a dummy as it may upset her milk flow and prevent her from producing sufficient quantities of milk. She can breastfeed discretely anywhere using a large scarf slung over her shoulder (to hide the baby and her midriff) or wearing nursing clothes.
- Explain the benefits of co-sleeping. As you probably know, this is now considered a safe practice as long as neither the mother nor father have drunk alcohol or taken drugs.
- Tell her about the risk of smothering her baby while she's breastfeeding on the sofa, in particular since she's very likely to fall asleep at some point. However, explain that the risks are minimised if she always keeps her baby on the edge of the sofa (under the crook of her arm) because then the worst that can happen is the baby would fall off!
- Explain the wonders of rocking chairs... They may well help her to relax with her baby, especially if she has a breastfeeding cushion to raise her baby to a good position.
- Encourage her to read *Breast is Best* (Pan Books 2005) or *The Womanly Art of Breastfeeding* (Plume Books 2004, available from La Leche League). Also tell her about new mother get-togethers organised by local health services, La Leche League and the NCT and the phone helplines.
- If ever she experiences problems encourage her to immediately seek help—either from a book, from an experienced breastfeeding mother or from a breastfeeding counsellor (e.g. trained by La Leche League or the NCT). With her baby correctly positioned, your client should soon find breastfeeding a painfree experience. Tell her to get info from: www.llli.org, www.laleche.org.uk, www.nct.org.uk and www.abm.me.uk—or from her local health services.

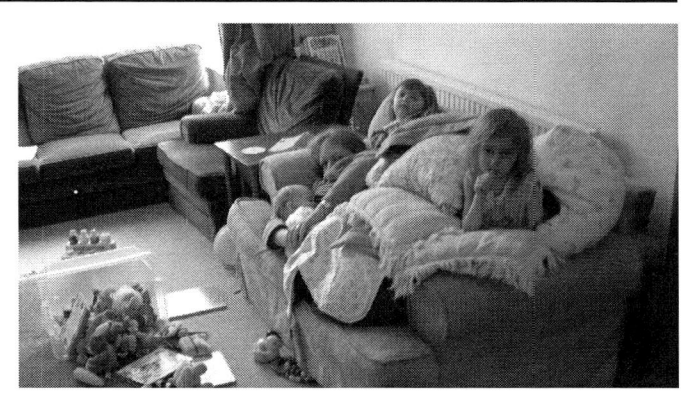

Breastfeeding on a sofa is fine if the baby's on the edge

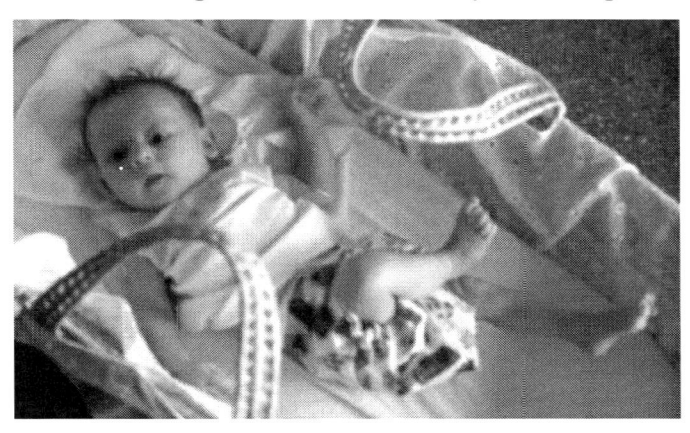

Remember that fully breastfed babies can have an altogether different growth pattern. As long as they're alert, their skin tone's good and they're producing wet nappies, it's OK if they're thin!

Breastfeeding helps mothers and babies

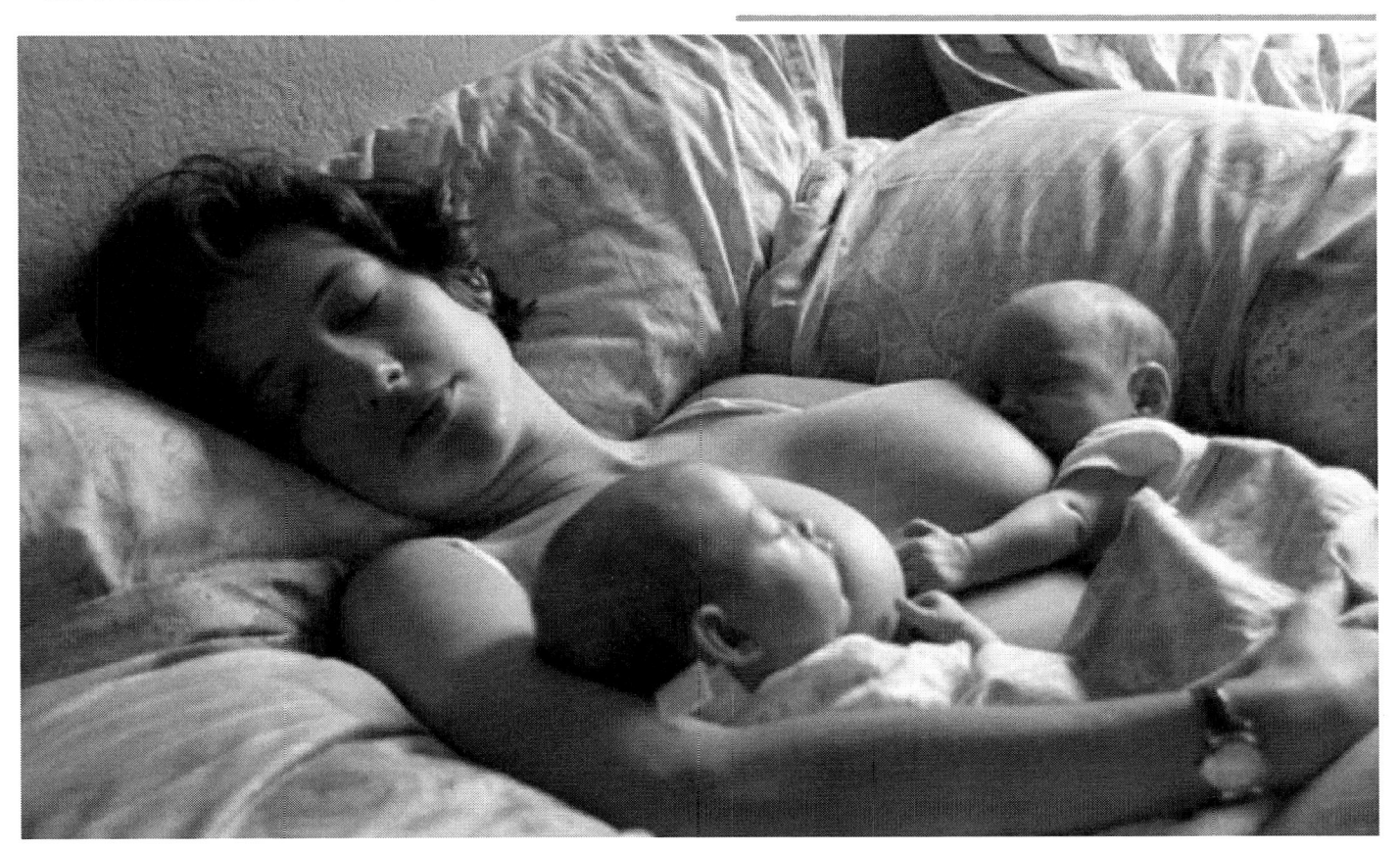

Olga Mellor breastfeeding her twins. Her full, completely natural birth story can be read in BIRTH: Countdown to Optimal.

Mothering

As you may know from your own experience, most new mothers feel diffident and overwhelmed by their new responsibilities. On top of this, their sudden change in lifestyle—often from full-time work to being a stay-at-home mum—throws them into both practical and psychological chaos. At the same time, new mothers may have high expectations of motherhood, which may soon become disillusionment if they don't have the right kind of guidance and support.

As the first professional in contact with the new mother you are in an excellent position to do something positive. Here are a few ideas on how you might relate to the new mothers in your care directly after the birth, based on my own experience of having physiological births:

- Even if you feel that all safety issues have been covered and that you've done enough cleaning up, please don't make the mother feel 'abandoned' by you. For the entire antenatal period she will hopefully have felt that you are her main source of support. She will feel betrayed and at sea if you leave too abruptly. Even if you can't spend 20 minutes or so with her while she's making her first, tentative steps into motherhood (or new motherhood if it's not her first baby) at least speak to her extremely sensitively while you're with her. Above all, *listen* well.
- Don't be brisk or disrespectful. Whether or not you're religious, since important bonding processes are taking place, you have to admit there is a certain sacredness about this time. The better the mother is made to feel, the more likely it is she will relax and be able to forge a good bond with her new baby.
- Aim to get a good balance between support and deference. The new mother—with all those wonderful hormones coursing through her body—really does know the best things to do for her baby. If she feels she doesn't, she probably just needs a little encouragement and reassurance. Inspire her to have faith in her own ability to mother her baby and tell her she'll learn quickly!
- Encourage her to see her baby as a person with feelings and a sense of self. He or she will need to be treated with respect at all times. Explain to the mother that whenever possible she needs to give her baby choices—even when he or she is just a few days old! She will be surprised by how well her baby is able to respond and communicate.
- Remind your client that she will need to be kind to herself. Although for many weeks she will be focused on her new baby's needs, she must also remember her own. This may mean forcing herself to get dressed in the mornings, allowing herself the 'luxury' of having a shower while her baby cries in a Moses basket on the bathroom floor... Or it may mean getting organised and going out to meet some friends, probably with her baby in tow!
- Encourage your client to explore environmentally-friendly nappy options or to find out about 'elimination communication', i.e. ways of doing without nappies altogether. Information can be obtained from www.natural-wisdom.com or www.White-Boucke.com/ifpt.html. Although it may be necessary to ease new mothers into baby care with a few disposables initially, in later days it would be wonderful if new mothers could be encouraged and taught how to tune into their babies' weeing and pooing needs... It's not only important so as to minimise landfill, but also for aesthetic reasons.

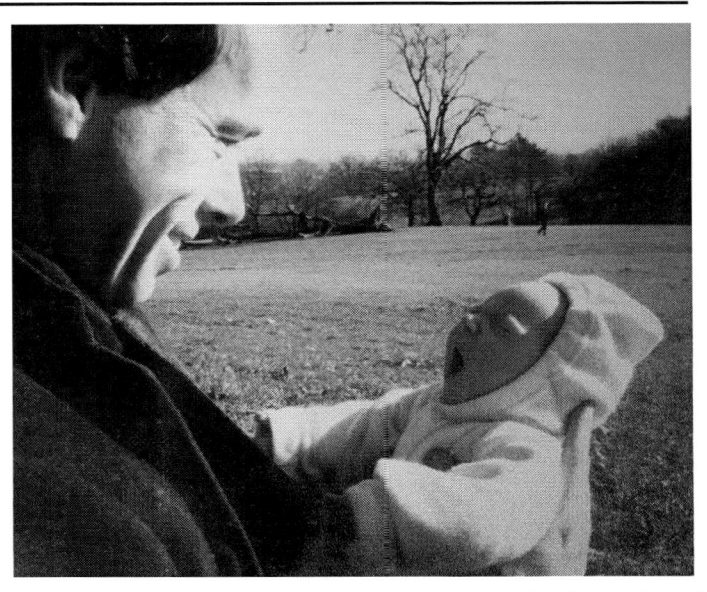

Also encourage new mums to get their partner to give them a break!

Postnatal lifestyle adjustment

Finally, since postnatal depression is so much in the news these days and since lifestyle adjustment is such a crucial issue to optimality, I would like to ask you to reflect on how you can help your clients to move beyond birth, breastfeeding and early motherhood into their new role as mothers and postpartum partners, as it were.

BONDING, BREASTFEEDING & MOTHERING

1. In what ways can a midwife interfere with mother-infant bonding? How can she facilitate it?
2. What kind of behaviour from midwives supports breastfeeding? What inhibits it?
3. To what extent do you feel new mothers value privacy over practical help?
4. To what extent do you feel they value advice? How can it be given successfully and sensitively?
5. How can you discretely find out about a mother's insecurities and empower her in these areas?
6. How can you discover and bring out a woman's natural mothering strengths?

PRACTICAL, PSYCHOLOGICAL & SEXUAL SUPPORT

1. What kind of advice would you personally want to give?
2. What can you say to women postnatally in order to help them avoid depression in a few weeks' or months' time?
3. Is it important to discuss sex and postnatal marital relationships, beyond a discussion of contraception?

PROFESSIONALISM IN RELATIONSHIPS

1. What could you do to extend your relationships with clients into the future... and is this a good idea?
2. Where should the dividing line come between professionalism and friendship?
3. How long do you feel a midwife-mother relationship should ideally be extended through official visits?
4. What can facilitate communication between midwives and mothers or between midwives and health visitors?

Birthframe 36

The issues discussed in this final birthframe are central to the way in which women re-evaluate themselves postnatally. How could you prepare women antenatally, perhaps in liaison with health visitors, to promote postnatal lifestyle optimality?

When I was blessed a few years back with a baby boy, I had a vision. My life would go on much as before, only with a tiny baby keeping me company, smiling and gurgling as I went through the routines of daily living. That vision was almost immediately replaced by a reality where I barely maintained my sanity while struggling to meet the needs of one who, while adorable, was a tyrant. Any time of the day and especially at night I answered his clarion calls for "Milk, milk, milk, and step on it!" In those early weeks I was oblivious to everything but mastering this new role of motherhood.

It was then that I began to notice that not only had my world changed, but also I had changed. Namely, there seemed to be a lot more of me. Twenty-four pounds more, to be exact. I told myself it was all in my breasts, but that myth was dispelled after my husband pointed out that I was wearing maternity jeans. Embarrassed, I packed them away, and was left with a wardrobe of sweatpants and tight T-shirts.

I told my doctor, "I think I have a glandular problem. All the other breastfeeding mothers are losing weight, but I hardly eat anything and I haven't lost an ounce!" She smiled gently and said, "If you burn more calories than you take in, you'll lose weight." She didn't believe me! I left her office in a huff, grumbling about the unfairness of it all. When did I, a new mother, ever have time for a meal? Most nights it was all I could do to grab a spoon and a pint of ice cream while my little one was nestled at my breast.

I tried to ignore the growing problem of the larger me by avoiding full-length mirrors and clothes in general, but my new pounds fairly shouted for attention. They stood out in all sorts of awkward bulges, as if they'd been lobbed at me from some distance away and stuck fast. My ankles were thick and my feet were plump, my knees had a double chin and my midsection, well, let's just say I got tired of people asking me when my next baby was due. My upper torso was dominated by 'The Milk Factory', but the novelty of being well endowed quickly wore off. I wanted my old body back and was willing to try anything to get it.

"I'll exercise," I declared. The local gym was advertising an aerobics class for new mothers. Babies were welcome. I signed up right away. On class day, I struggled to get out of the house on time, lugging my son in a car seat that seemed to weigh 100 pounds. I couldn't find parking nearby, so I walked a few blocks with the car seat bashing into my shins. By the time I reached the gym, I was sweating profusely. Class had already started, led by a boyish woman with a body fat percentage of 3.0. She whipped the class through a routine of jumping, step climbing and marching that hurt every part of my body. The other women moved smoothly through the programme while I focused on not looking like a fool, but I was always a step or three behind. Everyone was kind. I was glad, though, that my son slept through the entire pathetic performance. We went home and I weighed myself. I had lost a pound.

I went to my second class a few days later. This time I managed to keep up somewhat, and even to throw some verve into my moves. As I leapt onto my step and threw my right foot out, I lost my balance and fell, knocking over the woman in front of me. Red-faced, I finished the class and went home to weigh myself. I had gained a pound.

I decided aerobics was not my 'thing'. Instead I bought a fancy jogging buggy, intending to zip around the block a few times a week with my baby riding in style. I had been an enthusiastic runner before my pregnancy, thinking nothing of knocking off two or three miles every other day. It wouldn't take long to fall back into my old habits.

Everything went fine with my new programme until I came to my first hill and then I fell apart. It may as well have been Mount Rainier for all the gasping, grunting, and perspiring that went on—and that was just the first 20 yards. [Mount Rainier is a 14,410ft mountain in Washington State, USA.] I felt awkward not having my hands free and altogether discouraged with my outing. "My running days are over," I thought dispiritedly.

Right about then I decided to leave my fat where it was for a while and tackle another problem that had been bothering me—loneliness. My old friends didn't seem to understand my new life very well and sometimes blanched when I whipped out a breast to feed my son. I hadn't really gotten around to making new friends. So, despite my innate shyness, I dragged myself to a La Leche League meeting.

It was astonishing to see so many women brought together by a common interest, cheerfully breastfeeding their babies and discussing the changes motherhood had brought as if they actually relished their new lives. I really enjoyed my first meeting. I met someone there, a woman with a baby girl, who happened to live in my neighbourhood. Before long we had arranged to push our buggies around the lake a couple of times a week. She was such good company and we had so much in common that I really looked forward to these outings.

After a few weeks she suggested that we jog a little way each time we did our three-mile route, and it seemed like a good idea. The pace was never so strenuous that we couldn't keep talking. One day we were so engrossed in our subject (I think it was spit-up) that we jogged the whole three miles. It wasn't long after that that I put my sweatpants and my scales away.

My jogging and mothering buddy lives 600 miles away now... If I had any advice to give to other women in my shoes, it would be this: you are so much more than the sum of your parts. You're somebody's mother, for crying out loud! Life will never be the same, and neither will your body. It will be better. Miraculously, you're nourishing a baby in the best way possible, using only your body, so despite its obvious flaws, strange bulges and odd sagging areas it's amazing. Focus instead on building and nurturing relationships with your child, your partner and especially other mothers. Have a 'tribe' with which to hang out, share stories, gripe, go to the park, exercise, talk parenting or any other subject... it'll make all the difference. The first year of new motherhood is tough. Establish a support network. You'll be glad you did when you discover how tough the second year is... and the third, fourth, fifth, etc. That would be my advice. As far as my own weight goes, the less I think about it, the happier I am! I don't look like a model but I feel great: fit, healthy and occasionally like Supermum. I didn't get my old body back... I got a more fun version with bigger boobs! I still exercise regularly and I'm still breastfeeding—my second baby now!

Sarah Hobart

# YOUR INPUT!

Now that I've been through my view on The What, The Why & The How, I'd like to invite you to contribute your view. If you would like to help me improve this book or add to it for a future edition, please do make contact. Email me at sylvie@freshheartpublishing.co.uk. I am interested in:

- Feedback and opinions based on your experience
- Corrections, additional information or photographs
- Additional birthframes or comments from women, midwives and obstetricians, not to mention other staff
- Advice you would give to other midwives attending women who have chosen to have physiological births
- Ideas for improving the plight of women in developing countries, who face difficulties for all the wrong reasons

Thank you to Nina Klose for the beautiful photos below and right

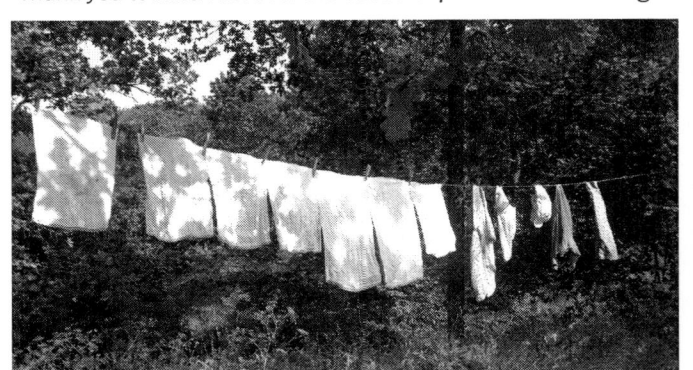

Visit www.freshheartpublishing.co.uk for more information on recent publications

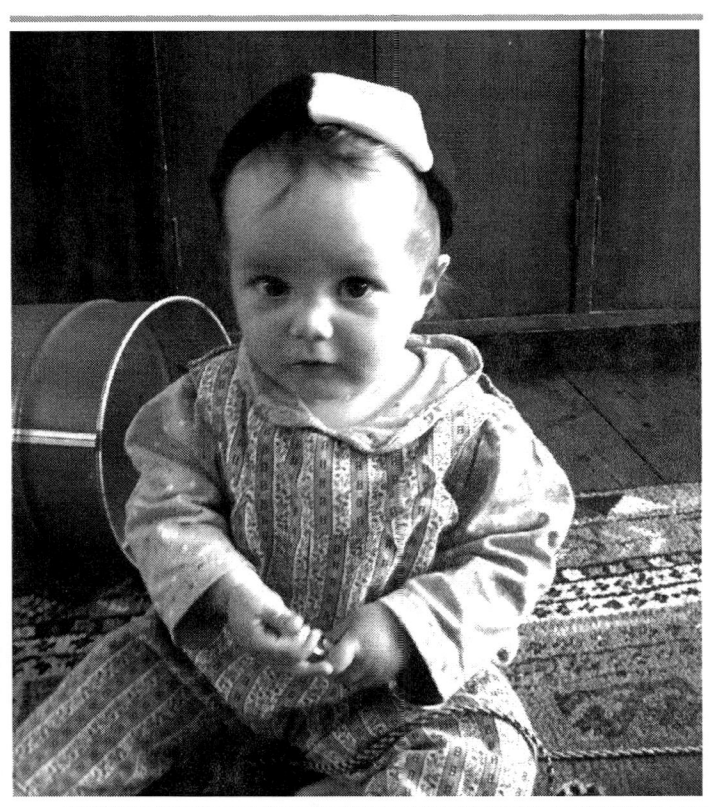

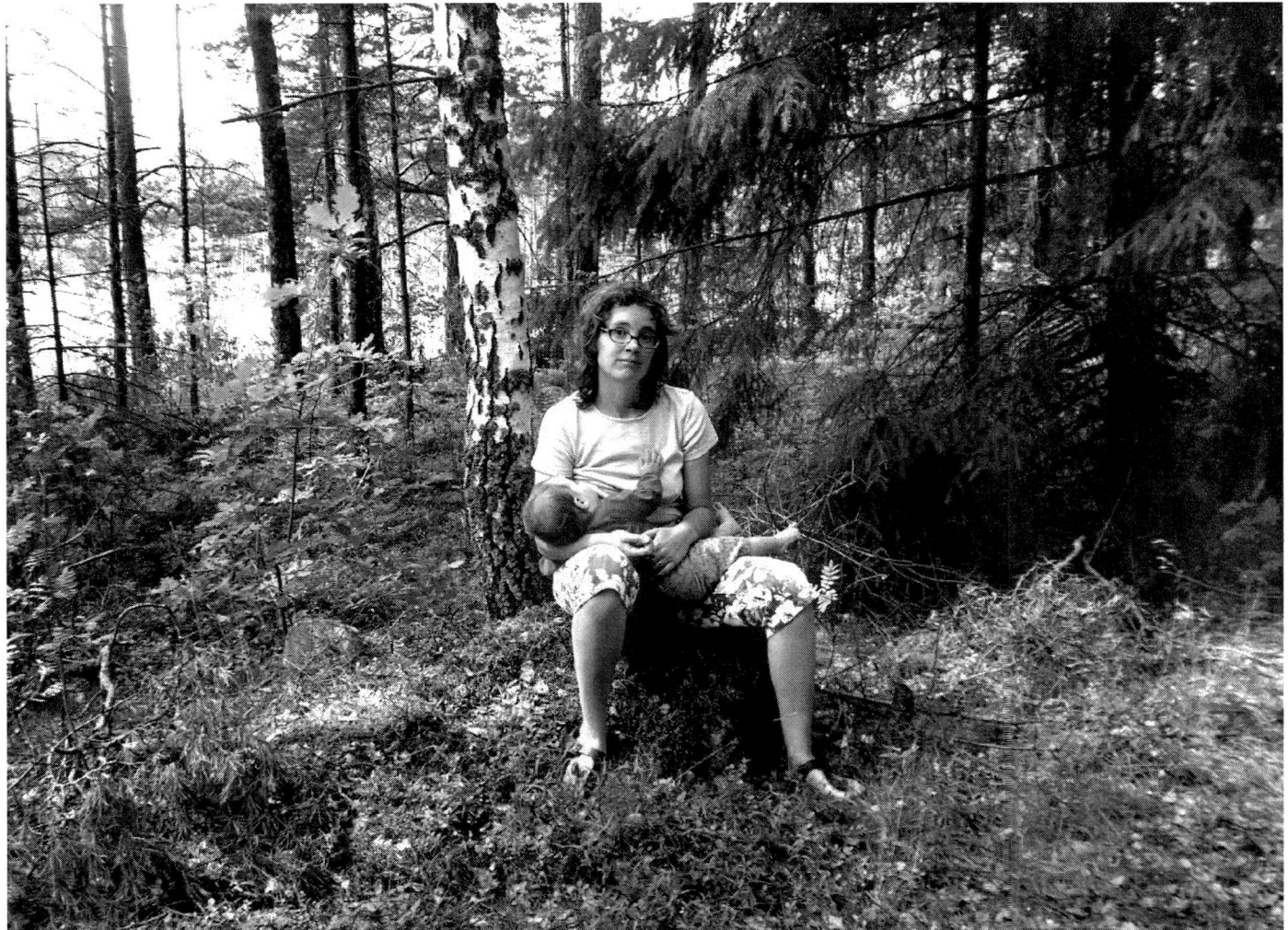

BIRTHFRAMES INDEX

No.	Name	Features	Page
1	Sylvie Donna	Posterior lie, face-to-pubis optimal birth in Sri Lanka	32
2	Sylvie Donna	Fetal ejection reflex experienced with Michel Odent in attendance	33
3	Sylvie Donna	Birthing optimally, with controversial support from the NHS	35
4	Maria Shanahan	Optimal birth despite extreme fear after a bad first birth experience	36
5	Rachel Urbach	The 'natural norm' experienced by a primagravida who was undisturbed	38
6	Anonymous	Life-saving intervention because of high risk of haemorrhage	39
7	Tina C from the UK	Management of persistent hyperemesis	39
8	Jo Siebert	Appropriate intervention of obstetric cholestasis in a twin pregnancy	41
9	Liliana Lammers	Appropriate intervention—an in-labour caesarean	42
10	Anonymous	NHS optimal twin birth, achieved as a result of thorough planning	42
11	Debbie Brindley	Arranging for minimal disturbance during a twin hospital birth	43
12	Nina Klose	The emotional memory of a caesarean section	47
13	Anonymous	Postnatal experiences after caesareans	48
14	Anonymous	A positive experience of a caesarean	48
15	Anonymous	A failed VBAC, despite excellent midwifery support	50
16	Michel Odent	A successful VBAC	51
17	Anonymous	Anger about treatment	57
18	Christina from the UK	Over-cautious intervention, then successful non-interventionist births	58
19	Sylvie Donna	Intervention refused, based on research and second opinions	60
20	Liliana Lammers	A first disturbed birth, followed by three undisturbed straightforward ones	62
21	Clare O'Ryan	A birth which was very disturbed by lack of continuity of care	63
22	Fiona Lucy Stoppard	The dignity and beauty of 'going to another planet' in labour	69
23	Pauline Farrance	Optimal birth after managed first birth	69
22	Anonymous	A disappointing, disempowering first antenatal appointment	76
23	Anonymous	A triplet birth which could have been much better in terms of relationships	88
24	Jenny Sanderson	Two completely undisturbed births with Michel Odent in attendance	92
25	Anonymous	A twin birth which was adversely affected by unnecessary interventions	95
26	Michel Odent	Encouraging women to tune into their 'mammalian self' to give birth	96
27	Michel Odent	The 'birthing pool test' in practice	100
28	Anonymous	Helping a woman deal with psychological issues—if it's not too late	100
29	Nuala OSullivan	A physiological birth which included postnatal life-saving intervention	101
30	Sarah-Jane Forder	The role of a doula in facilitating a smooth hospital birth	103
31	Natalie Meddings	A doula helping a woman 'go to another planet' at home	104
32	Ruth Clark	An expectedly straightforward and fast birth before the midwives arrived	106
33	Sylvie Donna	A birth which 'went wrong' in all kinds of ways, which was also 'optimal'	108
34	Ashley Marshall	A lotus birth (i.e. a birth with no cord cutting postnatally)	110
35	Krisanne Collard	Premature birth and kangaroo care	112
36	Sarah Hobart	Dealing with a few key issues a couple of months after giving birth	119

Note:
A hundred birthframes are included in the companion volume for pregnant women *BIRTH: Countdown to Optimal* (Fresh Heart 2008) and the ones in this book just represent a selection. 180 comments are also included (i.e. a lot more than in this book). The ones chosen for this edition were considered of particular interest, from your perspective as a midwife.

If you would like to contribute other birthframes, comments or research for possible inclusion in a future edition, please do not hesitate to contact the publisher via www.freshheartpublishing.co.uk. If any of your clients are interested in contributing their own experiences, please reassure them that they will have the opportunity to check how their accounts will be presented before publication and of course they would be able to choose to be named or anonymous.

Even though it's vital that practices are research-based, we also need to recognise that certain areas can never be researched. For this reason, we need to acknowledge the value of first-hand accounts which can sometimes give us enormous insight, not to mention inspiration or ideas.

USEFUL CONTACTS

AIMS (Association for Improvements in the Maternity Services) – www.aims.org.uk
Chair: Beverley Lawrence Beech. 5 Ann's Court, Grove Road, Surbiton, Surrey KT6 4BE. Tel: 0870 765 1453.
Vice Chair: Nadine Edwards. 40 Leamington Terrace, Edinburgh, EH10 4JL. Tel: 0870 765 1449.
Homebirth Support Co-ordinator. Tel: 0870 765 1447.
Support and information about parents' rights and choices. Provides information on complaints procedures.

Active Birth Centre – www.activebirthcentre.com
25 Bickerton Road, London N19 5JT. Tel: 020 7281 6760.
Classes for mothers interested in active, physiological birth. Can put women in touch with local groups. Supplier of pools.

Association of Breastfeeding Mothers – www.abm.me.uk
ABM, PO Box 207, Bridgwater, Somerset, TA6 7YT. Tel: 08444 122 948. Helpline: 08444 122 949.
Telephone and email advice. Support groups for breastfeeding mothers.

Association of Radical Midwives – www.radmid.demon.co.uk
Sarah Montagu. Tel: 01243 671673.
Support for midwives. Helpline for mums-to-be.

Back in Action – www.backinaction.co.uk
Tel: 020 7930 8309 (London), 01494 434343 (Amersham), 01628 477177 (Marlow) or 0117 922 6377 (Bristol).
Suppliers of chairs and products for good back health. They also supply pregnancy rockers, called 'kneeling chairs'.

BLISS – www.bliss.org.uk
2nd and 3rd floors, 9 Holyrood Street, London SE1 2EL. Tel: 020 7378 1122. Helpline: 0500 618140 Mon-Fri 10am-5pm.
Practical and emotional support for parents of premature babies.

Caesarean Support Network – www.ukselfhelp.info/caesarean
Yvonne Williams, 55 Cooil Drive, Douglas, Isle of Man IM2 2HF. Tel: 01624 661 269.
Emotional support and practical advice for women who have had or may need a caesarean delivery.

Care for the Family – www.careforthefamily.org.uk
Garth House, Leon Avenue, Cardiff CF15 7RG. Tel: 029 2081 0800.
Support for families and marriages in good and bad times.

Down's Syndrome Association – www.downs-syndrome.org.uk
Langdon Down Centre, 2a Langdon Park, Teddington, TW11 9PS. Tel; 0845 230 0372.
Information and support for parents of babies or children with Down's syndrome.

Doula UK – www.doula.org.uk
PO Box 26678, London N14 4WB. Tel: 0871 433 3103.
Information about birth and postnatal doulas. Can provide a list of doulas working in a particular area.

Foresight – www.foresight-preconception.org.uk
178 Hawthorn Road, West Bognor, W Sussex PO21 2UY. Tel: 01243 868001.
Information on preconceptual care and nutrition during pregnancy. [SAE required.]

Independent Midwives Association – www.independentmidwives.org.uk
PO Box 539, Abingdon OX14 9DF. Tel: 0845 4600 105 (leave message on answering machine).
Association for independent midwives. Can provide a list of independent midwives experienced in homebirth.

Informed Parent – www.informedparent.co.uk
PO Box 4481, Worthing, W Sussex BN11 2WH. Tel: 01903 212969.
Information about vaccinations to help women reach decisions. [SAE required.]

La Leche League Great Britain – www.laleche.org.uk
PO Box 29, West Bridgford, Nottingham. Tel: 0845 456 1855 (Mon-Thurs, answering machine at other times).
Support and information for pregnant women and breastfeeding mothers. Network of informal support groups.

Meet-a-Mum Association (MAMA) – www.mama.co.uk
54 Lillington Road, Radstock, BA3 3NR. Tel: 0845 120 6162. Helpline: 0845 120 3746 Mon-Fri 7pm-10pm.
Support for mothers who feel lonely, isolated or depressed. Puts mothers in touch with other mothers in a similar situation.

Miscarriage Association – www.miscarriageassociation.org.uk
C/o Clayton Hospital, Northgate, Wakefield, W Yorks WF1 3JS. Helpline: 01924 200799 Mon-Fri, 9am-4pm.
Support for mothers who have experienced miscarriage. Also information on cervical stitches and ectopic pregnancies.

The National Childbirth Trust (NCT) – www.nct.org.uk
Alexandra House, Oldham Terrace, Acton, London W3 6NH. Tel: 0870 444 8707 or 020 8992 8637.
Maternity sales: 0141 636 0600. Pregnancy and birth line: 0870 444 8708.
Information and support for all aspects of pregnancy and birth. Antenatal classes and network of informal postnatal groups.

Neal's Yard Remedies – www.nealsyardremedies.com
Mail Order, Peacemarsh, Gillingham, Dorset SP8 4EU. Tel: 0845 262 3145.
Mail order sales of a wide range of herbs and homeopathic remedies. Will send them anywhere in the world.

Parentalk – www.parentalk.co.uk
1 Kennington Road, London SE1 7QP. Tel: 020 7921 4234.
Support for parents in the workplace, as well as for employers and professionals who support parents.

Patients' Association – www.patients-association.org.uk
PO Box 935, Harrow, Middlesex HA1 3YJ. Tel: 020 8423 9111. Helpline: 0845 608 4455.
Forum for NHS users to raise concerns or share experiences about health care.

Primal Health Research Centre – www.birthworks.org/primalhealth
72 Savernake Road, London NW3 2JR.
Information on various aspects of primal health. Publishes a quarterly newsletter (available by subscription).

Rebirthing – www.re-birth.uk.com, www.ecstaticbirth.com, www.thehillthatbreathes.com
- Pat Bennaceur, Hove, E Sussex BN3 3PF. Tel: 01273 727588.
- Binnie A Dansby, Ecstatic Birth, 6 Court Lodge, Lamberhurst, Kent, TN3 8DU. Tel: 01 892 890614.
- Gaia Pollini. La Collina Che Respira, Localita Girfalco, Via Ca Loreto, 3, 61029, Urbino, Italy. Tel: 0870 609 2690.

Courses for pregnant women or new mothers and families.

Society for Teachers of the Alexander Technique (STAT) – www.stat.org.uk
1st floor, Linton House, 39-51 Highgate Road, London NW5 1RS. Tel: 020 7482 5135.
Information on classes. Can put women in touch with a teacher or group in their area.

Stillbirth and Neonatal Death Society (SANDS) – www.uk-sands.org
28 Portland Place, London W1B 1LY. Tel: 020 7436 7940. Helpline: 020 7436 5881 or email support@uk-sands.org
Support and information for bereaved parents.

The Carrying Kind – www.thecarryingkind.com
Units 12-15 Wood Street Market, 102a Wood Street, Walthamstow, London E17 3HX. Tel: 020 8509 1660.
Suppliers of a wide range of different baby carriers.

Twins and Multiples Births Association (TAMBA) – www.tamba.org.uk
2 The Willows, Gardner Road, Guildford, GU1 4PG. Tel: 01483 304 442. Helpline: 0800 138 0509.
Encouragement and support for parents of twins or more.

VBAC Information and Support (no website)
50 Whiteways, North Bersted, Bognor Regis, W Sussex PO22 9AS. Tel: 01243 868440.
Information and support for women who wish to avoid a repeat caesarean.

What Doctors Don't Tell You – www.wddty.com
WDDTY, Unit 10, Woodman Works, 204 Durnsford Road, London SW19 8DR. Tel: 0870 444 9886.
Information on medicine and health. Publishes WDDTY newsletter, 'Mothers Know Best', 'Proof!', and many booklets.

Wilkinet Baby Carriers – www.wilkinet.co.uk
P.O. Box 4521, Southam, CV47 4AS. Tel: 0800 2550 247 (anytime).
Suppliers of Wilkinet baby carriers.

Working Families – www.workingfamilies.org.uk
1-3 Berry Street, London EC1V 0AA. Tel: 020 7253 7243. Helpline: 0800 013 0313.
Support for parents and families who want to find a better work-life balance.

BIBLIOGRAPHY

Arms, S. *Immaculate Deception II.* Celestial Arts 1994. ISBN: 978 0 890876 33 6.

Block, J. *Pushed: The Painful Truth about Childbirth and Modern Maternity Care.* Da Capo 2007. ISBN: 978 0 738210 73 5.

Blumfield, W. *Life After Birth.* Element Books 1992. ISBN: 978 1 852303 51 8.

Bryson, B. *Bill Bryson's African Diary.* Doubleday 2002. ISBN: 978 0 385605 14 4.

Buckley, S. *Gentle Birth, Gentle Mothering: The wisdom and science of gentle choices in pregnancy, birth, and parenting.* One Moon Press 2005. Available from www.gentlebirthgentlemothering.com.

Caldwell Sorel, N. *Ever Since Eve.* Oxford University Press 1984. ISBN: 978 0 195034 60 8.

Campbell, S and C Lees. *Obstetrics by Ten Teachers.* Hodder Arnold 2000. ISBN: 978 0 340719 86 2.

Chamberlain, D. *Babies Remember Birth.* Ballantine Books 1990. ISBN: 978 3 45364 11 1.

Donna, S. *BIRTH: Countdown to Optimal.* Fresh Heart 2008. ISBN: 978 1 906619 00 8.

Downe, S. *Normal Childbirth: Evidence and Debate.* Churchill Livingstone 2004. ISBN: 978 0 443073 85 4.

Enkin, M et al. *A Guide to Effective Care in Pregnancy and Childbirth.* Oxford University Press 2000. ISBN: 978 0 192631 73 2.

Gaskin, I M. *Spiritual Midwifery.* Book Publishing Company 2002. ISBN: 978 1 570671 04 3.

Jadad, AR and M Enkin. *Randomized Controlled Trials: Questions, Answers and Musings.* Blackwell 2007. ISBN: 978 1 405132 66 4.

Kitzinger, S. *Birth Crisis.* Routledge 2006. ISBN: 978 0 415372 66 4.

Kitzinger, S. *New Pregnancy and Childbirth: Choices and Challenges* (Dorling Kindersley 2003). ISBN: 978 0 751364 38 5.

Kitzinger, S. *Ourselves as Mothers: Universal Experience of Motherhood.* Doubleday 1992. ISBN: 978 0 385403 20 7.

Leboyer, F. *Birth Without Violence.* Inner Traditions Bear and Company 2002. ISBN: 978 0 892819 83 6.

Metland, D (ed.) *The Complete Book of Pregnancy.* HarperCollins 2000. ISBN: 978 0 004140 99 5.

Myles, M. *Myles Textbook for Midwives.* Churchill Livingstone 1999. ISBN: 978 0 443055 86 7.

Odent, M and J Vincent-Priya. *Birth Traditions and Modern Pregnancy Care.* Element Books 1992. ISBN: 978 1 852303 21 1.

Odent, M. *Birth and Breastfeeding.* Clairview Books 2003. ISBN: 978 1 902636 48 1.

Odent, M. *Birth Reborn.* Souvenir Press 1994. ISBN: 978 0 285631 94 6.

Odent, M. *Primal Health*, Clairview Books 2007. ISBN: 978 1 905570 08 9.

Odent, M. *The Caesarean.* Free Association Books 2004. ISBN: 978 1 853437 18 2.

Odent, M. *The Scientification of Love.* Free Association Books 1999. ISBN: 978 1 853434 76 1.

Odent, M. *Water and Sexuality.* Penguin (Canada) 1990. ISBN: 978 0 140191 94 3.

Rank, O. *The Trauma of Birth.* Routledge 1999. ISBN: 978 0 415211 04 8.

Rix, J. *Is there sex after childbirth?* Thorsons 1995. ISBN: 978 0 722529 57 7.

Staff, D A. *Our Bodies, Ourselves.* Touchstone Books 2005. ISBN: 978 0 844672793.

Stanway, Penny. *Breast is Best.* Pan Books 2005. ISBN: 978 0 330436 30 4.

Sutton, J and P Scott. *Optimal Foetal Positioning.* Birth Concepts 1996. (No ISBN available.)

Torgus, Judy (ed.) *The Womanly Art of Breastfeeding.* Plume Books 2004. ISBN: 978 0 452285 80 4.

Wagner, M. *Born in the USA: How a broken maternity system must be fixed to put women and children first.* University of California Press 2006. ISBN: 978 0 520245 96 9.

Walker, A. *Possessing the Secret of Joy.* Vintage 1993. ISBN: 978 0 099224 11 2.

Wesson, N. *Home Birth: A Practical Guide.* Pinter & Martin 2007. ISBN: 978 1 905177 06 6.

RECOMMENDED READING

Most of the following books are readily available. If you have trouble finding any, you can do a search on the website www.bookfinder.com. Alternatively, contact the publisher directly or order any book via a bookshop, using its ISBN number.

Armstrong, P and S Feldman. *A Wise Birth*. Pinter & Martin 2007. ISBN: 978 1 905177 03 5.

Balaskas, J and A Sieveking. *Easy Exercises for Pregnancy*. Frances Lincoln Publishers 1997. ISBN: 978 0 711210 48 6.

Bauer, I. *Diaper Free! The Gentle Wisdom of Natural Infant Hygiene*. Natural Wisdom Press 2001. ISBN: 978 0 452287 77 8.

Block, J. *Pushed: The Painful Truth about Childbirth and Modern Maternity Care*. Da Capo Lifelong 2007. ISBN: 978 0 738210 73 5.

Castro, M. *Mother and Baby*. Pan Books 1996. ISBN: 978 0 330349 25 3.

Chamberlain, D. *Babies Remember Birth*. Ballantine Books 1990. ISBN: 978 3 45364 11 1.

Cohen, N and L Estner. *Silent Knife: Caesarean Prevention and Vaginal Birth After Caesarean*. Greenwood Press 1983. ISBN: 978 0 897890 27 4.

Donna, S. *BIRTH: Countdown to Optimal*. Fresh Heart 2008. ISBN: 978 1 906619 00 8.

Downe, S (ed.) *Normal Childbirth: Evidence and Debate*. Churchill Livingstone 2004. ISBN: 978 0 443073 85 4.

Enkin, M et al. *A Guide to Effective Care in Pregnancy and Childbirth*. Oxford University Press 2000. ISBN: 978 0 192631 73 2.

Jackson, D. *Three in a Bed: The Benefits of Sleeping with Your Baby*. Bloomsbury 2003 [first published in 1989]. ISBN: 978 0 747565 75 8.

Kitzinger, S. *Birth Crisis*. Routledge 2006. ISBN: 978 0 415372 66 4.

Leboyer, F. *Birth Without Violence*. Inner Traditions Bear and Company 2002 [first published in 1974]. ISBN: 978 0 892819 83 6.

McKenna, J. *Sleeping with Your Baby: A Parent's Guide to Cosleeping*. Platypus Media 2007. ISBN: 978 1 930775 34 3.

Odent, M and J Vincent-Priya. *Birth Traditions and Modern Pregnancy Care*. Element Books 1992. ISBN: 978 1 852303 21 1.

Odent, M. *Birth and Breastfeeding*. Clairview Books 2003 [first published in 1992]. ISBN: 978 1 902636 48 1.

Odent, M. *Birth Reborn*. Souvenir Press 1994 [first published in 1984]. ISBN: 978 0 285631 94 6.

Odent, M. *Entering the World: The De-medicalization of Childbirth*. Marion Boyars Books 1984. ISBN: 978 0 714528 00 5.

Odent, M. *The Caesarean*. Free Association Books 2004. ISBN: 978 1 853437 18 2.

Odent, M. *The Farmer and the Obstetrician*. Free Association Books 2002. ISBN: 978 1 853435 65 2.

Odent, M. *The Scientification of Love*. Free Association Books 1999. ISBN: 978 1 853434 76 1.

Rix, J. *Is There Sex After Childbirth?* HarperCollins 1995. ISBN: 978 0 722529 57 0.

Sears, W and M. *The Attachment Parenting Book*. Imported Little, Brown USA Titles 2001. ISBN: 978 0 316778 09 1.

Sears, W and M. *The Birth Book*. Little Brown and Company 1994. ISBN: 978 0 316779 08 1.

Stanway, P. *Breast is Best*. Pan Books 2005. ISBN: 978 0 330436 30 4.

Sutton, J and P Scott. *Optimal Foetal Positioning*. Birth Concepts 1996. Available from Jill Sutton, for £6.00. Please send cheque payable to J Sutton with an A5 stamped addressed envelope to: 95 Beech Rd, Feltham, TW14 8AJ.

Torgus, J (ed.). *The Womanly Art of Breastfeeding*. Plume Books 2004. ISBN: 978 0 452285 80 4.

Wagner, M. *Born in the USA: How a broken maternity system must be fixed to put women and children first*. University of California Press 2006. ISBN: 978 0 520245 96 9.

Wesson, N. *Home Birth: A Practical Guide*. Pinter & Martin 2006. ISBN: 978 1 905177 06 6.

Yntema, S. *Vegetarian Pregnancy: Definitive Nutritional Guide*. McBooks Press 2004. ISBN: 978 0 935526 21 9.

INDEX

abortion 66, 75, 80, 83, 86, **87**
Active Birth 36, 76, 92, 122, 130
acupuncture 3, 67
adrenaline 5, 59, **61**, 84, 111, 130
Africa 36, 56, 66, **79-81**, 120
afterpains 30, 108
alertness 3, 25, **27**, **28**, **30**, 31, 32, 34, **46**, 54, 58, 60, 69, 71, 97
Alexander Technique 123
amniocentesis 66, 83
amniotic fluid 10, 11, **15**, 19, 33, 45, 60, 61, 75, 84
amniotomy **38**, 58, 64, 67, 70, 95, 96, 97
amphetamines 55
anaemia 5, 52, **87**
anaesthesia —also see 'epidurals' and 'spinals' 5, **27**, 39, 44, **45**, 46, 47, 50, 51, 53, 55, 58, 60, 64, 65, 66, 67, 68, 69, 96
analgesia —also see specific drugs by name 5, **27**, 46, 47, 55, 60, **65**, 67, 69, 99
anorexia 55
antenatal care 43, 44, 50, 65, 74, **75-77**, 83, **84-89**, 92
antenatal checks 12, 23, 66, 70, 74, 75, **76**, 77, **84**, **87**, 88
antenatal classes 70, 72, **87**, 88, 123
antenatal tests 66, 70, 74, 75, 77, **83**, 84, **87**, 88
anterior position 16, 17, 18, 33
Apgar score **97**
ARM—see 'amniotomy'
arnica 4
aromatherapy **67**
asthma 55
augmentation of labour 22, 44, 52, 53, 54, 59, 60, 65, 66, 67, 77, 82, 94, 100
auscultation 12, 17, 24, 33, 42, 43, 74, 77, **84**, 91, 92, **97**—also see 'Pinard' and 'Sonicaid'
author's pregnancies and births **32-35**, 60, 82, 105
autism 55
baby carriers 34, 123
backache labour—see 'posterior position'
Balaskas, Janet 130
barbiturates 55
baths 12, 64, 92, **99**, 108—also see 'waterbirth'
birth **24-29**, 52, 57, **61**, 69—also see all birthframes
birthframes **32**—also see Birthframes index on p121
birthing pool—see 'waterbirth'
birthing pool test **100**
birth plans—called 'care guides' in this book—32, 36, 43, 49, **90**, 106-108
birth stories—see Birthframes index on p121
bleeding **27**, 30, 36, 39, 40, 43, 46, 65, 75, 78, 80, 112
blood pressure 32, 34, 40, 43, 45, 46, 47, 53, 70, 75, 76, 80, **84**
bonding 3, **27**, **28**, 29, 30, 31, 34, 37, 39, 44, 47, 50, 52, **53**, **54**, **56**, 58, **60**, **61**, **62**, 63, **69**, 70, 86, 87, **88-89**, 91, **95**, 103, **111**, **112-117**, **118**
Braxton Hicks contractions 11, 15, 33
breastfeeding 3, 18, 19, 25, **27**, **28**, 29, 30, 32, 33, 34, 35, 37, 38, 46, **49**, 52, 53, 54, 56, 57, 58, 60, 61, 62, 64, 68, 69, 70, 71, 76, 82, 88-89, 103, 106, 108, **109**, **116-117**, **118**, 122
breathing difficulties 28, 39, 45, 46, 47, 53, 54, 55, 61, 68, 102, 110, 113, 115, 116

breathing in labour **67**, 106
breech position 17, 19, 24, 42, **82**, 85, 106
caesareans 3, 37, 38, 39, 41, 42, **44-51**, 53, 55, 57, 58, 59, 60, 65, **66**, 68, 70, 94, 96, **100**, 112, 122, 123
camcorders 22, 91, 95, 96
cameras 22, 91, 96
care guides **90**—also see 'birth plans'
cascade of interventions 27, 36-37, 38, 52, 57, **58-60**, 62, 63, **69-72**, 75, **91**, 94, 95
catching the baby 25, 26, **28**, **34**, 36, 37, **55**, 92, 106, 108
Chamberlain, David 54
chorionic villus sampling 66, 83
commanded pushing **27**, 28, 32, **52**, 53, 63, 67—also see 'pushing'
complementary therapies 3, **4**, 5, 67
conception **6**, 32, 36, **78**, 83, 122
continuity of care 32, **38**, **52**, 62, **63**, 74, 75, 88-89, 92
continuous monitoring—see 'EFM' and 'monitoring'
contractions, 22, 23, **24**, 25, 32, 33, 35, 37, 38, 39, 50, 53, **59**, 61, 63, 69, 70-71, 77, 92, 95, 99, 100, 101, 102, 103, 104, 106—also see all other birthframes
control ix, 27, 35, **47**, 53, 57, **59**, **60**, **61**, 63, 67, **69**, 70, 72, **73**, 74, 75, 76, **77**, 83, 86, **91**, 96, 118
cord clamping—see 'cutting the cord'
cord prolapse 33, 42
cutting the cord **27**, 28, 29, 34, 37, 43, 45, 54, 62, 71, 107, 108, **110**, **111**
delivery rooms **32**, 43
depression—see 'postnatal scenarios'
developing countries **56**, **79-81**, 118, 30, 36, 37, **66**
diagnosis of labour **22**, **71**, 92—also see 'onset of labour' and 'false labour'
diamorphine 3, **53**
dilation 20, 22, 23, **24**, 34, 39, 50, 63, 74, **99**, 100, 112
disturbance 3, 5, 19, 20, 22, 23, 24, **27**, **28**, 30, 32, **33**, **34**, 35, 38, 43, **51**, **52**, 55, 56, **59**, 60, **61**, 62, **63**, 64, **67**, 69, 72, 73, 75, **82**, 84, **91**, 92, **94-97**, 100, 101, 107, 108, **111**, **116-117**, **118**, 130—also see 'going to another planet' and 'watchful waiting'
Donna, Sylvie—see 'author's pregnancies and births'
Doppler machine 85-86, 92—also see 'Sonicaid'
doulas 51, 62, 73, 90, **103-104**, 110, 122, 130
Down's syndrome 83, 85, 122
drug addiction 53, **55**
drugs 1, 10, 14, 21, 28, 34, 39, 39-41, 42, 47, 48, 51, **53**, 54, 55, 56, 58, 60, 64, **65**, **66**, 67, 69, 70, 72, 74, 81, 82, 91, 103, 111
due dates —also see 'ultrasound' 5, 15, 19, 20, 21, 23, 36, 37, 38, 41, 47, 58, 60, 63, 70, 75, **78**, 83, 92, 104, 106, 112
dystocia—see 'failure to progress' or 'shoulder dystocia'
eclampsia **83**, 84
ectopic pregnancy 39, 44, 123
EFM (electronic fetal monitoring) 39, 42, 43, 50, **51**, 52, 53, 58, 59, 62, **65**, **67**, **84**, 91, 93, 96, 112—also see 'monitoring', 'fetal scalp monitoring' and 'ultrasound'
elderly primagravida 32, 42, **82**, 83—also see 'older mothers'

elective caesarean **39**, 44, **48-49**—also see 'caesareans'
emergency caesareans 42, 48, 50, 53, 57, 58-59—also see 'caesareans'
emotions 5, 14, 17, 19, 24, 25, 27, 28, 29, 31, 32, 33, 34, 35, 36-37, **38**, 39, 40, 41, 42, 44, **47**, 48, 49, 50, 51, **52**, 54, 55, 57, 58, 59, 60, 62, 66, **67**, 68, 69, 70, 72, 74, 75, 76, **77**, 78, 79, **82**, 83, 84, 85, 86, **87-88**, 90, 91, 92, 94, 96, 97, 99, 100, 101, 102, 103, 107, 112, 115, 130
endorphins 3, 7, 28, 38, 53, 54, 57, **61**, 62, 68
enemas 25, 64, **97**
Entonox—see 'gas and air'
epidurals 3, 32, 39, 41, 43, 46, 47, 50, **53**, 58, 62, 63, **65**, 66, 68, 94, 96—also see 'anaesthesia'
episiotomy 52, 60, 62, **65**, 66, 67, 93, 95, 96
ergometrine 43
eye contact 62, 104
face-to-pubis births 32, 101
failure to progress 3, **22**, 51, 52, 58, 59, 64, 67, 70, 80, **99**, **100**
false labour **22**, 23, 32, 63, 100—also see 'failure to progress'
false negatives and positives 85, 86
fast labour 23, 25, 30, 33-34, 38, 60, 62, 74, 92, 103, 106, **107**, 108, 130
female circumcision 56, 66, 79
female incision 66, 79
fetal distress 12, 17, 33, 37, 44, 51, 53, 54, 58, 68, **84**, 86, 94, 96, 98, 99, 100
fetal monitoring—see 'fetal scalp monitoring', 'Sonicaid' and 'Pinard'
fetal scalp monitoring 51, 54, 58, **67**
fetal stethoscope—see 'Pinard'
fetus ejection reflex 4, **24**, 25, 33-34, **52**, **61**, **111**
first stage 3, 5, 22, 24, **61**
first trimester **6-8**, 75
fistula **80**
folic acid **4**, 75
footling breech **42**, 106
forceps 3, 36, 51, 52, 54, 55, 60, 62, 64, **65**, 66, 67, 95, 100
Friedman curve **22**, 52
gas and air 3, 32, 36, **53**, 55, 67
Gaskin, Ina May 100
gestational diabetes 52, 75, **87**
glucose 94, 104
going to another planet 22, 23, **24**, **27**, 28, 34, **38**, **51**, **53**, **61**, **69**, 72, **91**, 97, 103, 104
glucose tolerance testing **87**
haemoglobin levels **87**
haemorrhage 39, 44, 80, 90—also see 'PPH'
herbs 4, 123
high risk pregnancies and labours 42, **43**, **82**, 85, **87**, **97**
home birth 19, 33-34, 35, 38, 42, 43, 58, 59, 62, 63, 65, 70, 72, 74, **81**, 82, 92, 104, 106-107, 108, 110, 111, 122
homeopathy 3, 4, 123
hormones 4, 5, 6, 8, 10, 19, 20, **24**, **27**, **28**, 44, 51, **52**, 56, 57, 59, 60, **61**, **62**, 68, **77**, 82, 84, 87, 91, 94, 104, 116, 118
hospital birth 32, 36, 38, 39-41, 42, 43, **56**, 57, 58, 59, **62**, 63, 64, **65**, 67, 68, 69, 72, 74, 81, 82, 88, 93, 100, 103, 112-116
hyperemesis 39-41
hypertension—see 'blood pressure'
hypnosis 38, 54
incontinence 44, 60, 80
induction 21, 22, 37, 41, 44, 54, 55, **58**, 59, 60, 65, 66, 67, 69, 70, 78, 82, 83, 84, **94**, 104
infection 44, 53, 58, 59, 60, 61, 68, 72, 81, 96, 112
infertility 39, **44**, 59, 62
infibulation 66, 79
internal examinations 24, 42, 51, 59, 60, 91, 93, 96, 97
intervention 1, 3, 5, 21, 24, 28, **30**, 32, 35, 36, 38, **39-51**, **52**, **54**, **55**, **56**, 57, 58, 59, 60, 63, **65**, **64-68**, 69-72, 75, 79, 82, 83, 84, 87, 88-89, **91**, 92, 94, 95, 96, 99, 101, **102**, 103, **110**, 111, 123, 130
invasive tests **83**—also see 'antenatal tests'
iron supplements **87**
kangaroo care 13, 68, 89, **112-116**
Kitzinger, Sheila 30, 58, 64, 77, 103, 130
labour **22-24**, 43, 52, **61**, 66, 69—also see all birthframes
Lammers, Liliana 42, 56, 62, 69, 103, 104, 130
Leboyer, Frederick 54
legal issues 5, **35**, 38, 42, 46, 52, **73**, 75, 95
lithotomy position 43, 52. 67
lochia 30, 46
lotus birth **110**
low blood pressure—see 'blood pressure'
low-lying placenta —also see 'placenta praevia'
mammals 38, 57, **61**, 68, 86, 91, **96**, 97, **130**
massage 32
maternal mortality 1, 39, 44, **50**, **51**, 52, 56, 64, **68**, **79-80**. 94, **97**, 111, 120
miscarriage 32, 39, 40, 83, 86, 112, 123
monitoring 22, 24, 28, 33, 39, 41, 43, 47, 50, 53, 59, 63, 67, **73**, **84**, 85, 92, 96, 97, 99, 102, 104, 113—also see 'watchful waiting'
mortality rate—see 'maternal mortality' and 'neonatal death'
MS (multiple sclerosis) 82
multiple birth—see 'twins' and 'triplets'
negligence 57, 94—also see 'watchful waiting' and 'disturbance'
neonatal death 39, 44, **50**, **51**, 52, 79, **68**, 83, 85, 86, **92**, 94, 112, 123
new natural 3, **68**
nitrous oxide 53, 55—also see 'gas and air'
nocebo effect **52**, 57, 59, 63, 66, **67**, 72, **76**, **77**, **82**, **83**, 84, 86, 87, 90, 96
noise in labour 23, 24, 25, 33, **37**, 38, 51, 53, 71, 72, **91**, 101
nuchal translucency testing 66
number of people at the birth **28**, 32, 34, 43, **62**, **63**, 64, **71**, 92, 101-102
obstetric cholestasis 41
Odent, Michel 22, 24, 27, 28, 33-34, 36, 38, 42, 44, 51, 52, 53, 55, 56, 58, 60, 62, 68, 69, 70-72, 74, 77, 82, 83, 84, 85, 87, 91, 92, **94**, 96, 97, 100, 101-102, 108, 111, 130
old natural 3
older mothers 32-35, 38, 42
Omega-3 supplements **4**
onset of labour **22**, 32, 33, 51, 57, 58, **61**, 62, 64, 69, 70, 77, 88, 92, 106—also see 'false labour', 'SRM' and 'contractions'
opiates 4, **27**, 46, **53**, 55, 64, 65
optimal fetal positioning 12, **16**, 18, 84, 97, 122, 123
oxytocin (or 'oxytocics') 5, 20, 22, 23, 27, 30, 36, 43, 44, 52, 53, 54, 56, 57, 58, 59, 60, **61**, **62**, 65, 66, 67, 70, 77, 80, 84, 94, 100, 111

pain 1, 3, 4, 18, **22**, **24**, 25, **27**, 30, 32, 33, 35, 37, 38, 45, 46, 47, 48, **53**, 57, 58, 60, **61**, 65, **68**, 70, 90, 95, 96, **104**, 106, 108, 122, 123
pain relief 1, 3, **27**, 33, **38**, 41, 46, 47, **51**, 52, **53**, 54, 60, 64, **65**, 66, 67, 73, 82, 90, 91, **99**, 103, 108, 113
palpation 33, 37, 43, 75, 77, **84**, 85, 92
pethidine 3, 32, **53**, 65
photographs 22, 24, 96, 107, 120
physiological processes **5-35**, 44, 60, **61-63**, 64, 67, 68, 73, 82, 109, 116-117, 130
physiological third stage 30, 33, 34, 37, 43, 58, 65, 71, 90, 92, 95, **97**, 103, 107, 109, **111**—also see 'third stage'
Pinard 10, 33, 43, 74, 75, 84, **97**
placenta praevia **39**, 44, 75, 85
positions (for labour or birth) 23, **24**, 25, **27**, 33, 34, 35, 36, 37, 43, 50, **51**, 52, **53**, 58, 62, **67**, 96, **98**, **99**, **105**, 106, 108
posterior position 12, 16, 18, 23, 32, 33, 101-102
postmaturity 19, 37, 38, 41, 57, **58**, 78
postnatal care 30, 31, 34, 37, 92, **109-119**
postnatal depression 44, **57**, **89**, **118**, 122, 123
postnatal scenarios 3, 19, **27**, **28**, 29, **30-31**, 32, 34, 35, 37, 39, 42, 43, **44**, 46, 47, 48, 49, 50, 52, **53**, 54, 57, 58, 60, **62**, 63, **68**, 69, 70, 72, 71, 88, 96, 107, 108, **109**, 110, **116-117**, **118**, **119**, 122, 123
PPH (postpartum haemorrhage) 22, **27**, **56**, **62**, **64**, 65, 74, **90**, **97**, **111**
pre-eclampsia 55, 80, 84, 87
pregnancy 5, **6-21**, 52, **61**, 66, 69, **75-90**
premature labour—see 'prematurity' and 'kangaroo care'
prematurity 9, 11, 13, 14, 19, 68, 78, 86, 87, 88-89, 106, **112-116**, 122—also see 'kangaroo care'
primal health 3, 4, 9, 44, 52, **53**, **54**, **55-56**, **68**, 123
Primal Health Research Data Bank **55**
primiparas (first-time mothers) 32, 38, 58, 79, **82**, 92, 96
privacy **91**, 94, **96**, 101, 111, 116, 118—also see 'disturbance'
protocols 22, 27, 30, 34, 37, 42, 43, 44, 49, 52, 54, 58, 63, **65**, **67**, **68**, **73**, 74, **82**, 83, **84**, **87**, 91, 92, **95**, 99
psychological difficulties 21, 38, **44**, 52, 59, 66, 75, 82, **87**, 100, 116-117, **118**, 123
pushing **25**, **34**, 37, 50, 58, **61**, 62, 63, **67**, 71, 92, 95, 96, 102, **104**—also see 'commanded pushing'
randomised controlled trials 4, **44**, 57, **73**, 81, 83, 84, 85, 86, 97, 111, 130—also see 'watchful waiting'
Rank, Otto 54
raspberry leaf tea **4**
rebirthing 82, 123
reflexology 104
rest-and-be-thankful phase **24**, 99
ring of fire 18, 24, 25, **34**, 71
risk 3, 44, **47**, 55, 56, 58, 59, 60, 65, 70, 74, **75**, 76, 79, **82**, 83, 87, 90, 94
risk assessment 38, 74, 75, 79, **82**, 97
safety 1, 43, 44, **51**, 57, 60, 65, **68**, 73, 74, 77, **79-81**, 82, 91, 95, **107**
sanitation 79, 81—also see 'developing countries'
scans 9, **39**, 40, 41, 43, 52, 66, 75, 76, 82, 83, 84, **85-86**, 88, 112—also see 'ultrasound'
schizophrenia 55
screening tests—see 'antenatal tests'
second stage 22, **24-28**, **34**, 37, 51, 58, 92, 95, 106—also see all birthframes

second trimester **9-14**
sepsis **64**, 65, 80
sex 44, **47**, 48, 91, 118, 130
sexual abuse 38
SGA—see 'small for gestational age'
shiatsu 3
short labour—see 'fast labour'
shoulder dystocia 63, 87
side-effects 1, **27**, 40, 43, 51, **53**, 56, 64, 83, 84, 85, 87, 130
skin-to-skin contact 26, 29, 45, 54, 58, **62**, **89**, 113, 116—also see 'kangaroo care' and 'bonding'
slow labour—see 'failure to progress', 'disturbance' and 'number of people at the birth'
small for gestational age 52, 84, 85, **86**, 87
Sonicaid 10, 24, 43, 66, 75, 84, **85**, **86**, **97**
spinal 95, 96
SRM (spontaneous rupture of the membranes) 22, 23, 42, 58, 60, 69, 79, 102
stillbirth 12, 123
stitches 30, 33, 45, 47, 48, 49, **50**
Stoppard, Miriam 58
stress 15, 77
stress incontinence 60
sucking reflex **27**, 32, **53**, 54, 56
suicide 55
supplements **4**
sweeping membranes (or cervix) 58, 59, 67, 104
syntocinon 43, 59, 66
syntometrine 30, 36, 43, 65, 66, **90**, 93
talking in labour and birth **27**, 33, **56**, 74, **91**, 94, **97**, **104**, **111**
tandem feeding 32, 58
tearing 3, 25, **27**, 30, 33, 34, 37, 44, 52, 58, 80, 93, **99**
TENS 36, 41, 67, 106
tests 83—also see 'antenatal tests' and 'antenatal checks'
third stage 22, 25, **27**, 30, 32, 33, 34, 36, 37, 43, 56, 58, 64, 66, 71, 80, 90, 95, 97, 103, 107, 109, 111—also see all birthframes
third trimester **15-21**
transition 62, **63**, 95, 102
trial of labour 51
triplets 68, 75, **82**, 85, 88-89, 123
twins 18, 23, 38, 41, 42, 43, 68, 74, 75, **82**, 85, 94, 95-96, 117, 123
ultrasound 9, **39**, 43, 52, **65**, 66, 75, 76, 82, 84, **85-86**, 97, 112—also see 'scans'
unassisted birth 42, 82, 106-107, 107
urine testing 40, 75, **84**
vacuum extraction—see 'ventouse'
vaginal breech birth—see 'breech position'
vaginal examinations—see 'internal examinations'
VBAC **44**, **48**, **50**, **51**, 59, 82, 123
ventouse 52, 55, 65, 67
Vincent-Priya, Jacqueline 64
visualisation 38
vomiting 23, 33, 39-41, 43, 45, 53, 88, 108
washing the baby **30**, 54, 69
watchful waiting 22, **27**, **28**, 33, **36-37**, 38, 42, 51, **58**, 62, **69**, 69-72, 74, **91**, 92-93, 96, **97**, 100, 101-102, 103, 104, 110
waterbirth 24, 36, 37, 38, 42, 43, 58, 92, **97**, **99**, 101, 102, 104, 108
weighing the baby 49, 54, 56
X-rays 9, 85

Would you like to share this book with your colleagues and clients?

You can order more copies of this book and the companion volume for pregnant women directly from Fresh Heart. Simply complete the form below and send it to: Fresh Heart Publishing, PO Box 225, Chester le Street, DH3 9BQ, UK. Alternatively, visit www.freshheartpublishing.co.uk and click on 'Online shop', where you may find special offers.

ORDER FORM

I would like _____ copies of *Optimal Birth: The What, The Why & The How* [midwives' edition]
ISBN 978 1 906619 04 6 (£12.99 each)

I would like _____ copies of *BIRTH: Countdown to Optimal* [edition for pregnant women]
ISBN 978 1 906619 00 8 (£18.99 each)

I enclose a UK bank cheque or postal order, payable to Fresh Heart for £ _____.

[Note that P&P is free in the UK only. Overseas rates are available on request.]

NAME: _____

POSITION: _____

ADDRESS: _____
_____

POSTCODE: _____

Email: _____

Telephone: _____

DELIVERY NAME & ADDRESS (if different):

NAME: _____

POSITION: _____

ADDRESS: _____
_____

POSTCODE: _____

Email: _____

Telephone: _____

Please allow 28 days for delivery. Do not send cash. Offer subject to availability. We do not share or sell our customers' details. Please tick box if you would like to receive further information from Fresh Heart Publishing about other products. ☐

Comments from three well-known figures, referring to *BIRTH: Countdown to Optimal*...

Sheila Kitzinger, author of *Birth Crisis* (Routledge 2006) and *New Pregnancy and Childbirth* (Dorling Kindersley 2003), as well as many other books on birth:

It is difficult to write a book about birth drawing on research, analysing the effects and side-effects of interventions and also acknowledging that in the right setting and with loving, sensitive and unobtrusive support birth is a psycho-sexual process which can bring ecstasy. Sylvie has achieved this splendidly. She writes with energy and passion. Her book is rich with women's accounts of pregnancy, birth and after. Readers who do not relish childbirth may find it hard to take it all on board, but the tone, both of the women whom she quotes lavishly, and her own enthusiasm, is so compelling that many could be converted to a radically different view of birth. If they are brave enough to explore what she has to say, with another pregnancy birth may turn out to be a very much better experience.

This is a book that can help its readers be adventurous. Breaking the barrier involves not only getting information on which to base choices, or of acquiring the knowledge to make a birth plan, but also getting our inner confidence to grow and blossom!

Michel Odent, author, researcher, surgeon and midwife (see facing page for more information):

There are many reasons why this book is special. One of them is that Sylvie has become a real expert in childbirth. Thanks to her first-hand experience, she is immune to the countless received ideas that abound in magazines, newspapers and books.

Often women who talk a lot about the birth of their babies are those who had a difficult birth, problems and so on. And women who had a very easy birth tend not to talk about that. I have a very good example: my daughter, who has three children. Although she has a strong intellect—she's a professor of medical genetics—she would never talk about the birth of her babies. Never! Because for her it has always been so simple. The last one: contractions begin at 7 o'clock, baby born at 7.55. So I think it might be good to say somewhere that this book is special. It's full of accounts we can learn from.

I must admit, though, that I was sceptical when I first heard of her idea to write a book. My immediate and tacit reaction was: "Yet another book about natural childbirth. If I had kept all the manuscripts and books that have been sent to me over the last twenty years, I would need to have an extension built onto my study!"

It was only after several conversations with Sylvie that I started to change my mind. I realised that, thanks to her personal experience, Sylvie was aware of what very few people have understood. Here she tells you what she's learnt... In this book you'll absorb some authentic knowledge transmitted by an authentic expert.

> *Sylvie has become a real expert in childbirth. She is aware of what very few people have understood.*

> *This is a book that can help its readers develop confidence and be adventurous*

Janet Balaskas, author and founder of the Active Birth Centre in London, talking about this book:

BIRTH: Countdown to Optimal is a wonderful book for a pregnant woman (and her partner and family) to dip into. Written in a deliberately user-friendly style, it's a bit like a really juicy magazine. It's pitched just right for pregnancy reading. There is nothing to frighten a pregnant woman or cause her undue anxiety—nothing to stimulate her mind or her adrenal glands!

This is a book that absolutely celebrates the normality of birth and the joy of welcoming a new life into family and community. It is completely authentic, full of personal stories and evidence that lots of families and the author herself have truly experienced. For me this speaks volumes and means so much more than an analysis of randomised controlled trials, where there are so many hidden variables. This is about human experience rather than data or evidence-based practice! Yet the book is so much more than a collection of anecdotes. It is a truly scholarly work that weaves in the universal truths of birth physiology and research evidence while encouraging, inspiring and informing women. Professionals, as well as families, have so much to gain from its pages.

> *This is a book that absolutely celebrates the normality of birth. Professionals, as well as families have so much to gain from its pages.*

It is a huge endorsement of the work and essential message of Michel Odent and his partner, the doula Liliana Lammers, that women know how to give birth and do not usually need any help. This is true as long as people around the labouring woman are able to trust her and keep their distance. There is so much for practitioners still to understand about what this means. Reading the accounts in this book will help us all to better understand the discretion we need to have around the pregnant and birthing mother, so as not to disturb her highly sensitive physiological responses and the delicate hormonal secretions that characterise birth amongst all mammals, including humans. We would know and respect this around a mother cat or dog giving birth and would certainly hesitate to disturb what was going on, but we are ignorant of this around human mothers. This is a symptom of how alienated we have become from our essentially animal nature.

When you hold this book in your hands the cover photograph invites you to walk down a path in the woods between the trees, to sense and smell the earth underneath you and be in tune with the compassionate ever-presence of Mother Nature. This is exactly what optimal birth is like when mothers have the opportunity to be quietly in contact with the earth and let go to the forces of nature. When you open the book at first it's like opening a happy family album. Loving and joyful faces illuminate the text, like snapshots rather than commissioned birth photographs. The warmth of home and hearth as the best place for most women to give birth is clear. This gives us more than a clue that the true nature of birth is essentially wrapped within the love of mother and father, in happy families and healthy communities.

This is a very important book for our times, when we sure have got this whole process of birth wrong. I heartily congratulate Sylvie for her passion and all the work that went into compiling and writing this book.

WHO IS SYLVIE DONNA? WHO IS MICHEL ODENT?

About the author

Before she started having children, Sylvie Donna worked in companies or taught English, mostly to working adults. She also trained teachers, or managed courses, departments—or a whole language centre in one case. She taught or organised courses for middle and top-level managers (as well as clerical or research staff) in Europe, North Africa, South Asia, South East Asia, the Middle East and the Far East. Her first book—*Teach Business English* (Cambridge University Press 2000)—is a synthesis of her experience in this field. Since having children, Sylvie has worked from home, writing and editing, or marking Distance MA assignments. She still does some teaching and university lecturing.

> *Sylvie started researching pregnancy and childbirth when she conceived her first child at the age of 37*

Sylvie started researching issues surrounding pregnancy and childbirth when she conceived her first child at the age of 37. A few days after the birth she read *Birth Reborn* by Michel Odent and it struck a note of recognition in her—for the first time she was reading about the kind of birth she had just experienced. She then felt fortunate to have Dr Odent agree to attend the birth of her second child. The experience of birthing with him in attendance prompted her to think through more issues, which she was then also able to put to the test in a very modest way when she gave birth to her third child.

Despite being a busy work-from-home mother, she was determined to offer the book for pregnant women (*BIRTH: Countdown to Optimal*) to other women so as to help inform and inspire them to give birth as naturally as possible. This book then came as a natural consequence. Both books were researched around her family commitments. Her contributors and several key midwives and Heads of Midwifery, not to mention a couple of obstetricians and GPs, helped to sustain her belief that normal, physiological birth is what mothers and babies need if we are to build harmonious and happy families and societies, and a constructive future for humankind.

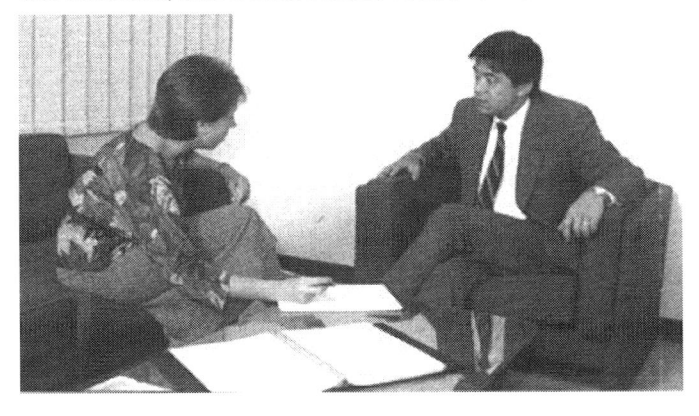

Sylvie when she was working as a Business English courses co-ordinator in Singapore

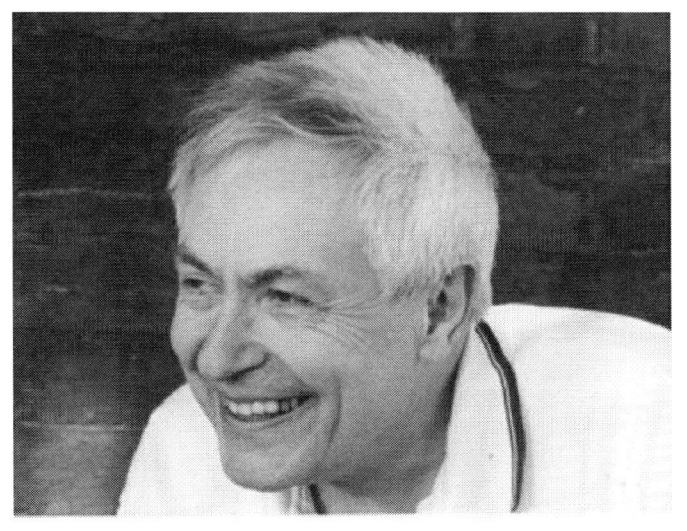

Michel in his Pithiviers days

About Michel Odent

Born in 1930, Michel Odent initially qualified and worked as a general surgeon. He gradually became more and more interested in issues surrounding childbirth, after being put in charge of a government maternity hospital in Pithiviers, near Paris, in the 1960s and '70s.

> *Coming new to the field, Michel was fortunate to have both a freshly-trained and an 'old-school' midwife to assist him*

Coming new to the field and fortunate to have both a freshly-trained and an 'old-school' midwife to assist him, he soon realised that pregnancy and childbirth were not things with easy or clear-cut answers. This led him to develop various practices which he later checked out through extensive research, both within the field of obstetrics and on a cross-disciplinary basis. As the years progressed, he came to feel more and more that childbirth was at its safest when the normal physiological processes were left to take place undisturbed.

In the 1980s he moved to London, where he set up the Primal Health Research Centre and practised as a homebirth midwife. His research has spanned topics such as preconceptional and antenatal care, nutrition in pregnancy, childbirth itself, breastfeeding and childhood vaccinations.

Frequently interviewed on television, in radio programmes and in the popular press, he has become known as the pioneer of the use of water during labour and homelike hospital birthing rooms. He is the author of numerous scientific papers and twelve books, including *The Caesarean*, *The Farmer and the Obstetrician*, *The Scientification of Love*, *Birth and Breastfeeding*, *Primal Health*, *Water and Sexuality* and perhaps his most well-known title: *Birth Reborn*.

Fresh ♥ Heart
PUBLISHING

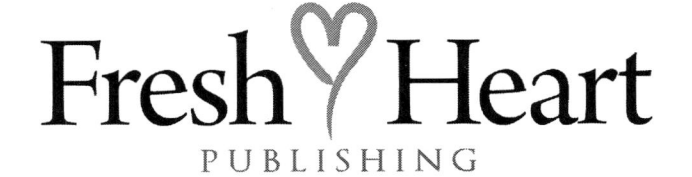

Check out www.freshheartpublishing.co.uk!

Contact us   Online shop

FAQs   Does 'optimal' mean 'natural'?   Is it safe?   But what about the pain?!   Quick tips   News

Why this book?

Too many women are traumatised temporarily, if not for the rest of their lives, after having a baby. Sadly, the memory of giving birth leaves some women feeling disappointed, alienated or betrayed. Their partners and families are affected too.

While researching childbirth over the last twelve years I came across quite a few parents whose experience of pregnancy and birth was negative. For many, pregnancy was more of an obstacle course of tests and worries, than a time of wonder and waiting. Somehow, amongst all the antenatal appointments, risk assessment and birthing pool hire, the baby-to-be got thrown out with the as yet non-existent bath water. And many women told me how the birth they'd planned went wrong in the end. From some of the women, who were the 'statistics' of care gone wrong, I heard horrendous stories of pain and trauma. Many simply spoke of their feelings of disempowerment as they were 'managed' through the maternity system. For others it was just the breastfeeding or the bonding which didn't work out...

What was it, I wondered, that made things go wrong? Listening carefully to countless women I started making connections between behaviour in pregnancy and birth and outcomes. I realised that things often start going wrong in pregnancy for no good reason, other than fear. I also discovered—through women's personal accounts—that pain relief often ended up causing more pain than it ever relieved, if postnatal pain was counted too.

While I was realising these things, I also became increasingly aware that very few women see the chain of events which they set up for themselves by accepting or even requesting certain treatment while they're pregnant, in labour, giving birth and even afterwards. For example, how many women would choose to have pethidine or diamorphine while they're giving birth if they knew it would dramatically decrease their chances of breastfeeding successfully? (And how many even know that 'diamorphine' is just another name for 'heroin'?) Amongst the women who couldn't care less about breastfeeding, how many of them would use pethidine or diamorphine if they knew it might increase the chances of their child becoming a drug addict in adulthood? How many have found out about and thought through the potentially harmful effects of an epidural, or gas and air?

Most importantly, I wondered how many women know that a great deal of antenatal and in-labour care still flies in the face of research recommendations, even though this is no longer supposed to be the case, given recent NICE guidelines... Of course, there's also the problem that some interventions cannot ever be tested in controlled research conditions.

A book or two were definitely needed. By networking with other women and midwives I soon discovered that in some places things are going very well indeed...

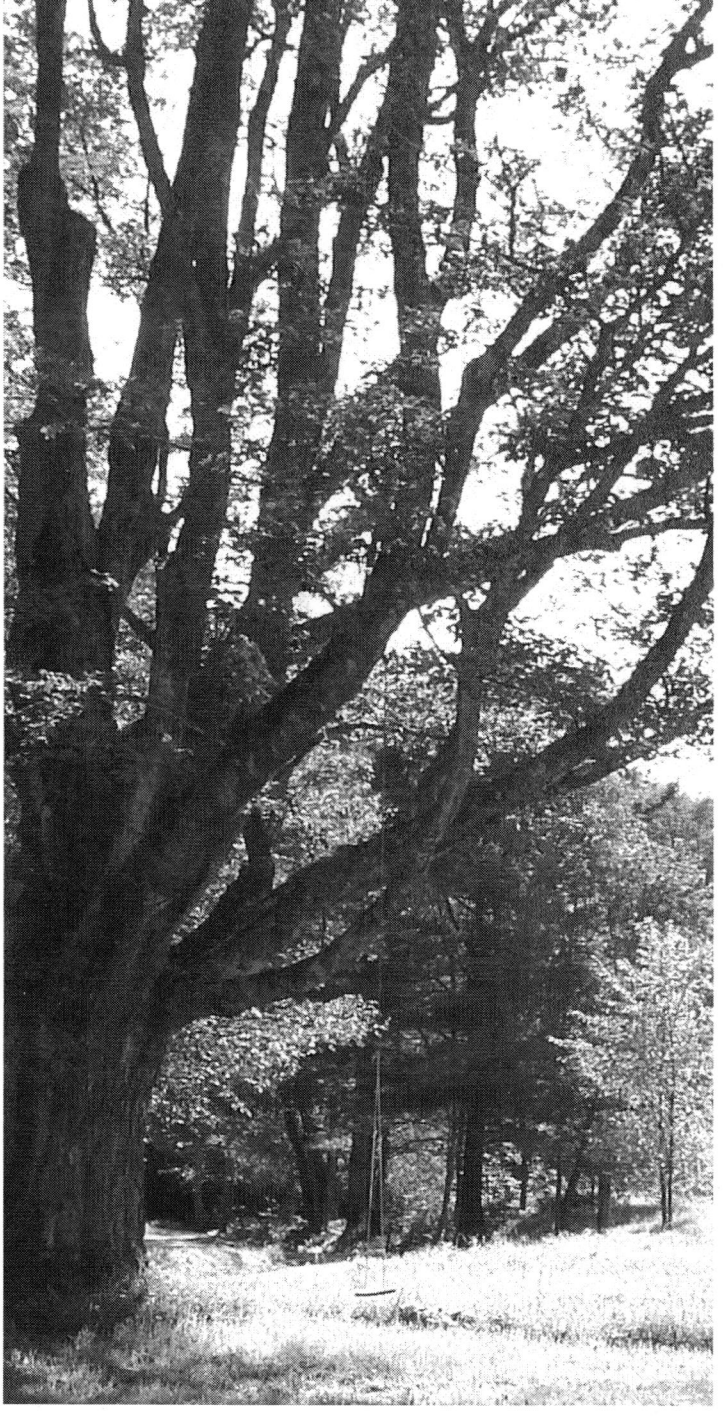

It's as if the world has forgotten the art of giving birth